Cases in Emergency Airway
Management

D0797176

Cases in Emergency Airway Management

Edited by

Lauren C. Berkow
Associate Professor of Anesthesia and Critical Care Medicine
at Johns Hopkins School of Medicine, Baltimore, Maryland, USA

John C. Sakles
Professor of Emergency Medicine at the University of Arizona College of Medicine,
Tucson, Arizona, USA

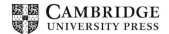

CAMBRIDGE
UNIVERSITY PRESS

CAMBRIDGE
UNIVERSITY PRESS

University Printing House, Cambridge CB2 8BS, United Kingdom

Cambridge University Press is part of the University of Cambridge.

It furthers the University's mission by disseminating knowledge in the pursuit of
education, learning, and research at the highest international levels of excellence.

www.cambridge.org
Information on this title: www.cambridge.org/9781107437449

© Cambridge University Press 2015

First published 2015

Printed in the United Kingdom by TJ International Ltd. Padstow Cornwall

A catalogue record for this publication is available from the British Library

Library of Congress Cataloguing-in-Publication Data
Cases in emergency airway management / edited by Lauren C. Berkow, John C. Sakles.
   p. ; cm.
Includes bibliographical references and index.
ISBN 978-1-107-43744-9 (paperback)
I. Berkow, Lauren C., 1968–, editor.   II. Sakles, John C., 1963–, editor.
[DNLM: 1. Airway Management – methods.   2. Emergencies.   WF 145]
RC87.9
615.8′36–dc23

                                                                    2015026755

ISBN 978-1-107-43744-9 Paperback

Contents

Contributors

Basem Abdelmalak, MD
Associate Professor of Anesthesiology, Cleveland Clinic Lerner College of Medicine of Case Western Reserve University, Cleveland, Ohio, USA

Director, Anesthesia for Bronchoscopic Surgery, Departments of General Anesthesiology and Outcomes Research, Anesthesiology Institute, Cleveland Clinic, Cleveland, Ohio, USA

Mohammed A. Abdel-Rahim, MD
Clinical Instructor, Department of Anesthesiology and Critical Care Medicine, Johns Hopkins School of Medicine, Baltimore, Maryland, USA

Mueen Ahmad, MD
Department of Otolaryngology, Head and Neck Surgery, Johns Hopkins School of Medicine, Baltimore, Maryland, USA

Carlos A. Artime, MD
Associate Professor, Department of Anesthesiology, University of Texas Medical School at Houston, Houston, Texas, USA

Aaron E. Bair, MD, MS, FAAEM, FACEP
Professor, Emergency Medicine, Associate Dean, Continuing Medical Education, Medical Director, Centers for Health and Technology & Virtual Care University of California, Davis, Sacramento, California, USA

Medical Director, Emergency Medical Services, Solano County, California, USA

Paul Baker, MD, MBChB, FANZCA
Clinical Senior Lecturer, Department of Anaesthesiology, University of Auckland, Auckland, New Zealand

Nasir Bhatti, MD, MHS
Associate Professor, Otolaryngology/Head and Neck Surgery, and Anesthesiology & Critical Care Medicine, Johns Hopkins School of Medicine, Baltimore, Maryland, USA

Director, Johns Hopkins Adult Tracheostomy and Airway Service, Johns Hopkins University, Baltimore, Maryland, USA

Calvin A. Brown III, MD
Assistant Professor of Emergency Medicine, Brigham and Women's Hospital, Boston, Massachusetts, USA

Kenneth H. Butler, DO, FACEP, FAAEM, FACOEP
Department of Emergency Medicine, University of Maryland School of Medicine, Baltimore, Maryland, USA

Davide Cattano, MD, PhD
Associate Professor, Director of Clinical Research, Department of Anesthesiology, University of Texas Medical School at Houston, Houston, Texas, USA

Medical Director Anesthesia Clinic, Anesthesia Service Chief for Head and Neck Surgery, Memorial Hermann Hospital, Texas Medical Center, Houston, Texas, USA

Adjunct Clinical Instructor of
Anesthesiology, Case Western Reserve
University, Cleveland, Ohio, USA

Richard M. Cooper, MD, FRCPC
Professor, University of Toronto, Toronto
General Hospital, Toronto, Ontario,
Canada

Ruggero M. Corso, MD
Operating Room Medical Director,
Department of Emergency Anesthesia and
Intensive Care Section, G. B. Morgagni
Hospital, Forlì, Italy

Nicholas M. Dalesio, MD
Department of Anesthesiology and Critical
Care Medicine, Division of Pediatric
Anesthesiology and Critical Care Medicine,
Department of Otolaryngology/Head and
Neck Surgery, Johns Hopkins School of
Medicine, Baltimore, Maryland, USA

Jaime Daly, MD
Department of Anesthesiology, Yale
University School of Medicine, New Haven,
Connecticut, USA

Peter M. C. DeBlieux, MD
Professor of Clinical Medicine, Director of
Resident and Faculty Development, Section
of Emergency Medicine, Louisiana State
University School of Medicine, New
Orleans, Louisiana, USA

Lorraine J. Foley, MD, MBA
Clinical Assistant Professor of Anesthesia,
Tufts School of Medicine, Boston
Massachusetts, Winchester Anesthesia
Associates, Winchester Hospital, Affiliate
of Lahey Health Winchester,
Massachusetts, USA

Oren A. Friedman, MD
Assistant Professor of Medicine,
Department of Medicine, Division of
Pulmonary and Critical Care Medicine,

Weill Cornell Medical College, New York,
New York, USA

Carin A. Hagberg, MD
Joseph C. Gabel Professor and Chair,
Department of Anesthesiology, University
of Texas Medical School at Houston,
Houston, Texas, USA

Narasimhan Jagannathan, MD
Attending Pediatric Anesthesiologist,
Department of Pediatric Anesthesia, Ann &
Robert H. Lurie Children's Hospital of
Chicago, Chicago, Illinois, USA
Director of Pediatric Anesthesia
Research, Associate Professor of
Anesthesiology, Northwestern University
Feinberg School of Medicine, Chicago,
Illinois, USA

P. Allan Klock, Jr., MD
Professor of Anesthesiology and Critical
Care, University of Chicago, Chicago,
Illinois, USA

Erik G. Laurin, MD
Professor and Vice Chair of Education,
Department of Emergency Medicine,
University of California, Davis,
Sacramento, California, USA

Seth Manoach, MD, CHCQM, FCCP
Assistant Professor of Medicine,
Department of Medicine, Division of
Pulmonary and Critical Care Medicine,
Weill Cornell Medical College, New York,
New York, USA

Lynette Mark, MD
Associate Professor of Anesthesiology
and Critical Care Medicine, and
Otolaryngology/Head and Neck
Surgery, Medical Director of
Weinberg Surgical Suite, Johns Hopkins
School of Medicine, Baltimore, Maryland,
USA

Marc L. Martel, MD
Emergency Physician, Department of Emergency Medicine, Hennepin County Medical Center, Minneapolis, Minnesota, USA
Associate Professor, Department of Emergency Medicine, University of Minnesota, Minneapolis, Minnesota, USA

Christina Miller, MD
Assistant Professor of Anesthesiology and Critical Care Medicine, Johns Hopkins School of Medicine, Baltimore, Maryland, USA

Neal Patrick Moehrle
Northwestern University Feinberg School of Medicine, Chicago, Illinois, USA

Athir H. Morad, MD
Assistant Professor, Departments of Anesthesiology, Critical Care Medicine and Neurology, Johns Hopkins School of Medicine, Baltimore, Maryland, USA

Jarrod M. Mosier, MD
Director of Emergency Medicine Critical Care, Assistant Professor of Emergency Medicine, Department of Emergency Medicine, University of Arizona, Tucson, Arizona, USA
Assistant Professor of Medicine, Department of Medicine, Section of Pulmonary, Critical Care, Allergy and Sleep, University of Arizona, Tucson, Arizona, USA

Jean-Pierre P. Ouanes, DO
Assistant Professor, Department of Anesthesiology and Critical Care Medicine, Johns Hopkins School of Medicine, Baltimore, Maryland, USA

Vinciya Pandian, PhD, RN
Assistant Professor, Division of Neuroanesthesia, Anesthesiology and Critical Care Medicine, Johns Hopkins

School of Medicine, Baltimore, Maryland, USA

Gail I. Randel, MD
Associate Professor, Northwestern University Feinberg School of Medicine, Chicago, Illinois, USA

Robert F. Reardon, MD
Department of Emergency Medicine, Hennepin County Medical Center, Minneapolis, Minnesota, USA
Associate Professor of Emergency Medicine, University of Minnesota Medical School, Minneapolis, Minnesota, USA

William Rosenblatt, MD
Professor of Anesthesiology, Yale University School of Medicine, New Haven, Connecticut, USA

Kenneth P. Rothfield, MD, MBA
Chairman, Department of Anesthesiology, Saint Agnes Hospital, Baltimore, Maryland, USA

Keith J. Ruskin, MD
Professor of Anesthesiology and Neurosurgery, Yale University School of Medicine, New Haven, Connecticut, USA

John C. Sakles, MD
Professor, Department of Emergency Medicine, University of Arizona College of Medicine, Tucson, Arizona, USA

Christa San Luis, MD
Division of Neuroanesthesiology and Neurocritical Care, Department of Anesthesiology and Critical Care Medicine, The Johns Hopkins School of Medicine, Baltimore, Maryland, USA

Adam Schiavi PhD, MD
Assistant Professor Anesthesiology and Critical Care Medicine, The Johns Hopkins School of Medicine, Baltimore, Maryland, USA

Michael Seltz Kristensen, MD
Head of Clinical Anaesthesia and Research,
Section for ENT-, Head-, Neck- and
Maxillofacial Surgery, Rigshospitalet,
University Hospital of Copenhagen,
Denmark

Tracey Straker, MD, MPH
Associate Professor Clinical
Anesthesiology, Montefiore Medical
Center, Albert Einstein College of
Medicine, Bronx, New York, USA

Sal J. Suau, MD
Emergency Medicine, Maimonides Medical
Center, Brooklyn, New York, USA

Lori Ann Suffredini, DO
Clinical Associate, Department of
Anesthesiology and Critical Care Medicine,
Johns Hopkins School of Medicine,
Baltimore, Maryland, USA

Wendy H. L. Teoh, MBBS, FANZCA, FAMS
Adj Assistant Professor, Dukes Uni-NUS
Graduate Medical School, Singapore

Senior Consultant Anaesthesiologist,
Department of Women's Anaesthesia,
KK Women's & Children's Hospital,
Singapore

Felipe Urdaneta, MD
Associate Professor in Anesthesiology,
University of Florida, Gainesville, Florida,
USA

Sage P. Whitmore, MD
Assistant Professor of Emergency
Medicine, Department of Emergency
Medicine, Division of Emergency Critical
Care, University of Michigan Health
System, Ann Arbor, Michigan, USA

Natasha Woodman, MBChB, BSc, FRCA
Fellow of Paediatric Anaesthesia, Starship
Children's Hospital, Auckland, New
Zealand

Preface

Emergent airway management, either inside or outside the operating room, can be a frightening challenge. The limited available history of the patient, the rapid need for action, the limited availability of equipment, and frequent lack of additional staff to assist are many of the reasons why complications in this arena are higher than in elective intubations. Both the American Society of Anesthesiologists closed claims analysis in the USA and the Fourth National Audit Project of the Royal College of Anaesthetists in the UK have demonstrated increased complication rates associated with airway management outside the operating room environment.

We created this book to remove many of the unknowns encountered, and to help prepare airway managers for these emergency situations. We strove to produce a volume that is part textbook and part handbook; providing both a scientific foundation about a variety of emergent clinical situations as well as suggested guidelines and algorithms to manage these patients safely. Many textbooks exist that cover the topic of airway management, and there are handbooks available as well. This is one of the few texts that covers specifically and solely airway management in the emergent setting.

This book covers a variety of scenarios in both the pediatric and adult populations that may require emergent airway management in the operating room, the intensive care unit, the emergency department, and on the wards. We hope that all clinicians who are tasked with the challenge of providing airway management in the emergent setting will be drawn to this volume, and that it will provide guidance to create airway management plans and gather appropriate equipment to turn a difficult situation into a smooth, elegantly managed one. We especially encourage physicians in training to read this book.

Many of our authors have created algorithms for specific airway management situations for which no algorithm previously existed. While some of these algorithms have not yet been validated, they are based on the available scientific evidence. Where previously published algorithms exist, they have been included here as well.

This book is dedicated to the front-line emergency airway managers, of all specialties, who work in the trenches and deal with these airway catastrophes on a daily basis.

The editors would like to thank Claire Levine, MS for her excellent and tireless editing.

Lauren C. Berkow and John C. Sakles
Baltimore, Maryland and Tucson, Arizona

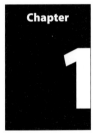

Chapter 1

Anatomic consideration for airway management

Gail I. Randel and Tracey Straker

Introduction

Surface structures of the head and neck that are relevant for airway management include the nose, mouth, and the cricothyroid area. These structures represent access points to the airway for mask ventilation, elective intubation, and emergent access for airway control (Figure 1.1). For most of the population, the nose, mouth, and oropharynx are easily identified. Identifying the cricothyroid membrane requires knowledge of the anterior neck and the skill set necessary for locating it. Ultrasound has improved the ability to identify the cricothyroid membrane.[1,2]

The nose and mouth, located on the anterior face, are easily accessed unless congenital anomalies, trauma, radiation, or prior surgery have complicated the anatomy. The cricothyroid membrane is located below the surface of the anterior neck.

This chapter will review the anatomy of the airway while highlighting surface and functional anatomy. The respiratory and digestive systems will also be discussed in regard to how they may impact airway management.

Nose

The nose participates in a number of functions – olfaction, phonation, humidification, respiration, and filtration.[3] The anatomy of the nose can be divided into two sections, the external nose and the nasal cavity including the septum.[4]

The upper one-third of the bony external nose connects the nasion to the forehead. The lower two-thirds is cartilaginous, consisting of two alar cartilages. The tip consists of fibrocartilage that helps to maintain the shape of the nose.

The nasal cavity encompasses the vestibule anteriorly and stretches to the nasopharynx posteriorly. This cavity is divided by the midline septum, which is composed of both cartilage and bone. The septum comprises the ethmoid bone descending from the cribriform plate, vomer, and septal cartilage. The lateral walls of the nasal cavity are composed of a series of turbinates – superior, middle, and inferior. The turbinates divide the nasal fossae into meatuses. The turbinates are lined by ciliated columnar epithelium, which aids in filtration and protection. The inferior turbinate determines the size of the endotracheal tube that may be passed nasally (Figure 1.2).

The end branches of the carotid arteries, both internal and external, supply the nose. The area above the middle turbinate is supplied by the anterior ethmoidal arteries. The remaining

Cases in Emergency Airway Management, ed. Lauren C. Berkow and John C. Sakles. Published by Cambridge University Press. © Cambridge University Press 2015.

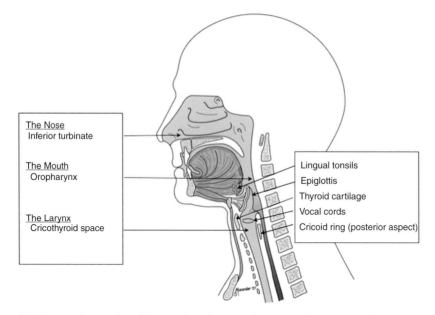

The Nose
Inferior turbinate

The Mouth
Oropharynx

The Larynx
Cricothyroid space

Lingual tonsils
Epiglottis
Thyroid cartilage
Vocal cords
Cricoid ring (posterior aspect)

Figure 1.1 The nose, the mouth, and the cricothyroid area are three potential access points for airway management. The cricothyroid membrane is not shown in this figure

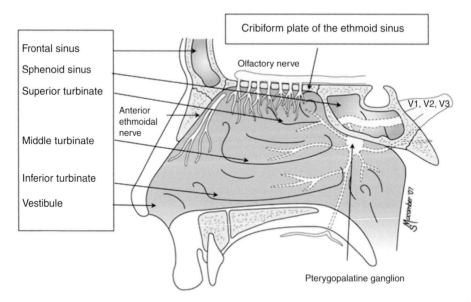

Cribiform plate of the ethmoid sinus

Frontal sinus

Sphenoid sinus

Superior turbinate

Middle turbinate

Inferior turbinate

Vestibule

Olfactory nerve

Anterior
ethmoidal
nerve

V1, V2, V3

Pterygopalatine ganglion

Figure 1.2 Lateral view and innervation of the nasopharynx

regions are supplied by the sphenopalatine, palatine, and labial arteries. This extremely vascular area, known as Kiesselbach's plexus, is the source of epistaxis and hemorrhage.

Non-olfactory areas of the nose are innervated primarily by the maxillary division of the trigeminal nerve – anterior ethmoid and sphenopalatine (pterygopalatine) nerves

(Figure 1.2). The vidian nerve supplies the secretory glands, and the parasympathetic and sympathetic systems supply the nasal vasculature.

The paranasal sinuses – maxillary, frontal, ethmoid, and sphenoid – drain into the nasal cavity. They are paired, pneumatic spaces that extend from the nasal cavity into the skull. The frontal sinus is not present at birth and, when it is fully developed, the anterior cranial fossa and the orbit border the frontal sinus.

The maxillary sinus continues to develop until the third decade. Structures bordering the maxillary sinus include orbit, cheek, nasal cavity, and teeth. The extremely thin walls of the ethmoid sinus are located in the superior and lateral aspects of the nose. The thin walls allow for easy spread of infection and tumor. The sphenoid sinus abuts several significant structures – optic nerve, internal carotid artery, pituitary fossa, and the cavernous sinus. The cavernous sinus contains branches of the trigeminal, oculomotor, abducens, and trochlear nerves.[4]

Nasal intubations can have serious complications. Severe facial trauma, such as Leforte fractures II and III, and basilar skull fractures are contraindications to nasal intubation. Nasal intubations in patients with these conditions may penetrate the brain via the orbit and cribriform plate. The cribriform plate is a part of the ethmoid bone, which separates the brain from the nasal cavity. It attaches to the frontal bone of the skull known as the ethmoidal notch. The roof of this structure also connects to the nasal cavities in the skull.[5] Nasal intubation, if attempted in patients with skull and facial fractures, is safest with fiberoptic assistance.[6]

Mouth

The mouth is involved with deglutition and speech articulation. It is functionally divided into two continuous areas: the oral cavity and the oropharynx (Figure 1.3).[7] Anatomically, the oral cavity starts at the lips, with the vermillion-skin borders extending posteriorly, and

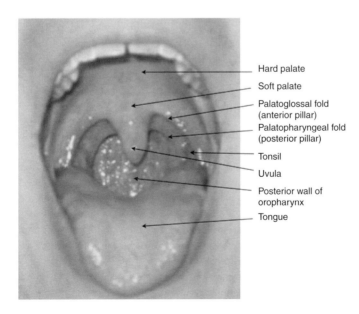

Figure 1.3 Structures of the oral cavity and oropharynx

Hard palate

Soft palate

Palatoglossal fold (anterior pillar)

Palatopharyngeal fold (posterior pillar)

Tonsil

Uvula

Posterior wall of oropharynx

Tongue

ends superiorly at the soft palate. Inferiorly, it includes the anterior two-thirds of the tongue. The oral cavity is, therefore, bounded superiorly by the hard palate, posteriorly by the oropharynx, inferiorly by the tongue, and anteriorly by the lips, with the maxillary and mandibular alveolar ridges/teeth and gingivae extending laterally and including the buccal mucosa and retromolar trigone (Figure 1.3).

Tongue

The tongue is involved with speech articulation and deglutition.[7] The anterior two-thirds of the tongue resides in the oral cavity, and the posterior third resides in the oropharynx. The intrinsic muscles of the tongue control its movement and the shape while the extrinsic muscles fix the tongue to bony landmarks for support. The following extrinsic muscles attach the tongue to the mandible (genioglossus), the hyoid (hyoglossus), the styloid process (styloglossus), and the soft palate (palatoglossus). When a supine patient loses consciousness, these muscles relax the tongue into the oropharynx and may produce airway obstruction. Applying the simple airway maneuver of a jaw thrust pulls the tongue forward by the action of the genioglossus muscle, which is attached to the symphysis menti of the mandible.[8] As a result, the pathway opens for airflow into the oropharynx. The tongue musculature is innervated by the hypoglossal nerve (CN XII), and taste to the anterior two-thirds of the tongue is provided by the lingual nerve (CN V_3).

Pharynx

The pharynx is a continuous and dynamic structure, conceptualized as a musculofascial distensible tube connecting the nasal and oral cavities with the lower larynx and esophagus.[8] The pharynx serves as a conduit for air and food while providing protection from pathogens and preventing entrance by foreign bodies. The adult pharynx is approximately 12–15 cm in length. It is functionally divided into three parts: nasopharynx, oropharynx, and hypopharynx (Figure 1.4).

The nasopharynx serves an important role in the respiratory system by warming and humidifying incoming air. The nasopharynx is located posterior to the nasal septum and extends to the level of the soft palate. The nasal choanae, eustachian tubes, and oropharynx converge into the nasopharynx. In this area, a ring of lymphoid tissue (palatine, lingual, tubal, and nasopharyngeal tonsils (adenoids)) is known as the Ring of Waldeyer. Suspended inhaled particles enter through the nose, reach the tonsils, and become sequestered. The tonsils serve as a defense against pathogens entering the body. As the lymphoid tissues enlarge, particularly the palatine tonsils, they may impede passage of air during mask ventilation or placement of a nasopharyngeal airway or endotracheal tube.[5] The lingual tonsils are located between the tongue and epiglottis, thereby precluding detection under routine airway examination (Figure 1.1). Enlarged lingual tonsils are often asymptomatic and have been a source for unanticipated difficult intubation and reported death during induction of anesthesia.[9]

The oropharynx has a role in both the digestive and respiratory systems. It is located between the soft palate superiorly and ends at the superior edge of the epiglottis. Functionally, it prevents food from entering the larynx.

The hypopharynx is situated behind the larynx and often is referred to as the laryngopharynx. It begins at the cervical vertebra C4 and ends at C6. It includes the epiglottis and extends to the inferior border of the cricoid cartilage, becoming continuous with the

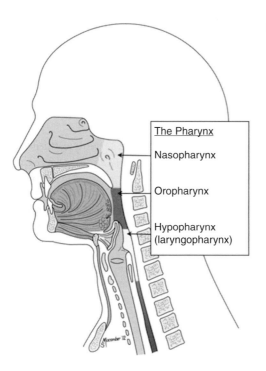

Figure 1.4 Lateral view of the pharynx

The Pharynx

Nasopharynx

Oropharynx

Hypopharynx
(laryngopharynx)

esophagus. The role of the hypopharynx is to channel air to the trachea and food to the esophagus.

Larynx

The larynx starts at the base of the tongue and ends at the trachea.[4,7,8] The U-shaped hyoid bone suspends and anchors the larynx during respiration and phonation. The laryngeal skeletal framework is formed by three unpaired cartilages (thyroid, cricoid, and epiglottis) and three paired cartilages (arytenoid, corniculate, cuneiform), which are joined by membranes, synovial joints, and ligaments. The ligaments are covered with mucous membranes and referred to as folds. The thyroid cartilage is the largest of the laryngeal structures and is embryologically fused in the midline, forming a V-shaped shield in the anterior neck. The laryngeal prominence in men is referred to as the "Adam's apple," whereas in women it is less prominent. On the inside of the thyroid laminae are the vestibular ligaments and below that, the vocal ligaments. The cricoid cartilage is the lower limit of the larynx and connects to the trachea.

Two membranes attach to the thyroid: the thyrohyoid membrane and cricothyroid membrane. The thyrohyoid membrane connects the thyroid cartilage to the hyoid bone whereas the cricothyroid membrane connects the cricoid to the thyroid cartilage (Figure 1.5).

The cricoid cartilage is a signet-shaped ring with the anterior side shorter (5–7 mm) and posterior side taller (2–3 cm); it is the only complete cartilaginous ring in the airway.[8] It serves several functions: anatomically, it provides posterior support of the larynx; clinically, it is used as a landmark to identify the cricothyroid membrane for emergency airway access. Cricoid pressure is used during emergency placement of an endotracheal tube in patients with a high risk of aspiration. The action of pressing the cricoid ring downward, thereby

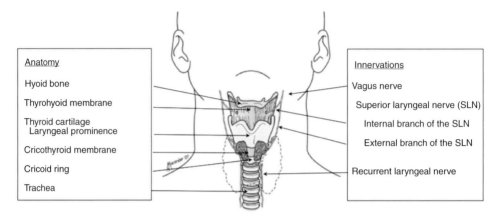

Figure 1.5 Anterior view of larynx with landmarks and innervation of the larynx

compressing the esophagus against the cervical vertebrae, is thought to prevent passive regurgitation without creating airway obstruction. Particularly in an airway emergency, the cricothyroid membrane is an important landmark to identify.

When other points of entry to the airway are not available, the cricothyroid membrane serves as a window and allows entry into the respiratory tract below the glottis.[10,11] The cricothyroid membrane is located superficially below the skin in the anterior neck and is situated between the thyroid cartilage and cricoid ring. It covers the cricothyroid space, which averages 9 mm in height and 3 cm in width in adults. The cricothyroid space is palpable as an indentation or soft spot at the inferior edge of the thyroid cartilage (particularly in men) and/or superior to the cricoid cartilage (in women).[7] The vocal cords, which are protected by the thyroid cartilage, are located approximately a centimeter above the cricothyroid space (Figure 1.1).

During endoscopy, the larynx can be seen beginning at the base of the tongue. The initial view is of the epiglottis, which is a flexible, fibroelastic, omega-shaped cartilage. The epiglottis serves as a protective structure and acts to guide food away from the larynx. The epiglottis is attached to the tongue by the medial glossoepiglottic fold and lateral glossoepiglottic folds. The area between these folds is termed the valleculae. The tip of the Macintosh blade is placed at this site for direct laryngoscopy. The paired arytenoids articulate with the posterior aspect of the cricoid cartilage. This is a synovial joint that can be affected by rheumatoid arthritis. The arytenoids control the vocal cord movement. The vocal cords (folds) project from the arytenoids in a posterior to anterior plane and attach to the inner surface of the thyroid cartilage. The epiglottis is also connected to the arytenoids laterally by the aryepiglottic ligaments and folds. Within these folds, paired fibroelastic cartilages – the cuneiform and the corniculate – reinforce the support of the aryepiglottic fold and aid arytenoid movement. The glottic opening is bounded by the epiglottis, the aryepiglottic fold, and the corniculate cartilages (Figure 1.6).

Two muscle groups control movement of the larynx. The extrinsic muscle group modifies the larynx position by its attachment to the hyoid bone and other anatomic structures. The extrinsic muscles include the sternohyoid, sternothyroid, thyrohyoid, thyroepiglottic, stylopharyngeus, and inferior pharyngeal constrictor. The intrinsic muscles directly affect the glottic movement by facilitating movement of the laryngeal cartilages.

Table 1.1 The larynx intrinsic muscles: action and innervation

Muscle	Action	Innervation
Transverse arytenoid	Adducts arytenoids	Recurrent laryngeal nerve
Lateral cricoarytenoids	Adducts arytenoids, closes glottis	Recurrent laryngeal nerve
Posterior arytenoids	Abducts vocal cords	Recurrent laryngeal nerve
Thyroarytenoids	Relaxes tension on vocal cords	Recurrent laryngeal nerve
Vocalis	Relaxes vocal cord	Recurrent laryngeal nerve
Oblique arytenoid	Closes the glottis	Recurrent laryngeal nerve
Aryepiglottic	Closes the glottis	Recurrent laryngeal nerve
Cricothyroid	Tensor of the vocal cords	External branch of the superior laryngeal nerve

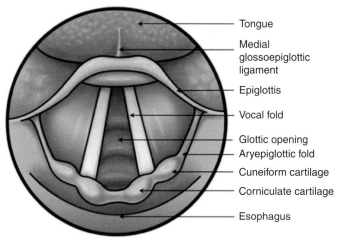

Tongue

Medial glossoepiglottic ligament

Epiglottis

Vocal fold

Glottic opening
Aryepiglottic fold

Cuneiform cartilage

Corniculate cartilage

Esophagus

Figure 1.6 Endoscopic view of the larynx

The intrinsic muscles include posterior cricoarytenoid, lateral cricoarytenoid, transverse arytenoid, oblique arytenoid, aryepiglottic, vocalis, thyroarytenoid, and cricothyroid muscles. The intrinsic muscles coordinate movement of the vocal cords to facilitate respiration, deglutition, and phonation (Table 1.1).[4]

The vagus nerve (CN X) and its branches innervate the larynx (Figure 1.5). Just inferior to the hyoid bone, the vagus nerve branches into the superior laryngeal nerve, which further bifurcates into external and internal branches. The internal branch pierces the thyrohyoid membrane, carrying sensory input from the laryngeal mucosa to the area above the vocal cords. The recurrent laryngeal nerve, a branch of the vagus, supplies sensory input to the larynx below the vocal cords and motor innervation to all intrinsic muscles of the larynx except the cricothyroid muscle. The external branch of the vagus supplies motor innervation to the cricothyroid muscle. The laryngeal branches of the superior and inferior thyroid arteries supply the larynx. Clinically, injury to one recurrent laryngeal nerve may present asymptomatically or as a slight change in voice quality. Damage to both recurrent laryngeal

Table 1.2 Comparative airway anatomy

Anatomic location	Infant	Adult	Clinical impact
Head	Large occiput to body ratio	Proportional occiput to body	Adults require blankets to achieve sniffing position for intubation; infants naturally in sniffing position, no blankets required
Tongue	Relatively large related to submandibular space	Usually proportionate to submandibular space	Infants are obligate nasal breathers until 6 months
Epiglottis	Increased vagal tone Floppy, long, omega- or U-shaped	Normal vagal tone Flexible, tear-drop shape	In infants, bradycardia more likely to occur compared to adults In infants, better view of vocal cords with Miller blade
Larynx Position	C2–C3 until age 6 years	C4–C5	Airway obstruction more likely in children
Shape	Funnel shape	Cylinder shape	
Vocal cord	Angled	Horizontal	
Narrowest part	Cricoid cartilage	Level of the vocal cords	Use uncuffed endotracheal tubes in infants

nerves presents as a dire emergency due to total airway obstruction since the vocal cords cannot abduct and allow passage of air into the lungs.

The pediatric airway

Pediatric patients are more prone to airway obstruction than adults due to the size, shape, and position of the anatomic parts of the airway. The tonsils are small in newborns and become adult size by ages 4 to 7 years old, which may make mask ventilation difficult as well as obscure the view of the larynx.[12–14] In an unconscious child, the tongue falls back in the oropharynx blocking the flow of air.

Infants desaturate faster than adults with upper airway obstruction due to smaller lung volumes and a more compliant chest wall. The pediatric airway has several distinctive features. The larynx is positioned more rostrally in children than in adults, making the tongue size relatively large in relation to the oropharynx. The vocal cords are angled and protected by a posterior angled U-shaped epiglottis. Most important, the narrowest part of the airway is at the level of the cricoid cartilage, and the diameter of the trachea is smaller and shorter than that of adults. Table 1.2 describes the differences between the infant and adult airway and highlights the effect on clinical practice.

Conclusion

The nose, mouth, pharynx, and larynx comprise a complex array of structures designed to give us the "human airway." These highly integrated structures permit breathing, protect the airway from foreign bodies, protect the body from pathogens, enable taste and phonation, and assist in food intake and emergency airway access. Mastery of the anatomy and understanding the function and innervation of the "human airway" facilitates an approach for safe elective and emergent airway management.

References

1. Elliott DSJ, Baker PA, Scott MR, Birch CW, Thompson JMD. Accuracy of surface landmark identification for cannula cricothyroidotomy. *Anaesthesia.* 2010;**65**:889–94.

2. Kristensen MS. Ultrasonography in the management of the airway. *Acta Anaesthesiol. Scand.* 2011;**55**:1160–61. PubMed PMID: 22092121.

3. Dhillon RS, East CA, *Nose and Paranasal Sinuses, Ear, Nose and Throat and Head and Neck Surgery*, Elsevier, 2013, pp. 29–54.

4. Krohner R, Ramanathan S. Functional anatomy of the airway. In Hagberg C, editor, *Benumof's Airway Management*, 2nd edn., Mosby Elsevier, 2007, pp. 3–21.

5. Hall CE, Shutt LE. Nasotracheal intubation for head and neck surgery. *Anaesthesia.* 2003;**58**:249–56.

6. Hagberg C, Rainer G, Krier C. Complications of managing the airway. In Hagberg C, editor, *Benumof's Airway Management*, 2nd edn., Mosby Elsevier, 2007, p. 1193.

7. Fowler N, Scharpf J. Clinical head and neck anatomy for the anesthesiologist. In Abdelmalak B, Doyle D, editors, *Anesthesia for Otolaryngologic Surgery*, Cambridge University Press, 2013, pp. 1–10.

8. Redden R. Anatomic airway considerations in anesthesia. In Hagberg C, editor, *Handbook of Difficult Airway Management*, Churchill Livingstone, 2000, pp. 1–13.

9. Ovassapian A, Glassenberg R, Randel GI, Klock A, Mesnick PS, Klafta JM. The unexpected difficult airway and lingual tonsil hyperplasia: a case series and a review of the literature. *Anesthesiology.* 2002;**97**:124–32.

10. Goumas P, Kokkinis K, Petrocheilos J, Naxakis S, Mochloulis G. Cricothyroidotomy and the anatomy of the cricothyroid space. An autopsy study. *J. Laryngol. Otol.* 1997;**111**:354–6.

11. Melker R, Florete F. Cricothyrotomy review and debate. *Anesthesiol. Clin. N. Am.* 1995;**13**:565–83.

12. Rabb M, Szmuk P. The difficult pediatric airway. In Hagberg C, editor, *Benumof's Airway Management*, 2nd edn, Mosby Elsevier, 2007, pp. 783–5.

13. Wheeler M. The difficult pediatric airway. In Hagberg C, editor, *Handbook of Difficult Airway Management*, Churchill Livingstone, 2000, pp. 257–300.

14. Sunder RA, Haile DT, Farrell PT, Sharma A. Pediatric airway management: current practices and future directions. *Paediatr. Anaesth.* 2012;**22**:1008–15. PubMed PMID: 22967160. Epub 2012/09/13.

Airway algorithms and guidelines

Carlos A. Artime and Carin A. Hagberg

Introduction

Over the last 30 years, thousands of clinical practice guidelines have been developed in the field of medicine. The Institute of Medicine defines clinical practice guidelines as "system- atically developed statements to assist practitioner and patient decisions about appropriate healthcare for specific clinical circumstances."[1] For the clinician involved in airway manage- ment, the difficult airway remains one of the most relevant and challenging clinical circumstances because the implications of failing to establish a patent airway are potentially grave. As such, numerous practice guidelines have been developed to assist clinicians in managing the difficult airway, and a number of algorithms have been devised to assimilate these guidelines into stepwise decision trees that a practitioner can use when faced with this clinical situation.

The American Society of Anesthesiologists (ASA) Practice Guidelines for Management of the Difficult Airway

In a 1990 analysis of the ASA Closed Claims database, Caplan *et al.* reported that adverse respiratory events were responsible for a plurality (34%) of settled or awarded claims related to unfavorable anesthetic outcomes and that death or hypoxic brain damage occurred in 85% of these cases.[2] Although a majority (72%) of these cases were deemed to be preventable with better monitoring (i.e. pulse oximetry and capnography), only 36% of cases involving difficulty with tracheal intubation were found to be as easily preventable. These findings suggested that clinicians needed a broad-based approach to tackle the issue of difficulty with tracheal intubation. In response, the ASA formed a Task Force on Management of the Difficult Airway that same year.

The product of that task force was the 1993 ASA Practice Guidelines for Management of the Difficult Airway, which sought to "facilitate the management of the difficult airway and reduce the likelihood of adverse outcomes."[3] These guidelines delineated recommendations for evaluation of the airway, basic preparation for difficult airway management, and a strategy for intubating the difficult airway centered on a difficult airway algorithm (DAA). The Practice Guidelines have since undergone two revisions: first in 2003, which, among other changes, incorporated use of the laryngeal mask airway (LMA) into the algorithm; and most recently in 2013.[4] Among the most recent modifications are the replacement of LMAs with supraglottic airways (SGAs) to reflect the growing number of SGAs available in clinical

Cases in Emergency Airway Management, ed. Lauren C. Berkow and John C. Sakles. Published by Cambridge University Press. © Cambridge University Press 2015.

practice and the addition of video laryngoscopy (VL) as both an initial approach to intubation (awake or following induction of general anesthesia) and after failed intubation when facemask or SGA ventilation is adequate.

A prominent focus of the ASA Practice Guidelines is the formation of organized, preplanned strategies for airway management, including a preemptive evaluation of the airway meant to detect a potentially difficult airway ahead of time. Advanced recognition enables the practitioner to formulate a specific management plan for the patient and provides an opportunity to secure the airway before induction of general anesthesia (i.e. awake intubation). Per the ASA Practice Guidelines, evaluation of the airway should include a detailed airway history, examination of previous anesthetic records (if applicable), and a physical examination of the airway that focuses on multiple different airway features. The information gathered is then used to assess the likelihood of difficulty with one or more of the following: patient cooperation or consent, mask ventilation, SGA placement, laryngoscopy, intubation, and surgical airway access.

The guidelines recommend making the following basic preparations for difficult airway management: have a specialized portable storage unit available with equipment for management of a difficult airway, inform the patient with a known or suspected difficult airway, ensure that a skilled individual is immediately available to provide assistance when a difficult airway is encountered, provide adequate preoxygenation by facemask, and administer supplemental oxygen throughout the process of difficult airway management.

The ASA DAA (Figure 2.1) is the Practice Guidelines' recommended strategy for intubation of the difficult airway. It begins with a consideration of the relative clinical merits and feasibility of four basic management choices: (1) awake intubation versus intubation after induction of general anesthesia, (2) noninvasive versus invasive techniques (i.e. surgical or percutaneous airway) for the initial approach to intubation, (3) VL as an initial approach to intubation, and (4) preservation versus ablation of spontaneous ventilation.

The ASA DAA can appear confusing at first glance because it does not follow a linear decision-making tree, as the advanced cardiovascular life support algorithms do. However, it can be better understood and remembered by considering it as three separate scenarios: (1) predicted difficult airway (awake intubation), (2) difficult intubation with adequate ventilation, and (3) difficult intubation without adequate ventilation (the "cannot intubate, cannot oxygenate" (CICO) scenario).

In the predicted difficult airway, awake intubation is generally indicated for the following reasons: (1) patency of the airway is maintained through upper pharyngeal muscle tone, (2) spontaneous ventilation is maintained, and (3) the awake patient is easier to intubate because after anesthesia induction the larynx moves to a more anterior position. Awake intubation may be attempted through noninvasive or invasive methods (e.g. surgical airway, percutaneous airway, or retrograde intubation). In the ASA DAA, several options are suggested if awake intubation fails, including canceling and postponing surgery, performing surgery using facemask or SGA ventilation (if these are not predicted to be difficult), using a regional anesthetic technique, or establishing invasive airway access.

When awake intubation is not feasible despite a predicted difficult airway (e.g. in an uncooperative or pediatric patient) or when initial attempts at intubation after induction of general anesthesia are unsuccessful (the unanticipated difficult airway), the intubation strategy depends on whether or not facemask or SGA ventilation is adequate. This is a major decision point in the ASA DAA; ability to ventilate directs the practitioner to the "nonemergency" pathway, whereas an inability to ventilate directs the practitioner to the

American Society of Anesthesiologists®

DIFFICULT AIRWAY ALGORITHM

1. **Assess the likelihood and clinical impact of basic management problems:**
   - **Difficulty with patient cooperation or consent**
   - **Difficult mask ventilation**
   - **Difficult supraglottic airway placement**
   - **Difficult laryngoscopy**
   - **Difficult intubation**
   - **Difficult surgical airway access**

2. **Actively pursue opportunities to deliver supplemental oxygen throughout the process of difficult airway management.**

3. **Consider the relative merits and feasibility of basic management choices:**
   - **Awake intubation vs. intubation after induction of general anesthesia**
   - **Noninvasive technique vs. invasive techniques for the initial approach to intubation**
   - **Video-assisted laryngoscopy as an initial approach to intubation**
   - **Preservation vs. ablation of spontaneous ventilation**

4. **Develop primary and alternative strategies:**

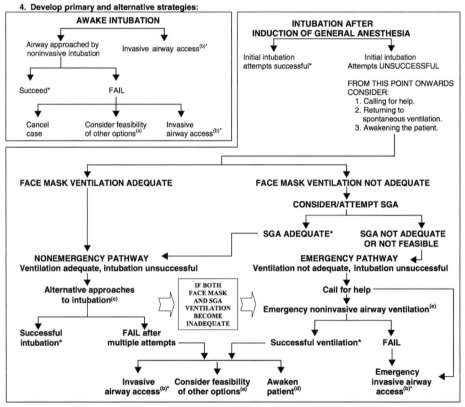

*Confirm ventilation, tracheal intubation, or SGA placement with exhaled CO_2.

a. Other options include (but are not limited to): surgery utilizing face mask or supraglottic airway (SGA) anesthesia (e.g. LMA, ILMA, laryngeal tube), local anesthesia infiltration or regional nerve blockade. Pursuit of these options usually implies that mask ventilation will not be problematic. Therefore, these options may be of limited value if this step in the algorithm has been reached via the Emergency Pathway.

b. Invasive airway access includes surgical or percutaneous airway, jet ventilation, and retrograde intubation.

c. Alternative difficult intubation approaches include (but are not limited to): video-assisted laryngoscopy, alternative laryngoscope blades, SGA (e.g. LMA or ILMA) as an intubation conduit (with or without fiberoptic guidance), fiberoptic intubation, intubating stylet or tube changer, light wand, and blind oral or nasal intubation.

d. Consider re-preparation of the patient for awake intubation or canceling surgery.

e. Emergency noninvasive airway ventilation consists of a SGA.

Figure 2.1 The American Society of Anesthesiologists' difficult airway algorithm. (From Apfelbaum JL, Hagberg CA, Caplan RA, et al.: Practice Guidelines for Management of the Difficult Airway: An updated report by the American Society of Anesthesiologists Task Force on Management of the Difficult Airway. Anesthesiology 2013;118:251–270.)

"emergency" pathway. In either case, the practitioner should call for help and consider allowing the return of spontaneous ventilation and/or awakening the patient, if practical.

In the nonemergency pathway, alternative approaches to intubation can be considered, including VL, alternative laryngoscope blades, intubation using an SGA as a conduit, flexible scope intubation, use of an intubating stylet, transillumination, and blind intubation techniques. It is important that the same approach to intubation not be repeated multiple times, especially with laryngoscopy, as doing so can worsen airway integrity. If intubation fails after multiple attempts with alternative approaches, options include awakening the patient (with preparation for awake intubation or surgery cancellation), invasive airway access, or consideration of alternative anesthetic options to enable surgery (e.g. using facemask or SGA as the primary airway, or using a regional anesthetic technique). If ventilation via facemask or SGA becomes inadequate at any time during airway management, the emergency pathway should be followed.

The CICO scenario is a life-threatening situation that requires immediate action. In the ASA DAA, CICO directs the practitioner to the emergency pathway. Practitioners are recommended to call for help immediately and to attempt emergency noninvasive ventilation with an alternative SGA if feasible (i.e. if the patient has not developed life-threatening hypoxemia). If SGA placement is not successful or practical, the ASA DAA recommends obtaining emergency invasive airway access (i.e. surgical or percutaneous airway, or transtracheal jet ventilation).

The ASA Practice Guidelines also recommend considerations and strategies for extubation of the difficult airway, which are discussed later in this chapter. In addition, measures for appropriate follow-up care after difficult airway management are delineated, including thorough documentation of the difficulty in the medical record and a debriefing with the patient or responsible person regarding the nature of the difficulty encountered and any possible complications.

The ASA Practice Guidelines and the ASA DAA have been subject to criticism for various reasons, particularly for the difficulty users have following the multiple decision points. The broad, comprehensive nature of the recommended techniques at various points in the algorithm has also been critiqued as being insufficiently specific to be of use in a true airway emergency. These guidelines, however, are intended to be basic recommendations and not standards of care or absolute requirements.[5] Rather, the recommendations found in the ASA Practice Guidelines should be used to help formulate a plan for airway management and should be adapted to reflect the specific skill set of the practitioner as well as individual patient factors.

The ASA DAA has also been criticized for beginning with a failure to intubate, in effect assuming that the primary intention of the airway practitioner is to intubate the trachea.[6] Considering that difficulty with facemask ventilation or SGA placement is often the initial difficulty encountered, the algorithm may then direct the practitioner toward interventions that have already proven ineffective. Other criticisms include a lack of recommendations for assessment of aspiration risk and various other minor inconsistencies, such as the inclusion of retrograde intubation as an option for emergency invasive airway access in the emergency pathway.[7]

Other national anesthesia society guidelines

In addition to the ASA, several different national anesthesia societies have published their own guidelines for managing the difficult airway, including the Difficult Airway Society (DAS) from the UK, the Canadian Airway Focus Group (CAFG), the French Society of

Anesthesia and Intensive Care (SFAR), the German Society of Anesthesiology and Intensive Care Medicine (DGAI), and the Italian Society for Anesthesia and Intensive Care (SIAARTI).

Except for the DAS guidelines, all of these include recommendations for predicting the difficult airway and suggest awake intubation as a management strategy. All of the practice guidelines include algorithms for both unanticipated difficult intubation with adequate oxygenation and the CICO scenario. Commonalities include a focus on awakening the patient if intubation is difficult but ventilation is adequate, using an LMA as a rescue for difficult mask ventilation, and performing an emergency surgical airway in the CICO scenario. The primary differences in these algorithms are in specific details, such as the number of intubation attempts suggested, the specific alternate devices recommended for difficult intubation, and the organization of the algorithm. Like the ASA algorithm, the Italian, French, and German guidelines incorporate all scenarios into one algorithm, whereas the DAS and CAFG guidelines have distinct algorithms for specific scenarios.

The crash airway algorithm

The difficult airway guidelines and algorithms developed by anesthesia societies are focused primarily on the elective management of airways in the perioperative setting. Many of these recommended strategies make several assumptions that often do not apply in emergency or prehospital settings. In these circumstances, clinicians may not have the opportunity to perform a detailed assessment of the potential for a difficult airway (owing to the emergent need for intubation), patients may not be cooperative or stable enough to undergo awake intubation, patients are frequently unfasted, and awakening the patient is often not an option (e.g. the patient in extremis). As such, a number of DAAs have been developed for use in the emergency department or prehospital setting. For example, the algorithm developed by Drs. Walls and Murphy consists of four distinct algorithms for separate scenarios: the main algorithm, the crash airway algorithm (for the patient in extremis), the difficult airway algorithm (for the predicted difficult airway), and the failed airway algorithm (for the CICO scenario). These algorithms have many similarities to the anesthesia society algorithms, but they do not focus on awakening the patient. One notable difference is the recommendation to administer succinylcholine if the initial attempt at intubation is unsuccessful during a "crash" airway.

The ASA DAA itself has been modified for the trauma setting, as well. The 2003 DAA was modified in 2005 by W. C. Wilson,[8] who also developed specific algorithms for various trauma settings. The ASA Committee on Trauma and Emergency Preparedness has recently updated these modifications using the latest revisions to the DAA.[9] In addition to providing specific recommendations on cricoid pressure, manual in-line stabilization, and VL in the trauma setting, algorithms are suggested to aid in management of various difficult airway scenarios, including closed head injury, airway disruption, oral/maxillofacial trauma, cervical spine injury, and airway compression.

Institutional algorithms

A limitation of the guidelines and algorithms presented thus far is a lack of validation in a clinical trial. Although a recent analysis of the ASA Closed Claims Database showed that the incidence of adverse respiratory events at induction has decreased since the introduction of the ASA DAA,[10] it is difficult to assign sole benefit to the adoption of the ASA Practice Guidelines' recommendations.

Various institutional algorithms have been devised and many have been evaluated in clinical trials. These institutional algorithms differ from national society guidelines in that they are usually more specific with regard to the airway devices that are suggested at different points in the algorithm. This specificity accounts for usual institutional practices, the availability of particular airway adjuncts, and the familiarity of individual practitioners with different airway management techniques.

One of the most well-studied and commonly cited algorithms is the emergency airway algorithm developed at the R. Adams Cowley Shock Trauma Center at the University of Maryland.[11] This algorithm is a simplified version of the ASA DAA and focuses on rapid sequence intubation with up to three laryngoscopic attempts (utilizing a bougie, if indicated), followed by an attempt at LMA ventilation, and finally the performance of a surgical airway if ventilation has not been established. In a 10-year retrospective analysis of the use of this algorithm, in more than 30,000 patients, the overall rate of surgical airway was 0.1%, and no patients died from a failed airway.[11]

The Vortex approach

The Vortex approach, conceived by Dr. Nicholas Chrimes, a specialist anaesthetist in Melbourne, Australia, is a cognitive tool designed to facilitate management of the unanticipated difficult airway.[6] Rather than relying on complex algorithms that are based on decision trees, the Vortex model utilizes a visual aid in the shape of a funnel or vortex (Figure 2.2) to guide the airway practitioner through the three basic nonsurgical airway techniques (facemask ventilation, SGA, and endotracheal intubation (ETT)). If after an "optimal attempt" at each of these nonsurgical modalities, alveolar oxygen delivery has not been achieved, then one "travels down the vortex," and an emergency surgical airway is indicated.

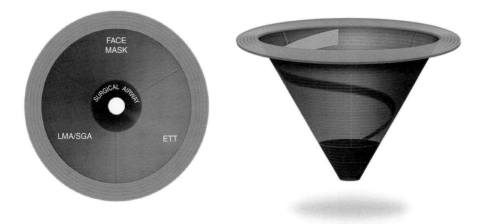

Figure 2.2 The Vortex approach. (From Chrimes N, Fritz P. *The Vortex Approach: Management of the Unanticipated Difficult Airway.* Los Gatos, CA: Smashwords; 2013.)

In the Vortex model, an "optimal attempt" is defined as no more than three attempts at any single modality, with special attention paid to various optimization strategies. The strategies are: (1) manipulation (e.g. jaw thrust, "sniffing" position, external laryngeal manipulation), (2) use of adjuncts (e.g. naso- or oropharyngeal airways, stylets, bougies), (3) changing the size or type of device, (4) suctioning the airway to remove blood, secretions, or foreign material, and (5) ensuring that muscle tone is allowing optimal attempts at nonsurgical airway management (i.e. ensuring adequate muscle relaxation if the prospect of spontaneous ventilation recovery is poor).

If one of the airway techniques results in confirmation of oxygen delivery, one moves out of the vortex into the "green zone." The "green zone" is conceptualized as an airway "time out" during which alternative options can be explored, including waking the patient or establishing a definitive airway via noninvasive or surgical means. If, on the other hand, the practitioner is unable to establish adequate oxygenation and ventilation by facemask, SGA, or ETT within three attempts at any technique, the practitioner proceeds down the vortex and should establish invasive airway access, such as a cricothyrotomy.

The benefits of the Vortex approach are its simplicity and flexibility. Because this strategic approach is more conceptual, it is simple enough to be utilized and recalled during a stressful airway emergency, but it can also be used to devise an airway management plan preemptively. Because the model is circular, it can be easily utilized in various scenarios, whether the primary airway plan was to mask ventilate, place an SGA, or intubate.

Extubation guidelines and algorithms

Although outcomes related to airway complications at the time of intubation have been improving over the last 20 years, the same does not hold true for extubation. As shown by the recent Fourth National Audit Project (NAP4) of the Royal College of Anaesthetists in the United Kingdom, one-third of major complications of airway management occurred at extubation or in the recovery room and were associated with a 5% mortality rate.[12] Findings such as these have highlighted the need to develop strategies for safe and successful extubation.

The ASA Practice Guidelines for Management of the Difficult Airway put forth the following recommendations regarding how to formulate an extubation plan for patients with a difficult airway:[4]

1. Consider the risks and benefits of awake extubation versus extubation in the deeply anesthetized state.
2. Carefully evaluate factors that could impair ventilation after extubation.
3. Formulate a plan to immediately regain control of the airway if adequate ventilation is not achieved after extubation.
4. Consider the short-term use of a stylet or airway exchange catheter to aid in reintubation and/or ventilation if extubation fails.

In 2012, DAS published the first comprehensive guidelines for management of tracheal extubation in adult perioperative practice.[13] These guidelines consider the presence of pre-existing airway difficulties (e.g. difficult initial airway management, obesity/obstructive sleep apnea, and elevated risk for aspiration of gastric contents), perioperative airway deterioration (anatomic distortion, edema, or hemorrhage caused by surgical or nonsurgical factors), and/or restricted airway access as risk factors for extubation failure. In patients at risk for extubation failure, particularly those with a difficult airway, one of several alternative strategies can be utilized. These include airway exchange catheter-assisted extubation, LMA-assisted extubation, and the use of remifentanil (an intravenous, ultrashort-acting opioid).

Summary

Despite the number of different practice guidelines available to assist practitioners with management of a difficult airway, no evidence supports one set of guidelines over another. It is clear, however, that they play an important role in patient safety. Even if not implemented exactly as written, the dissemination of these guidelines encourages airway practitioners to consider their strategies and formulate specific plans for management of a predicted or unexpected difficult airway.

The different algorithms and guidelines are highly variable owing to the lack of an optimal technologic solution for all difficult airway scenarios. The continued proliferation of airway devices designed to aid management of the difficult airway has the potential to improve outcomes but may leave the airway practitioner with unanswered questions regarding which device to use in which circumstance. Each device has unique properties that may be advantageous in certain situations, yet limiting in others. Specific airway management techniques are greatly influenced by individual disease and anatomy, and successful management may require a combination of devices and techniques. It is important, therefore, that practitioners develop their own individual strategies, founded on their own clinical experience and skills, and that any technique chosen is well rehearsed in patients with nonproblematic airways before it is implemented in those who are likely to be difficult.

References

1. Institute of Medicine. *Clinical Practice Guidelines: Directions for a New Program.* Washington, DC: National Academy Press; 1990.

2. Caplan RA, Posner KL, Ward RJ, Cheney FW. Adverse respiratory events in anesthesia: a closed claims analysis. *Anesthesiology.* 1990;**72**(5):828–33.

3. Practice Guidelines for Management of the Difficult Airway. A report by the American Society of Anesthesiologists Task Force on Management of the Difficult Airway. *Anesthesiology.* 1993;**78**(3):597–602.

4. Apfelbaum JL, Hagberg CA, Caplan RA, *et al.* Practice Guidelines for Management of the Difficult Airway. An updated report by the American Society of Anesthesiologists Task Force on Management of the Difficult Airway. *Anesthesiology.* 2013;**118**(2):251–70.

5. Caplan RA, Apfelbaum JL, Connis RT, Nickinovich DG. In reply. *Anesthesiology.* 2013;**119**(3):733.

6. Chrimes N, Fritz P. *The Vortex Approach: Management of the Unanticipated Difficult Airway.* Los Gatos, CA: Smashwords; 2013.

7. Levine AI, DeMaria S, Jr. An updated report by the American Society of Anesthesiologists Task Force on management of the difficult airway: where is the aspiration risk assessment? *Anesthesiology.* 2013;**119**(3):731–2.

8. Wilson WC. Trauma: airway management. *ASA Newsletter.* 2005;**69**(11):9–16.

9. Hagberg CA, Kaslow O. Difficult airway management algorithm in trauma updated by COTEP. *ASA Newsletter.* 2014;**78**(9):56–60.

10. Metzner J, Posner KL, Lam MS, Domino KB. Closed claims' analysis. *Best Prac Res Clin Anaesthesiol.* 2011;**25**(2):263–76.

11. Stephens CT, Kahntroff S, Dutton RP. The success of emergency endotracheal intubation in trauma patients: a 10-year experience at a major adult trauma referral center. *Anesth Analg.* 2009;**109**(3):866–72.

12. Cook TM, Woodall N, Frerk C. Major complications of airway management in the UK: results of the Fourth National Audit Project of the Royal College of Anaesthetists and the Difficult Airway Society. Part 1: anaesthesia. *Br J Anaesth.* 2011;**106**(5):617–31.

13. Popat M, Mitchell V, Dravid R, Patel A, Swampillai C, Higgs A. Difficult Airway Society guidelines for the management of tracheal extubation. *Anaesthesia.* 2012;**67**(3):318–40.

Chapter

3

A general approach to evaluation and management of the emergency airway

Adam Schiavi and Christina Miller

Introduction

You are on call as part of the emergency response team, or "code team," at your hospital. As a skilled airway manager, your responsibilities include responding to all emergency calls, anticipating that airway management may be necessary. You are asleep in the call room when the code pager alerts you to an emergency event ...

Subsequent chapters in this book will deal with defined airway pathology and how to manage each of these challenging situations effectively. This chapter, however, covers the general approach to emergency airway management (EAM). In this case, the challenge is the emergent nature of the situation rather than the specific pathology you may encounter. The case is intentionally vague because this event could be any patient, in any location, at any time, for any indication. Whenever the need for airway management is not elective, you will be operating at a deficit of information.

Airway management is not about placing an endotracheal tube on request. Airway management begins by evaluating the patient in order to decide whether or not intubation is appropriate – be a clinician, not a technician. Consider a patient who is experiencing increasing respiratory distress because of volume overload, which should be treated with diuresis rather than intubation and all of its ramifications. Airway management includes airway evaluation that aids in decision-making, even if the airway is not secured. Consider a patient who has an allergic reaction with isolated tongue and lip swelling but who does not have laryngeal edema when evaluated by nasopharyngoscopy. Forging ahead with intubation may be far more dangerous than providing supportive care and close monitoring. Airway management may lead to an intervention that can include manipulation of an existing airway device. For instance, a patient may have a dislodged tracheostomy tube or an endotracheal tube with a ruptured cuff that requires tube exchange. Finally, airway management may ultimately include securing the airway.

In contrast to the elective intubation in an operating room setting, where a preoperative assessment has been performed and the airway provider has access to airway equipment, medications, and skilled resources, emergent intubations on critically ill patients in remote locations can be quite complicated. Unfamiliarity with patient medical or intubation history; incomplete airway examination; inadequate monitoring, positioning, lighting, and equipment; and lack of knowledgeable personnel can all conspire against securing the airway successfully. These considerations are compounded by the fact that many patients who require

Cases in Emergency Airway Management, ed. Lauren C. Berkow and John C. Sakles. Published by Cambridge University Press. © Cambridge University Press 2015.

emergent intubation have abnormal or edematous airway anatomy, hemodynamic instability, limited pulmonary reserve, full stomachs, and metabolic or hematologic derangements.

Those responsible for managing emergency airways have many competing responsibilities. You may be responsible for covering many different locations in your facility, most of which are remote to where you are based. Your job may be to secure the airway and return to your primary service obligations, or you may be the code team leader and required to manage the entire event to its conclusion. Regardless of the specific situation, your job is clear. You must shift your focus to this patient and manage his or her airway as safely and efficiently as possible. This task requires you to be in a constant state of readiness and already prepared with a number of things. You need to know what material and personnel resources you have immediately available to help you; be able to get to the event quickly, assess the situation, and learn about the patient; have the necessary skill set to accomplish the task and manage the effects of doing so; support a patient with a secured airway; and transport the patient to a confirmed destination where he or she can be cared for appropriately.

Considering your resources and getting to the event

The emergency event is on a medicine ward in an adjoining building on the 10th floor. You get out of bed, turn on the light, find your glasses and shoes, gather your pagers and your code bag and hurry off to the event. (You have a code bag, right … ?)

The portable code bag should contain everything necessary to manage most airway situations. It should include a variety of laryngoscopes and endotracheal tube sizes. Other helpful adjuncts include malleable stylettes and Eschmann stylettes, or bougies. It should also contain equipment for assisting in ventilation should initial attempts at intubation fail, such as nasal trumpets, oral airways, supraglottic airways (SGAs) such as laryngeal mask airways (LMAs), and needle cricothyrotomy supplies. At the beginning of a call shift, test all of the equipment used for EAM and make sure laryngoscopes are functional. Check to make sure that all adjunct supplies are present and in usable condition. This process is also performed by nurses on the wards for the defibrillator and the contents of the code cart. Having a portable bag with you that contains basic tools is essential because others in the room may not be familiar with your equipment, thereby limiting their ability to help you. Additionally, knowing the location of other emergency equipment such as a flexible bronchoscope, or how to obtain assistance with a surgical airway, can save a difficult situation. Knowing how to contact those who can help with these techniques is crucial. If others are supposed to respond to these events with you, know how to contact them to coordinate your efforts.

As the technology of airway management continues to advance, new tools such as the video laryngoscope are more prevalent and may be part of the initial approach. A recent review of over 3,500 emergency airway events throughout the hospital at our institution revealed that video laryngoscopy (VL) is the most common technique after direct laryngoscopy (DL) for intubating the trachea successfully, as well as the most useful rescue method after failure of DL (personal communication, manuscript in preparation). Similarly, in the emergency department (ED), when DL is unsuccessful at securing the airway on the initial attempt, the use of VL is more successful on the second attempt at intubation (82.3%) than a second DL (61.7%).[1] In addition, it has also been shown in the ED that the use of VL is associated with increased success of tracheal intubation over DL when there are predictors of a difficult airway.[2] As a result of these findings, our institution now has a video laryngoscope present at nearly every emergency airway event. A caveat to this tenet is that advanced techniques require training to be proficient. Additionally, the more sophisticated the equipment, the more ways it can fail. Too much reliance on technology can lead to a false sense of security. It is worth considering having a video laryngoscope as standard equipment, but DL tools should always be immediately available and laryngoscopy skills maintained.

Although code carts may contain emergency medications, they are generally limited to advanced cardiac life support (ACLS) drugs. If EAM is needed, it is important to have immediate access to the necessary drugs, which may include hypnotic or paralytic agents. These drugs are usually dispensed from the pharmacy, which may delay management. Included in the portable EAM bag should be a drug box containing commonly used intravenous (IV) anesthesia drugs. Anesthetic agents such as propofol and etomidate, and paralytic agents such as succinylcholine and rocuronium are commonly used. Respiratory depression may be the result of narcotics, benzodiazepines, or residual paralytic agents, thus making the reversal agents naloxone, flumazenil, and neostigmine quite useful in correcting the indication for intubation. Additional emergency drugs for treating hemodynamic instability (pre-existing or iatrogenic) include atropine, glycopyrrolate, ephedrine, phenylephrine, epinephrine, esmolol, and labetalol. Rapidly acting drugs can temporarily stabilize the patient until more definitive treatment is initiated.

IV access is the preferred route of drug administration. If IV access is inadequate, it is helpful to have large- and small-bore catheters available, as well as a long 14-gauge IV catheter for needle decompression of a pneumothorax or a needle cricothyrotomy. Many institutions have moved away from gaining central IV access in a code situation in preference of intraosseous (IO) techniques when peripheral IV access is inadequate. If gaining IV access is difficult in a life-threatening situation, having a simple IO kit can allow medications to be given quickly.

Time is of the essence when dealing with EAM situations. Unfortunately, responders are rarely present at the bedside when an event occurs. The time from recognition of the event to presence at the bedside should be minimized. Know your way around the hospital and be familiar with the most direct route to hotspot areas, such as the intensive care unit (ICU) and the ED. A simple map can be of assistance if you are covering a large facility or are unfamiliar with the building. Move to the location quickly but safely and arrive fresh and ready for action. You are no good to the patient if you are wheezing and have a sprained ankle from running up 10 flights of stairs.

The location of the event matters. ICUs and EDs are better equipped to handle emergencies. Emergent intubations are common and providers in these locations are frequently trained in airway management. It is reasonable for any area that typically deals with acute care patients to be prepared with immediately accessible airway supplies in an EAM toolkit similar in contents to the portable bag carried by the code team. In addition, many EDs and ICUs are equipped with advanced tools for airway management such as a video laryngoscope and flexible bronchoscope. In comparison, public areas have no resuscitation equipment other than what the responding teams bring to the event.

Crowd control and getting to know your patient

You arrive on the ward and find a large crowd gathered at the end of the hall, hurriedly moving the crash cart into the area. You see a great deal of commotion, several medical students huddled in the doorway, nurses darting in and out of the room, and orders being shouted by several different people.

A patient in extremis can garner a lot of attention, especially if ACLS protocols have been implemented. Inevitably a crowd forms around the patient, making access to the head of the bed challenging. When you arrive at the scene, it is important to announce clearly who you are so you can gain access to provide a valuable service. Identify the team leader and let her know you are present and what skills you can provide; your level of training may also be important information. If you are responsible for being the team leader as well as managing the airway, it is appropriate to delegate leadership to another provider while you temporarily divert your attention to airway management. Delegation allows you to narrow your focus while someone else keeps track of the big picture.

Identify who can give you information about the patient so you can begin to make a plan about how to manage this airway. If the team leader is actively engaged in ACLS protocols, she may not be able to discuss the situation and should identify some other person knowledgeable about the medical history.

You find the patient in the midst of the action, tachypneic and somnolent

The more stable the patient is, the more time you have to ask relevant questions so as to make prudent decisions about management. If you are not well-informed, your airway management may be more dangerous than the patient's underlying disease process. Before you administer medications that may blunt airway reflexes, inhibit spontaneous respiration, cause hemodynamic instability, or trigger an allergic reaction, you must have a clear plan to support the patient safely. On the other hand, if the patient is already apneic or pulseless, you cannot do much to make the situation worse; the potential adverse effects of your management pose less of a risk than his current situation. If the patient's condition is rapidly deteriorating, spending too much time gathering details could also pose a threat. Striking a balance between the urgency of the situation and the time needed to gather information is a judgment call that must be made on the spot with the help of input from the primary team. Start with general information such as the admitting diagnosis. Essential information about the medical history for airway management includes reason for respiratory compromise, NPO (nil per os) status, allergies, weight, and a recent potassium level. Of particular interest is any prior airway management, such as history of difficult airway, airway surgery, lesions, or trauma.

Infectious risk determines the level of protection you may require; universal precautions are always appropriate. Gross contamination with blood or other bodily fluids may require a gown and face shield. Infectious diseases that are transmitted by droplets, such as influenza or tuberculosis, pose an additional risk to anyone in close proximity of the patient's airway during management.

If the patient's condition and time permit, a more extensive history is indicated. Focus on aspects of the history that are likely to influence your management decisions. Specifically learn about cardiac history, including functional status, heart failure, coronary artery disease or recent myocardial infarction, pulmonary hypertension, valve dysfunction, arrhythmias, or presence of devices such as pacemakers, implantable cardioverter defibrillators, or ventricular assist devices. Pertinent pulmonary history may include chronic obstructive pulmonary disease, pulmonary edema, hemorrhage, pneumonia, or aspiration; this may be an indicator of pulmonary reserve once the patient is no longer spontaneously ventilating. Renal insufficiency and associated hyperkalemia may influence the choice of muscle relaxant. Poor liver function or other coagulopathies increase the risk of airway bleeding, make nasal interventions less desirable, and may limit the number of attempts at securing the airway before visibility is impaired.

Similar to history, physical examination should be focused and based on the acuity of the patient. Begin with the basics – level of consciousness, presence or absence of a pulse, respiratory rate, effort and effectiveness of ventilation, and IV access. Look at any physiologic monitors in place for heart rate and rhythm, oxygen saturation, and blood pressure. A rapid assessment of the airway should also be performed, including oral excursion, ability to prognath, dentition (especially loose, missing, or removable teeth), thyromental distance, neck flexibility, and presence of secretions, to determine whether securing the airway may be challenging. Mallampati class alone can be misleading because the patient may be unable to cooperate. Clear the mouth of any foreign bodies, including removable dental appliances or piercings, before proceeding.

You maneuver through the crowded room with some difficulty to reach the head of the bed. You realize the patient has a 22-gauge IV in the hand, but no IV fluids are being infused.

Take everything you think you will need to manage the airway and make your way to the head of the bed. Ensure that you have working suction (a backup suction is useful in the event of large particulate or thick secretions); an oxygen source and bag-valve mask (BVM) for positive-pressure ventilation; your airway equipment, including endotracheal tubes, several types and sizes of laryngoscope blades, and stylettes; a rescue method for ventilating such as an oral airway and/or SGA; and a backup plan in mind. Bring any medications you may administer already drawn up and make sure you have a free-flowing IV with an injection port easily accessible from the head of the bed. If the patient is not on supplemental oxygen at this point ask to have high-flow oxygen delivered via facemask as soon as possible as you prepare to secure the airway.

Securing the airway
The bed is against the wall, and the room is rapidly filling with medical providers and monitoring equipment. The head of the bed is elevated, but the patient is slumped over in the middle of the bed, his chin on his chest.

Effective airway management is conducted from the head of the bed. Move the bed away from the wall to take this position. The initial attempt to secure the airway may be difficult. Even if the patient does not have a history of a difficult airway, you are participating in a complicated airway event because it is not elective and is in a remote location. The difficulty may not be the patient, but the limitations of the conditions in which you are compelled to function. Communicate any concerns you have as well as your primary and backup plans to others in the room; they will be more prepared to help you if they know what is coming next.

Your first attempt at securing the airway is the best attempt. With each subsequent manipulation of the airway, changes occur and conditions can deteriorate. Optimize intubating conditions before the first attempt to maximize the chance of success. Think ergonomically: you are strongest when you stand up straight, with your elbows close to your body and your arms bent at 90 degrees. Position the patient with his head at the top of the bed as close to you as possible to facilitate mask ventilation and laryngoscopy. This position allows you to perform those functions for a sustained period of time with less fatigue. Unless ACLS or other vital procedures are in progress, raise the bed to a comfortable height.

Laryngeal exposure is maximized by positioning the patient's head so that it is translated anteriorly compared to the rest of the body along the upper cervical spine and the neck is extended at the atlanto-occipital junction, in the classic "sniffing position." Support the head with a firm pillow or folded blanket, but avoid neck flexion. Create a horizontal plane between the external auditory meatus and the sternal notch. This head-up position, with the plane of the face parallel to the ceiling, facilitates viewing of the vocal cords during direct laryngoscopy by maximizing mouth opening and optimizing pharyngeal dimensions.[3] If the patient is obese and lying on a flat surface, adipose tissue in the upper back can contribute to hyperextension of the neck. In such cases, the patient's shoulders and upper back, as well as the head, need to be supported with a ramp to create similar axes and achieve optimal conditions for laryngoscopy.[4]

You place the pulse oximeter on the patient and find that oxygen saturation is 82%. With supplemental oxygen via a 100% non-rebreather facemask, it increases to 89%.

Preoxygenating the patient before securing his airway can significantly reduce the risk of hypoxia during periods of hypoventilation or apnea. Oxygen saturation below 70% increases the risk of cardiac dysrhythmias, hemodynamic instability, hypoxic brain injury, and death.[5] Delivering an increased oxygen fraction to a patient prior to intubation maximizes oxygen content, extends the length of time before desaturation or deleterious effects from hypoxia, and is especially important in patients with increased metabolic demands, anemia, or lung pathology. If the patient has poor ventilatory effort, apply a facemask with a tight seal and gently assist the patient's spontaneous efforts with positive ventilation pressure while he can still protect his airway. This approach reduces atelectasis, increases functional residual capacity, and bolsters the patient's reserve of oxygen prior to apnea. Similarly, delivering oxygen to the lungs passively via nasal cannula while securing the emergency airway significantly extends the time before oxygen desaturation.[6] Airway patency is necessary for this passive oxygenation to occur and can be achieved by using a nasal trumpet or jaw thrust during apneic periods.

You administer a small dose of propofol and 1 mg/kg succinylcholine. After 45 seconds, the patient fasciculates. You open the mouth, place your laryngoscope blade, and notice dark brown fluid pooling in the back of the oropharynx.

Rapid sequence intubation (RSI) is the standard approach for all urgent or emergent intubations in which the patient requires sedation. Most patients who require EAM are not appropriately fasted or are in extremis and have gastric contents due to physiologic stress and/or decreased gastric emptying. It should be assumed that these patients are at risk for regurgitation and aspiration. Classic RSI involves preoxygenation, cricoid pressure, and the use of rapidly acting hypnotic and paralytic agents administered sequentially without attempts at mask ventilation. The paralytic agent facilitates optimal positioning and intubating conditions, relaxes the vocal cords to permit atraumatic passage of an endotracheal tube, and inhibits the gag reflex, which can lead to active regurgitation. The application of cricoid pressure is believed to compress the esophagus and prevent passive regurgitation. The effectiveness of cricoid pressure in reducing the risk of aspiration is contested, but its use should be considered standard of care until definitive studies resolve this controversy.[7] From a medico-legal point of view, it is difficult to defend failure to apply cricoid pressure if a patient suffers from aspiration during intubation. Positive-pressure ventilation beyond 25 cm H_2O may exceed lower esophageal sphincter pressure, thus insufflating the stomach and increasing the risk of regurgitation and aspiration. In some cases, when hypoxia or hypercarbia are of paramount concern (the already hypoxemic patient, increased intracranial pressure, or severe pulmonary hypertension), it may be appropriate to mask ventilate gently after induction with pressures of less than 25 cm H_2O.

The choice and dose of hypnotic agents used to facilitate intubation depend on the experience of the provider administering the drugs and the patient's condition. First, determine if any pharmacologic agent is needed at all. Patients in cardiac arrest generally do not require any drugs for intubation. Consider the patient's level of consciousness when determining how much hypnotic to give, if any. The more awake a patient is, the greater his requirement. However, critical illness substantially reduces a patient's ability to tolerate these agents safely. Gentle sedation should be used cautiously if a patient is conscious but hemodynamically unstable. Many hypnotic agents cause vasodilation and depress cardiac output, thereby causing or exacerbating hemodynamic instability.

Only rapidly acting paralytic agents such as succinylcholine and rocuronium should be used to facilitate intubating conditions as quickly as possible and minimize apnea and risk for aspiration. Rocuronium 1.2 mg/kg achieves optimal relaxation as quickly as succinylcholine while avoiding fasciculations and is useful when succinylcholine is contraindicated, such as in patients with hyperkalemia, upper motor neuron injuries, and burns. However, the time to return of muscle tone and spontaneous ventilation with rocuronium is substantially longer. Use paralytics with caution if you have a concern for airway difficulty or if it is desirable for the patient to maintain spontaneous ventilation because positive-pressure ventilation could be detrimental.

After suctioning, you are able to see laryngeal structures and advance the endotracheal tube through what you believe to be the vocal cords. It is difficult to hear breath sounds.

Once an airway has been placed, its position in the trachea must be confirmed. The first indicator that an artificial airway is in place is visual confirmation. Confirmation may be made by using DL or VL to directly visualize the tip of the tube passing through the cords or by confirming bronchial rings and carina if a flexible bronchoscope is used for intubation. Confirmation by direct visualization in emergency situations may not be possible due to the presence of blood, secretions, or gastric contents. In an RSI, the epigastrum is auscultated during the first attempt at ventilation through the tube to exclude esophageal intubation before cricoid pressure is released. Other common methods of confirmation include fogging in the tube, chest rise, breath sounds, or resolution of cyanosis or hypoxia. These methods may be inaccurate in patients in extremis. Severe bronchospasm, obesity, pneumothorax, or other lung pathology can obscure physical examination findings, making them unreliable. The gold standard should be measurement of sustained end-tidal carbon dioxide either by a colorimetric technique or capnography.[8] It must be recognized that measurement of end-tidal carbon dioxide can be compromised by low cardiac output, so corroboration with multiple methods is ideal. False positive end-tidal carbon dioxide measurements can be attained if the patient received mouth-to-mouth resuscitation or recently consumed carbonated beverages. If there is any doubt as to proper placement of the tube, DL, VL, or bronchoscopy can be performed to confirm position.

Supportive care and transportation to a secured location

Once the airway has been secured, it is important to describe your interventions to whoever is recording information associated with the event. Information to be signed out includes the drugs used and doses given, the findings from laryngoscopic airway examination, the endotracheal tube size used, the measurement of its position in the mouth, and any complications you have noted.

You cycle the blood pressure cuff after intubation and find that the patient has a blood pressure of 85/43 mmHg.

You may be responsible for managing complications associated with securing the airway. Hypnotic agents commonly cause hypotension from vasodilation and/or depressed cardiac output. These effects are typically self-limited and can be temporized with short-acting agents such as phenylephrine or, in severe cases, epinephrine. If long-term vasopressor management is necessary, an infusion may be used. The stimulation of laryngoscopy or emergence from sedation can cause hypertension and tachycardia, which may be managed with additional sedation or short-acting beta blockers, depending on the etiology and severity. Bradycardia can result from increased vagal tone or severe hypoxia and may need to be addressed with anticholinergics (such as atropine or glycopyrrolate) or, in some severe cases, epinephrine.

Airway bleeding from laryngoscopy is usually superficial, isolated to the lip, tongue, or pharyngeal mucosa, and self-limited. If the bleeding is sustained because of coagulopathy, the underlying cause may need to be addressed. In cases of severe airway trauma, evaluation by otolaryngology may be warranted. Note any changes in dentition. If any teeth have been inadvertently dislodged, make sure they are accounted for and not still present in the airway.

A common complication of airway management is endobronchial intubation. Bilateral breath sounds and chest rise may have been noted immediately after intubation, but the tube can migrate. If hypoxia recurs, tube position should be reconfirmed with visual inspection and auscultation. Unilateral chest rise or breath sounds indicate the possibility of mainstem intubation, pneumothorax, or mucous plugging. Consider withdrawing the endotracheal tube carefully while listening for breath sounds, palpating inflation of the endotracheal tube cuff in the sternal notch, passing a soft suction catheter down the endotracheal tube, or obtaining a portable chest X-ray to check for tube position or other occult lung pathology.

You treat the patient's hypotension with phenylephrine and stabilize his vital signs. Now you are standing at the head of the bed manually ventilating the patient with a BVM, unsure of your next move.

After intubation, the patient will likely need continued ventilator support in a monitored setting. The patient may need to be transferred to an ICU, with manual ventilation via a BVM during transport or until ventilator support arrives. As the patient emerges from any sedating medications, he may become agitated. Additional sedation or opioid medications can blunt airway reflexes making the patient more comfortable and tolerant to the endotracheal tube. If the patient is to be transported, a plan for sedation is important so that he remains calm and does not endanger his safety by attempting to self-extubate en route.

If transport to another setting is indicated, it is important to have a detailed conversation with the person responsible for triage and admission of patients to that unit. Do not make any assumptions about her knowledge of the situation. If you need resources such as a ventilator or vasoactive infusion, alert her so that she has time to prepare. NEVER initiate transport of an intubated, critically ill patient unless you have confirmation that you will arrive at a secured location that is prepared to accept him. It is safer to stay where you are than to be in limbo during transport with limited resources. Before you leave your current location, make sure you have a full oxygen tank; a transport monitor with an electrocardiogram (EKG), blood pressure, and pulse oximetry capabilities; confirmed IV access; and a transport kit or code bag with emergency drugs and airway supplies in case the patient becomes unstable during transport. Know the most direct route. Do not attempt to transport an intubated patient alone. One person should be dedicated to supervising the airway and ventilating the patient; two people are preferable to manage steering the bed and handling other equipment such as ventilators or IV poles. If possible, have someone on the team accompanying you to call elevators, clear hallways, and open doors.

You arrive in the ICU, give a clear sign-out regarding the management you have just provided, heave a sigh of relief, and return to your call room for a well-deserved rest.

Conclusion

In this case, the situation poses the challenge rather than the patient. One is forced to make decisions and act despite incomplete information and unfavorable circumstances. Having a consistent approach to emergency airway situations will provide some order to what is frequently a chaotic event. This approach should be considered for any patient who needs airway management and is applicable to many, if not all, of the challenging airway cases described in the following chapters. Always be prepared – *Semper Paratus*!

References

1. Sakles J, Mosier J, Patanwala A, Dicken J, Kalin L, and Javedani P. The C-MAC® video laryngoscope is superior to the direct laryngoscope for the rescue of failed first-attempt intubations in the emergency department. *J Emerg Med.* 2015;**48**(3):280–6.

2. Sakles J, Patanwala A, Mosier J, and Dicken J. Comparison of video laryngoscopy to direct laryngoscopy for intubation of patients with difficult airway characteristics in the emergency department. *Intern Emerg Med.* 2014;**9**:93–8.

3. Levitan R, Mechem C, Ochrock E, *et al.* Head-elevated laryngoscopy position: improving laryngeal exposure during laryngoscopy by increasing head elevation. *Ann Emerg Med.* 2003;**41**:322–30.

4. Collins J, Lemmens H, Brodsky J, *et al.* Laryngoscopy and morbid obesity: a comparison of the "sniff" and "ramped" positions. *Obes Sur.* 2004;**14**:1171–5.

5. Mort T. The incidence and risk factors for cardiac arrest during emergency tracheal intubation: a justification for incorporating the ASA guidelines in the remote location. *J Clin Anesth.* 2004;**16**:508–16.

6. Weingart S and Levitan R. Preoxygenation and prevention of desaturation during emergency airway management. *Ann Emerg Med.* 2012;**59**:165–75.

7. Ellis D, Harris T, Zideman D. Cricoid pressure in emergency department rapid sequence tracheal intubations: a risk–benefit analysis. *Ann Emerg Med.* 2007;**50**:653–65.

8. Vukmir R, Heller M, Stein K. Confirmation of endotracheal tube placement: a miniaturized infrared qualitative carbon dioxide detector. *Ann Emerg Med.* 1991;**20**:726–9.

Management of patients with angioedema

Wendy H. L. Teoh and Michael Seltz Kristensen

Case presentation

A 58-year-old woman is brought to the emergency department with increasing swelling of her tongue and progressive dyspnea. The tongue is severely swollen and protrudes from her mouth. Arterial oxygen saturation is 97% on room air, pulse is 92 beats per minute, and respiratory rate is 22 breaths per minute. The patient has a subjective feeling of dyspnea but demonstrates no audible stridor. Her neck has no swelling. The patient is 163 cm tall and weighs 62 kg. No oropharyngeal structures are seen on inspection, and neck mobility is normal. The patient can protrude her lower jaw and her mouth opening is approximately 3.5 cm, of which 2 cm is occupied by the tongue.

The patient immediately gets oxygen via a non-rebreather facemask at an oxygen flow rate of 15 L/min. She is also given intravenous glucocorticoid and repeated doses of nebulized epinephrine (3 mL per dose, 1 mg/mL), but her clinical condition slowly worsens. The physicians decide to secure the airway. The patient receives 2 mL of nebulized cocaine (40 mg/mL) for local anesthesia via the right nostril followed by lidocaine gel. While the patient is receiving a mixture of 3 mL lidocaine 40 mg/mL and 3 mL epinephrine 1 mg/mL by inhalation, the practitioner threads a flexible video laryngoscope with an endotracheal tube that has an inner diameter of 6.0 mm. A remifentanil infusion (0.1 mcg/kg/min) is started, and the tip of the flexible optical scope is introduced via the right nostril until it is at the level of midtrachea. Subsequently, the endotracheal tube is railroaded until its tip is 5 cm above the carina. A direct laryngoscopy is performed after intubation and induction of anesthesia, but not even the epiglottis can be visualized. Inspection with a McGrath series V curved video laryngoscope permits a view of the posterior aspect of the vocal cords. The patient is transferred to the intensive care unit. Later, it is discovered that the patient had initiated angiotensin-converting-enzyme (ACE)-inhibitor treatment for arterial hypertension 2 weeks prior to the event. This treatment was changed, and the patient was successfully extubated 2 days later.

Pertinent review of the medical problem/condition and relevant literature review

Angioedema and urticaria consist of relatively short-lived edema in the skin. Individual lesions may persist for hours to days and can occur in conjunction with edema episodes of several organs.[1] Urticarial wheals and angioedema may be single or multiple. Angioedema is

---

a short-lived edema in the deep dermal layer of the skin and the subcutaneous tissue. Associated airway compromise can have fatal consequences.[2]

Vasodilation and increased vascular permeability are the main mechanisms in urticaria and angioedema.[3] The plasma passes through the vessel wall and becomes interstitial fluid. Endothelial cells control the movement of plasma constituents from blood to tissues. If the endothelium is permeable, blood constituents may pass through or between endothelial cells. The exact mechanism of edema formation and the mechanism of reabsorption of the fluid, after hours to days, is not fully known. Histamine might play a major role. Many patients who have angioedema that is associated with chronic spontaneous urticaria (CSU) respond partially or completely to treatment with antihistamines.

Diseases with urticaria combined with angioedema

Acute spontaneous urticaria

In acute spontaneous urticaria, angioedema usually occurs in the form of facial swelling, which usually responds to corticosteroids and antihistamines.

Chronic spontaneous urticaria

Angioedema is a frequent symptom of CSU.[3] It can be a considerable clinical problem when the angioedema affects the upper airway, especially the neck, pharynx, and/or tongue. Antihistamines may not work at low doses but may be effective at higher doses. Omalizumab is a chimeric monoclonal antibody that has shown efficacy for urticarial lesions and angioedema in patients with CSU who exhibit immunoglobulin E (IgE) against thyroperoxidase.

Other forms of disease in which urticaria and angioedema may occur simultaneously include cold urticaria, exercise-induced anaphylaxis/urticaria, episodic angioedema with eosinophilia (Gleich syndrome), and vibration-induced urticaria/angioedema.

Hereditary angioedema due to C1-inhibitor deficiency

Hereditary angioedema (HAE) caused by C1-inhibitor deficiency is a rare disease with an autosomal dominant pattern of inheritance.[3] During acute attacks of HAE, patients have elevated bradykinin, the main mediator of increased vascular permeability, and hence of the edema. Clinically, the condition is characterized by recurring swelling of the skin (extremities, face, genitals), gastrointestinal attacks (painful abdominal cramps, mostly accompanied by circulatory symptoms caused by hypotension, sometimes vomiting and diarrhea), and by edema of the larynx and other organs. Hereditary angioedema caused by C1-inhibitor deficiency is mainly seen in the first three decades of life, predominantly in the second decade. The tendency toward edema attacks can be greatly increased by ingestion of ACE inhibitors; these are contraindicated in patients with HAE. Angiotensin convertase II (ATII) receptor blockers can also increase a tendency for edema attacks.

Hereditary angioedema with normal C1-inhibitor (HAEnC1)

The clinical symptoms of HAEnC1 include recurrent skin swelling, abdominal pain attacks, tongue swelling, and laryngeal edema. Oral contraceptives, pregnancy, and hormone replacement therapy often play a particular role as triggering or aggravating factors. HAEnC1 has been observed predominantly in women, but male patients have been reported. Antihistamines and corticosteroids are not effective. Icatibant, a bradykinin-B2 receptor antagonist, and C1-inhibitor concentrate, as well as tranexamic acid and danazol, are effective, at least in some patients.

Angioedema caused by ACE inhibitors

Approximately 0.1% to 2.2% of patients treated with ACE inhibitors develop recurrent angioedema, often facial or lip swelling or edema of the tongue. Several patients are reported to have died from asphyxiation after their upper airways closed. The interval between the start of treatment with ACE inhibitors and the appearance of the first angioedema can vary greatly up to several years. ATII receptor blockers can also trigger the same forms of angioedema, though more rarely.

Angioedema with unknown cause (idiopathic angioedema)

Angioedema of unknown cause, or idiopathic angioedema, is one of the most frequent forms of angioedema and is therefore important in daily practice. Some such patients respond to antihistamines and corticosteroids, at either normal or higher doses. Clinically, massive edema of the tongue can cause airway compromise, and even without any externally visible edema, swelling of the pharynx can obstruct respiration.

Potential airway management scenarios and discussion

In the case described above, the pre-anesthetic airway examination indicated that direct laryngoscopy, video laryngoscopy, facemask ventilation, and supraglottic airway placement could be difficult or impossible. We considered three possible management strategies: (1) awake flexible optical intubation under ongoing inhalation of nebulized epinephrine and lidocaine mixture; (2) awake tracheostomy under ongoing inhalation of nebulized epinephrine and lidocaine mixture; and (3) awake intubation with a video laryngoscope.

We chose to use the awake flexible optical approach because it allowed us to keep the patient sitting up and maintain the inhalation of nebulized lidocaine (for local analgesia) and epinephrine. We could have performed an awake tracheostomy, but it would have been very difficult because the patient had difficulty lying down. Awake video laryngoscopy would have been equally challenging because the patient could not lie flat, and we were not sure that we would be able to visualize the vocal cords at all.

Algorithms/pathways to follow if indicated, alternate airway devices/resources to have emphasized

The swelling and airway compromise that result from angioedema are dynamic, progressive conditions that develop over time. Therefore, timing and clinical judgment are crucial elements in their management. It is extremely important to secure the airway before the angioedema can evolve into a health-threatening airway obstruction. Delay in securing the airway can result in airway edema that is so severe that even attempts at tracheostomy are unable to provide a patent airway.[2]

During the whole course of treatment, practitioners must have a plan for airway management, including a plan for rapidly gaining front-of-the neck airway access, should it become necessary. A stepwise approach has been suggested for airway management of patients with angioedema (Table 4.1).[1]

Table 4.1 Stepwise approach to airway management of angioedema

Symptoms	Features	Airway treatment	Pharmacologic treatment
Mild	Neck swelling Facial swelling Normal voice Normal swallowing	Conservative	Glucocorticoids Tranexamic acid Attenuated androgens
Moderate	Tongue fills mouth Altered voice Drooling Limited swallowing	Preventative – consider awake/spontaneous breathing flexible optical intubation	Fresh frozen plasma C1-inhibitor concentrate
Severe	Tongue outside mouth Cannot talk Cannot swallow Breathing difficulty Respiratory rate>20 SpO_2<95%(room air)	Supportive treatment – consider awake flexible optical intubation or awake tracheostomy	C1-inhibitor concentrate

Supplemented and modified from Cheng et al., 2007[1]

In addition to the management steps described in Table 4.1, practitioners should conduct a thorough airway evaluation to estimate the likelihood of success with the different ways to secure the airway, including percutaneous emergency airway access.[4,5] The trachea and cricothyroid membrane should be identified before any airway management is initiated. This examination can be supplemented with an ultrasound examination if the cricothyroid membrane cannot be located with inspection and palpation alone.[6,7] The size and shape of the tongue and floor of the mouth can also be evaluated with ultrasonography (Figure 4.1).[7] However, it is important to prioritize the clinical findings. If the respiratory distress is emergent, one should not delay treatment unnecessarily by obtaining images of the airway.

Tracheal intubation *after* induction of general anesthesia should be considered only when success with the chosen device(s) can be predicted![5] That means that if we cannot predict that intubation will be successful after induction of anesthesia then we should secure the airway while the patient is awake, or at least breathing spontaneously. Likewise, if our airway examination leaves us in doubt regarding our ability to perform percutaneous emergency airway access, we should also continue with awake intubation.

The airway of an awake patient can be secured by endotracheal intubation or with a cricothyrotomy or tracheostomy. Any known method for intubation can be used for awake intubation as well, but some are more suited than others. We suggest a flexible optical intubation if the patient needs to sit up and if we suspect that the edema extends beyond the glottic opening. Otherwise we can choose a video laryngoscope or an alternative technique (for example retrograde intubation) for intubation.

In the patient with no, or only a few, indicators of difficult laryngoscopy, it can be justified to induce general anesthesia before tracheal intubation. If the case is non-emergent, the patient can lay supine, and we induce anesthesia before intubation, we can use any of a

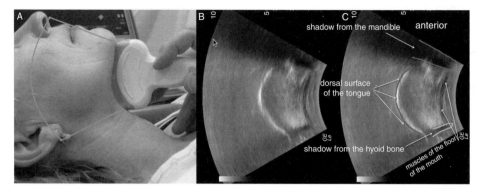

Figure 4.1 Ultrasonography for evaluation of the tongue before airway management. (A) The curved, low-frequency transducer and the area covered by the scanning (light blue). (B) The resulting ultrasound image. (C) The ultrasound image with labeling of the structures that are seen. The shadow from the mentum of the mandible (green). The muscles in the floor of the mouth (purple). The shadow from the hyoid bone (light orange). The dorsal surface of the tongue (red). Note the colors are not reproduced in the printed version of this book. For further reading see: Kristensen MS, Teoh WH, Graumann O, Laursen CB: Ultrasonography for clinical decision-making and intervention in airway management: from the mouth to the lungs and pleurae. *Insights Imaging* 2014;5:253–79.[7] Illustration from Kristensen MS: Ultrasonography in the management of the airway. *Acta Anaesthesiol Scand* 2011;55:1155–73

number of techniques, including video laryngoscopy, direct laryngoscopy, and intubating laryngeal mask.[2] In these cases the initial attempt at intubation can ideally be performed with a Macintosh-shaped video laryngoscope because it allows a lifting motion that may help to create space in the oral and pharyngeal cavity while also improving visibility of the glottis.[8] Immediate availability of both equipment and skill to perform emergency transcutaneous airway access via the front of the neck is mandatory.

Pharmacologic treatment of angioedema will not be covered in detail in this chapter, but for allergic and idiopathic angioedema, treatment includes antihistamines, glucocorticoids, and symptomatic treatment. For hereditary angioedema, one can give tranexamic acid and prophylactic treatment with C1-inhibitor concentrate before surgery. This prophylactic treatment is used to prevent attacks caused by the surgical trauma. C1-inhibitor concentrate can also be used to treat acute attacks. A whole range of new medications is currently becoming available for prevention and treatment of HAE.[9]

Post-management care and follow-up

Patients should be observed in the intensive care unit until airway compromise has resolved sufficiently. At discharge, patients with recidivating attacks of severe airway compromise should be equipped with relevant drugs to take in case they have a new attack.

References

1. Cheng WY, Smith WB, Russell WJ. Acute upper airway obstruction from acquired angioedema. *Emergency Medicine Australasia: EMA.* 2007;**19**(1):65–7.

2. Wood A, Choromanski D, Orlewicz M. Intubation of patients with angioedema: a retrospective study of different methods over three year period. *International Journal of Critical Illness and Injury Science.* 2013;**3**(2):108–12.

3. Bork K. Angioedema. *Immunology and Allergy Clinics of North America.* 2014;**34**(1):23–31.

4. Kristensen M. Predicting difficult intubation 2. *Anaesthesia.* 2002;**57**(6):612; discussion -3.

5. Law JA, Broemling N, Cooper RM, *et al.* The difficult airway with recommendations for management – part 2 – the anticipated difficult airway. *Canadian Journal of Anaesthesia (Journal canadien d'anesthesie).* 2013;**60**(11):1119–38.

6. Teoh WH, Kristensen MS. Ultrasonographic identification of the cricothyroid membrane. *Anaesthesia.* 2014;**69**(6):649–50.

7. Kristensen MS, Teoh WH, Graumann O, Laursen CB. Ultrasonography for clinical decision-making and intervention in airway management: from the mouth to the lungs and pleurae. *Insights Imaging.* 2014;**5**(2):253–79.

8. Teoh WH, Saxena S, Shah MK, Sia AT. Comparison of three videolaryngoscopes: Pentax Airway Scope, C-MAC, GlideScope vs. the Macintosh laryngoscope for tracheal intubation. *Anaesthesia.* 2010;**65**(11):1126–32.

9. Bhardwaj N, Craig TJ. Treatment of hereditary angioedema: a review (CME). *Transfusion.* 2014;**54**(11):2989–96.

Stridor due to upper airway obstruction/mass

Sage P. Whitmore

Case presentation

A 66-year-old woman with a history of obesity and chronic obstructive pulmonary disease (COPD), and a remote history of pharyngeal squamous cell carcinoma in remission, presents to the emergency department complaining of fatigue and shortness of breath. She is placed on noninvasive ventilation for increased work of breathing, and treated for suspected COPD exacerbation. Upon admission to the intensive care unit, she is having increased dyspnea. Physical examination reveals a somnolent but arousable patient with supraclavicular and suprasternal retractions. She has diminished breath sounds but no wheezing. Closer examination of the head and neck reveals harsh, raspy inspiratory sounds auscultated over the neck, as well as limited mouth opening and a firm, fixed, 2-cm right submandibular lymph node. Out of concern for upper airway obstruction and respiratory failure, the decision is made to secure her airway.

Introduction

Upper airway obstruction (UAO) is one of the most frightening and dire situations a clinician may encounter, and the decision regarding when and how to secure the airway is challenging. Patients with UAO present with symptoms of anxiety, shortness of breath, panic when lying supine, and occasionally dysphonia, dysphagia, or a subjective sensation of airway swelling. On examination, the patient may have visible anxiety and distress. Trismus, decreased neck movement, and inability to handle secretions may be present depending on the underlying pathology. Retractions and increased work of breathing are ominous signs of critical airway narrowing. Importantly, oxygen desaturation is a very late finding, and normal pulse oximetry or blood gas values do not rule out imminent respiratory collapse.

On physical examination, the hallmark finding of UAO is stridor, defined as a harsh, monotone airway sound produced during airflow through the obstructed airway.[1] This sound can be high or low pitched, may be audible at the bedside or only by auscultation of the neck, and may occur during inspiration or expiration. Stridor is not to be confused with stertor, the common snoring sound made by air passing through a partially obstructed nasal or oral cavity.

The characteristic sound of stridor is caused by the vibration of turbulent air rushing quickly through a narrowed airway.[1] By the time stridor develops, airway

Cases in Emergency Airway Management, ed. Lauren C. Berkow and John C. Sakles. Published by Cambridge University Press. © Cambridge University Press 2015.

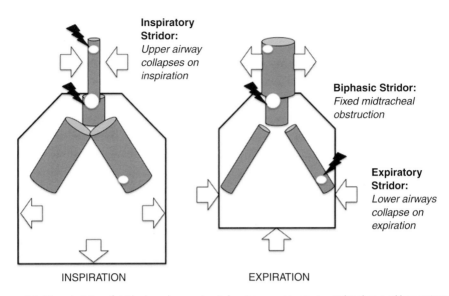

Figure 5.1 Characteristics of stridor based on anatomic location – upper airway, midtrachea, and lower airways

diameter has decreased by approximately 50%.[2] Gas flowing through an obstructed airway undergoes changes in speed and pressure. Specifically, flow increases and pressure decreases via the Venturi effect, causing a relative vacuum within the airway.[1] As a result, vigorous respiratory efforts such as gasping, crying, or coughing can lead to airway collapse because the pressure outside the airway is high relative to that inside the airway.

As detailed in Figure 5.1, the pattern of stridor can be used to approximate the level of airway obstruction, which may occur anywhere from the supraglottic structures of the posterior pharynx down to the large conducting airways within the thoracic cavity.[1] Supraglottic airway obstruction results in a loud, high-pitched stridor on inspiration when airway diameter decreases owing to the Venturi effect; on expiration, the pressure of exhaled gas increases the airway diameter and no stridor is heard. A fixed midtracheal obstruction, such as subglottic stenosis or mediastinal mass, typically produces a medium-pitched, biphasic stridor. If intrathoracic conducting airways are obstructed, such as by an endobronchial mass, the stridor is typically low pitched and heard best on expiration when the airways collapse under positive intrathoracic pressure; this resembles a wheeze except it is fixed in location and without the multiplicitous musical sounds typical of wheezing.

The differential diagnosis of stridor depends on the patient's age and history, as well as on the pattern of stridor detected on examination. Table 5.1 includes common causes of UAO by age. In adults, common causes of stridor include masses and malignancies, as well as infections; in the pediatric population, with the exception of congenital anomalies, stridor is much more likely to be related to infection than mass.[3] This chapter will focus on upper airway masses, as infections, angioedema, subglottic stenosis, midtracheal and mediastinal obstructions, burns, trauma, and congenital issues are discussed in other chapters.

Table 5.1 Potential causes of stridor based on age group and anatomic location

Anatomic location	Adult	Child
Glottic/supraglottic	Tumor Epiglottitis/supraglottitis Deep neck space infection Anaphylaxis Angioedema Inhalation injury Vocal cord dysfunction Vocal cord fixation (rheumatoid arthritis, relapsing polychondritis) Foreign body	Epiglottitis/supraglottitis Deep neck space infection Foreign body Anaphylaxis Angioedema Inhalational injury Tonsillar enlargement Congenital anomalies Vocal cord paralysis Mass
Subglottic/midtrachea	Subglottic stenosis Deep neck space infection Tumor Thyroid cancer Trauma Hematoma	Laryngotracheobronchitis Deep neck space infection Bacterial tracheitis Tracheomalacia Hemangioma Cyst Papillomatosis Congenital anomalies Vascular ring/sling Subglottic stenosis Mass Trauma Hematoma
Mediastinal/intrathoracic	Mediastinal mass Endobronchial mass Foreign body	Foreign body Mediastinal mass Endobronchial mass

Airway management

First principle: the clinical picture trumps the data

When gauging the severity of UAO, it cannot be overemphasized that the clinician should not wait for oxygen desaturation, blood gas abnormalities, or radiographic confirmation to act; the degree of respiratory effort and patient discomfort should guide action. UAO is unlikely to cause hypoxemia until respiratory arrest is imminent; in fact, in a patient with UAO who is adequately ventilating, hypoxemia should prompt a search for atelectasis, poor secretion clearance, poor cough, negative pressure pulmonary edema, and/or pneumonia.[2,4,5] Additionally, as long as respiratory rate and effort are adequate, patients with UAO are unlikely to exhibit a respiratory acidosis on blood gas testing until late in their course.[4] We strongly caution against sending a patient with symptomatic UAO to radiology or computed tomography, as lying flat with inadequate supervision may lead to sudden loss of the airway, respiratory arrest, and devastating neurologic outcomes as a result.

Table 5.2 Potential difficult airway characteristics in the patient with stridor and upper airway obstruction

Anticipated difficulty	Difficult airway characteristic	Related example
Difficult mask ventilation	Distorted facial/upper airway anatomy	Post-surgical changes
Difficult laryngoscopy	Distorted supraglottic anatomy Difficult mouth opening Difficult neck extension	Mass effect Post-surgical changes Post-radiation changes Rheumatoid arthritis Cervical fusion
Difficult supraglottic airway	Distorted supraglottic anatomy	Mass effect
Difficult surgical airway	Distorted neck anatomy Difficult tissue dissection Difficult tracheal cannulation	Post-radiation changes, scarring Subglottic stenosis
Difficult physiology	Hypoxemia Acidosis Hypotension	Pneumonia Atelectasis Pulmonary edema Hypoventilation Concurrent sepsis or bleeding

Second principle: avoid sedation and paralysis

When treating a patient with UAO, it is critically important *never to take away what cannot be given back*; that is, do not extinguish spontaneous respirations in a patient for whom intubation, bag-mask ventilation, and surgical rescue are likely to be difficult. One must assume myriad difficult airway characteristics to be present in a patient with UAO. While a full discussion of difficult airway algorithms is beyond the scope of this chapter, it is worth reiterating that all factors that contribute to an anticipated difficult airway may be present simultaneously in a patient with UAO (see Table 5.2); therefore we recommend against the routine use of sedation, intravenous anesthetics, neuromuscular blockade, and rapid sequence intubation in these cases. Anecdotally, even an otherwise benign dose of benzodiazepine or ketamine can result in complete apnea in an obstructed and exhausted patient.

Third principle: surgical management may be "Plan A"

A major feature of UAO management is that surgical intervention is now near or at the top of the algorithm and may be the preferred method for securing the airway. It is crucial to have all necessary surgical equipment at the ready and quickly to gather a coordinated, multidisciplinary team, including an emergency or critical care physician, anesthesiologist, and head and neck surgeon. The operating room (OR) may be the ideal environment for managing the obstructed airway, provided it is safe to transport the patient. The OR provides a controlled environment with dedicated surgical and anesthetic teams and equipment not readily available elsewhere, such as rigid ventilating bronchoscopes, instruments for endoscopic tumor debulking, open tracheostomy trays, cautery, jet ventilation equipment, and inhaled anesthetics.

Fourth principle: buy time while examining the airway

With the exception of an agonal patient, the starting point for airway management in patients with UAO is to visually inspect the upper airway as quickly as possible, usually via fiberoptic nasopharyngoscopy or another flexible endoscopic technique.[2,4,6–8] This visual examination provides crucial information for airway management planning, including obstruction severity, ease of visualization of the glottic opening, and clues to the diagnosis. Simultaneously, measures to temporize the patient and improve symptoms should be initiated. Seat the patient fully upright for comfort and efficiency of ventilation, place him/her in a care area with close monitoring, apply humidified high-flow oxygen, and consider nebulized racemic epinephrine and parenteral corticosteroids.[2,9] Helium–oxygen mixtures (heliox) may be effective in relieving stridor and improving work of breathing by providing a low-density gas that produces less turbulence and better laminar flow than room air or oxygen;[10] however, use of heliox is a temporizing measure that does not treat the obstruction and may mask deterioration.

Fifth principle: intubation technique is dictated by the airway examination

The method of intubation will depend on the information obtained during airway inspection (See Figure 5.2 for suggested algorithm). There are essentially three main options for intubating a patient with UAO, all of which include maintaining spontaneous respirations and having multiple surgical options at the ready: rigid (direct or video) laryngoscopy with inhaled induction or topical anesthesia, awake fiberoptic intubation (AFOI) with topical anesthesia, and awake tracheostomy with local anesthesia.[2,4,6,7,9]

If the upper airway examination reveals a mild to moderate obstruction, a mostly or partially visible glottic opening, and minimal anatomic difficulty, intubation by rigid laryngoscopy is reasonable. Rigid laryngoscopy may be accomplished with pharmacologic anxiolysis and topical anesthesia to the oropharynx, or in some cases it may be preferable to use inhaled anesthetic while maintaining spontaneous respirations.[2,6] If the patient has mild to moderate obstruction but has other difficult airway characteristics, such as limited jaw mobility, limited neck extension, postoperative or post-radiation changes to the head and neck, or morbid obesity, AFOI is useful.[6] In the case of severe obstruction, difficult or impossible visualization of the glottic opening, multiple difficult airway characteristics, and/or severe patient distress, one should proceed directly to awake tracheostomy with local anesthesia.[2,6,8,9] In all situations, the need for a smaller endotracheal tube (6.0 or smaller) should be anticipated.

Adjuncts and rescues

The use of AFOI for UAO is controversial. In the case of edematous or friable lesions directly about the glottic opening, railroading an endotracheal tube over a scope has the potential to worsen intubating conditions, leading to bleeding, swelling, and loss of the airway.[2,6] Furthermore, the presence of a scope between the vocal cords, along with topical anesthetic delivered to the cords, may lead to the sensation of suffocation and cause paroxysms of coughing, converting a partial obstruction into a total obstruction. Conversely, the use of AFOI is specifically advocated in cases of deep neck space infection, such as Ludwig's angina or retropharyngeal abscess, as the scope maneuvers easily through distorted anatomy while

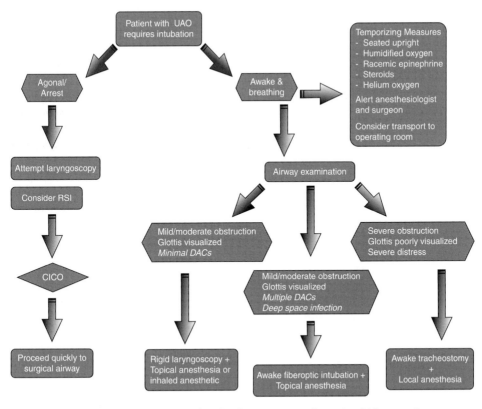

Figure 5.2 Suggested airway management algorithm for upper airway obstruction. UAO, upper airway obstruction; RSI, rapid sequence intubation; CICO, cannot intubate, cannot oxygenate; DACs, difficult airway characteristics (e.g. trismus, limited neck mobility, obesity, post-surgical or post-radiation changes)

maintaining spontaneous respirations and avoiding direct pressure on pus-filled spaces.[7] AFOI may also be preferred if the patient has a midtracheal or mediastinal mass.[2] In the former situation, cricothyrotomy or tracheostomy may be impossible; thus, it is critical to maintain spontaneous respirations while directly guiding the endotracheal tube past the obstruction. The latter situation takes advantage of spontaneous inspiration with negative intrathoracic pressure to keep the obstructed intrathoracic airway open.

Although advanced surgical techniques are beyond the scope of this chapter, it is worth mentioning several key rescue maneuvers that may be applied during airway management of UAO. If rigid laryngoscopy is attempted, it is possible that the practitioner may be able to visualize the glottis but be unable to insert the tube. In such cases, a ventilating rigid bronchoscope may enable the practitioner to access the airway and provide gas exchange during inspection.[2] If AFOI is attempted, it may be possible to pass a bronchoscope into the trachea but impossible to railroad the preselected endotracheal tube into position. If this occurs a stiff guidewire may be passed through the working channel of the bronchoscope, over which an airway exchange catheter can be placed for temporary oxygenation while a smaller tube is loaded over the exchange catheter.[9] If the patient cannot be intubated by any method and cannot be oxygenated, a surgical airway must be performed; however, if a surgical airway proves to be difficult or time-consuming, surgical access to the airway may be achieved via emergent cricothyrotomy or placement of a transcricothyroid or transtracheal catheter for jet ventilation.[9] Extreme caution is advised during jet ventilation, as a complete airway obstruction may cause rapid and severe air trapping that leads to barotrauma.[4]

Post-management care and follow-up

Routine post-intubation management should include adequate analgesia and sedation, chest radiography, ventilator management, and blood gas measurements. Patients intubated for UAO may develop post-obstructive pulmonary edema, also known as negative pressure pulmonary edema (NPPE), with an incidence of about 11–12%.[5] NPPE is a syndrome of dyspnea and hypoxemia caused by transudative alveolar filling that follows prolonged, forceful respiratory efforts against an obstructed airway (Type I) or the immediate relief of a chronic, partially obstructed airway (Type II). In adult patients, the most common causes are laryngospasm or upper airway masses, whereas children may develop NPPE during the course of severe croup or epiglottitis. The pathophysiology is not clearly elucidated but is thought to involve elevated hydrostatic pressures within the pulmonary vasculature from a combination of increased preload to the right heart, increased pulmonary blood volume, and increased afterload to the left heart resulting from excessively negative intrathoracic pressures during vigorous respiratory efforts. As this process is self-limiting, treatment is supportive and involves providing supplemental oxygen and/or increasing positive end-expiratory pressure. Routine use of diuretics is discouraged, as the problem is not one of overall volume overload.

Case resolution

In the presence of multiple difficult airway characteristics and a possible upper airway mass, the patient was kept sitting upright and awake. She was supported with supplemental humidified oxygen. Her blood gas indicated an early respiratory acidosis with adequate oxygenation. She underwent an oral endoscopic airway examination after the application of topical lidocaine. This examination revealed a large, friable, exophytic mass filling the entire hypopharyngeal/supraglottic space. Bubbles were tracking around the left side of the mass, but the practitioner was unable to maneuver the scope past the mass to visualize the glottic opening. Based on this information, an anesthesiologist and general surgeon were consulted, and the patient was taken emergently to the OR for awake tracheostomy. She was positioned sitting upright with her neck extended, and nasal continuous positive airway pressure was provided via anesthesia circuit and a pediatric mask held over her nose. Light dissociation and analgesia were achieved with 5–10 mg aliquots of intravenous ketamine every few minutes, while the anterior neck was prepped and anesthetized locally. An open tracheostomy was successfully performed without any adverse event, and the patient was returned to the intensive care unit in stable condition for airway monitoring and further workup.

References

1. J. H. Greinwald, R. T. Cotton. Pathophysiology of stridor and airway disease. In T. R. Ven de Water, H. Staeker, eds. *Otolaryngology: Basic Science and Clinical Review*. New York, Thieme Medical Publishers, 2006, pp. 212–19.

2. R. A. Mason, C. P. Fielder. [Editorial] The obstructed airway in head and neck surgery. *Anaesthesia* 1999;54:625–8.

3. J. Hammer. Acquired upper airway obstruction. *Paediatric Resp Rev* 2004;**5**:25–33.

4. P. J. Bradley. Treatment of the patient with upper airway obstruction caused by cancer of the larynx. *Otolaryngol Head Neck Surg* 1999;**120**(5):737–41.

5. A. Udeshi, S. M. Cantie, E. Pierre, *et al.* Post-obstructive pulmonary edema. *J Crit Care* 2010;**25**:508e1–5.

6. S. S. Moorthy, S. Gupta, B. Laurent, *et al.* Management of airway in patients with laryngeal tumors. *J Clin Anesth* 2005;**17**:604–9.

7. A. Ovassapian, M. Tuncbilek, E. K. Weitzel, C. W. Joshi. Airway management in adult patients with deep neck infections: a case series and review of the literature. *Anesth Analg* 2005;**100**:585–9.

8. J. E. Peters, C. J. Burke, V. H. Morris. Three cases of rheumatoid arthritis with laryngeal stridor. *Clin Rheumatol* 2011;**30**:723–7.

9. N. Choudhury, V. Perkins, R. Bhagrath, *et al.* Endoscopic airway management of acute upper airway obstruction. *Eur Arch Otorhinolaryngol* 2014;**271**:1191–7.

10. J. M. McGarvey, C. V. Pollack. Heliox in airway management. *Emerg Med Clin N Am* 2008;**26**:905–20.

Chapter 6

Tracheostomy-related airway emergencies

Vinciya Pandian, Mueen Ahmad, and Nasir Bhatti

Case presentation 1

A 51-year-old woman who had undergone partial hepatectomy with ileostomy closure and right hemicolectomy for liver cancer stemming from metatstatic lung adenocarcinoma presented with septic shock and acute respiratory failure that required intubation and mechanical ventilation. Because she had difficulty weaning off the ventilator, a size 8 tracheostomy tube was placed. Throughout her course, the patient was agitated and confused, and she attempted to pull out tubes. Three days post-tracheostomy, the tracheostomy tube is found lying on the patient's chest, and the monitor suggests hypoxia (oxygen saturation = 74%). The nurse attempts to replace the tracheostomy tube but is unable to reinsert it. The patient becomes agitated and tachycardic. Her heart rate increases to 145 beats per minute while the oxygen saturation continues to decrease. The nurse activates a code. When the code team arrives, the patient is intubated orally, stabilized, and then taken to the operating room (OR) for dilation of the tracheostomy stoma and reinsertion of a size 8 tracheostomy tube.

Review of the airway situation

The case described above is an emergent airway situation caused by accidental decannulation of the tracheostomy tube and difficulty to recannulate. Accidental decannulation refers to an unplanned and unexpected removal of the tracheostomy tube either by the patient or during patient care, such as while turning or ambulating the patient. A multicenter study reported that accidental decannulation occurred at a rate of 4.2/1,000 tracheostomies over a 7-month period.[1] Risk factors associated with accidental decannulation include mental status changes, increased airway secretions, change of shift, loose tracheostomy ties, and absence of limb restraints in confused patients.[1] Accidental decannulations are becoming increasingly common on wards where patients are relatively active and mobile and where the nurse staffing ratio is low.[2]

Airway management

The first rule in managing an accidental decannulation is to avoid panicking, because the provider's anxiety could impact the patient's anxiety level and in turn worsen the respiratory status of the patient. When an accidental decannulation has been identified, the provider who is present or arrives first at the scene should assess four key factors (Figure 6.1):

Cases in Emergency Airway Management, ed. Lauren C. Berkow and John C. Sakles. Published by Cambridge University Press. © Cambridge University Press 2015.

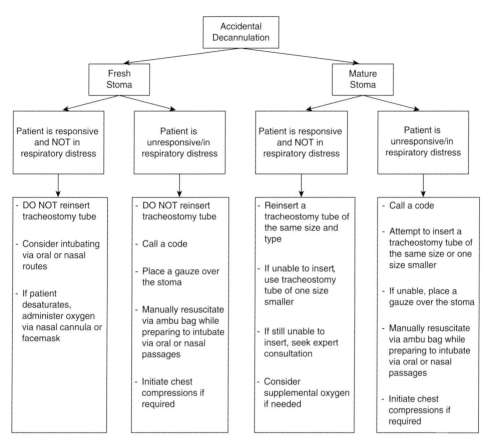

Figure 6.1 Algorithm for management of accidental decannulation

1. the patient's need for tracheostomy reinsertion
2. the patient's respiratory status
3. the patient's mental status
4. the age of the tracheostomy stoma.

If a patient requires a mechanical ventilator, or if the patient needs the tracheostomy tube for airway protection or patency, the provider should consider reinserting the tracheostomy tube. However, if the team has plans to cap the tracheostomy tube for potential decannulation or if the patient is already capped for decannulation, the provider must reassess whether the patient is stable from a respiratory standpoint and can tolerate being without the tracheostomy tube. This is the same principle that is used when an intubated patient self extubates. Not every extubated patient is reintubated immediately. However, the difference is that if the tracheostomy tube is not reinserted in a timely manner, the stoma may close. If that occurs, replacing the tracheostomy tube, should the patient need it, will become challenging, and the patient might require endotracheal intubation. If the patient's need for tracheostomy reinsertion is unknown, then it is best to replace it immediately.

It is vital to quickly assess the patient's respiratory status and mental status. If the patient is breathing comfortably, oxygenating adequately, and awake, then the provider may have adequate time to open a new, clean tracheostomy tube for insertion. However, if the patient is desaturating, the provider will need to make a quick clinical judgment regarding whether to replace the same tracheostomy tube if a clean one is not available within reach. Additionally, if the patient is in respiratory arrest and not responsive, then the first responder should call for help using the hospital's designated airway emergency number, or call emergency medical response if the patient is outside a hospital setting, and initiate manual bag resuscitation while seeking assistance from additional personnel to reinsert the tracheostomy tube.

It is also very important to investigate the age of the tracheostomy tube. A fresh or an established stoma will indicate whether the patient needs to be intubated from above or whether the tracheostomy tube can be reinserted safely. A stoma is considered to be established after the first planned tracheostomy tube change. Traditionally, this is considered to be approximately 7 days after an open tracheostomy or 14 days after a percutaneous dilational tracheostomy. Assessing the age of the stoma is vital because if it is fresh, the patient has a high risk of bleeding into the airway, which will worsen pulmonary status. Additionally, extensive bleeding can hinder a provider's ability to visualize the stoma, increasing the possibility of developing a false passage. If a patient has a fresh stoma, clinicians responding to the scene should focus on providing supplemental oxygen, ventilating the patient, or manually resuscitating based on clinical indications after calling the surgical team who placed the tracheostomy tube or a team who is capable of taking the patient to the OR for tracheostomy replacement. If the patient has an established stoma, then the first responder (nurse or respiratory therapist) can attempt insertion of a tracheostomy tube. The usual practice is that a tracheostomy tube of the same size is inserted first. If successful, it is secured in place with a necktie. If unable to insert the same size tracheostomy tube, then a tube one size smaller is attempted. If unable to insert the smaller size tube, then supplemental oxygen and ventilation should be provided and the surgical team should be contacted for additional help.

Post-management care

It is important to identify and address the etiology of accidental decannulation. If the tracheostomy tie was loose, the reinserted tube must be secured well. If the patient was confused and agitated, appropriate restraints, medications, and a bedside sitter should be considered to prevent future accidental decannulations. Increased secretions may stimulate vigorous coughing that can lead to accidental decannulations, especially if the tracheostomy ties are loose. In addition to securing the tube well, it is important to maintain an adequate suctioning regimen to avoid mucus buildup.

Case presentation 2

A 54-year-old woman with congestive heart failure (ejection fraction = 20%) and muscular dystrophy was admitted with cardiogenic and septic shock complicated by pulseless electrical activity arrest, a new cerebrovascular accident, and acute renal failure that required continuous veno-venous hemodialysis. The patient needed a tracheostomy tube for airway protection and chronic ventilator dependence. Because of her poor ejection fraction and uncorrectable thrombocytopenia (platelet count = 9), she was taken to the OR for an open tracheostomy. She had very minimal but constant oozing of blood from the tracheostomy site. Additional blood products were given as needed to correct the coagulopathy; however, 12 days after the tracheostomy, the patient had a significant bleed (~ 900 mL) via the tracheostomy tube. Computed tomographic (CT) angiography shows that the tracheostomy tube tip is causing physical irritation of the innominate artery. Interventional radiologists are able to embolize the area of irritation and stop the bleeding. An extended length tracheostomy tube is placed to bypass the source of bleeding.

Review of the airway situation

Bleeding is a common complication after a tracheostomy and can range from small to large volumes. Bleeding can be caused by aggressive suctioning, coagulopathy, stomal irritation, or physical injury to a blood vessel. Management usually includes gentle suctioning with a softer catheter, increasing humidification, and packing the stoma with hemostatic agents. Tracheoinnominate artery fistula bleeds are rare, with an incidence ranging from 0.3% to 0.79%,[3] but they are life-threatening without immediate intervention. A tracheoinnominate artery fistula usually develops from physical irritation of the tracheostomy tube against the innominate artery. It can occur immediately or even years after tracheostomy tube placement; however, it occurs most frequently between 7 and 14 days of placement.[4] In a meta-analysis of 127 documented cases worldwide, 72% of patients with a tracheoinnominate fistula were reported to have had the bleeding event within the first 3 weeks of tracheostomy tube placement.[5] Signs and symptoms of tracheoinnominate fistula, in addition to massive pulsatile bleeding, include those of hypovolemic shock. Bleeding may present as small amounts of gushing blood at intervals or massive hemorrhage. Often, clinical presentation is sufficient to diagnose the fistula, but bronchoscopic evaluation of the airway and CT angiography might serve to confirm the diagnosis. CT angiography is considered only if the patient is stable enough to be transported for radiologic testing.

Airway management

Once a tracheoinnominate fistula has been diagnosed, management must be immediate (Figure 6.2). The patient may require bedside intervention and/or emergent transfer to the OR or radiology suite. Therefore, surgical and radiological teams should be consulted promptly. Sometimes a thoracic and/or vascular surgeon might be necessary as well. A rapid response team, code team, or airway management team should also be activated to obtain adequate support personnel, experts, and equipment. While waiting for the appropriate personnel to arrive, medical providers should inflate the tracheostomy tube's cuff more to obtain a compressive pressure on the bleeding vessel. If bleeding does not stop, then the patient must be intubated from above. Then the tracheostomy tube should be decannulated and the bleeding site compressed with a finger. Because these patients could exsanguinate quickly, it is vital to ensure that the patient has adequate intravenous access (2 large-bore IVs – 16 or 18 gauge) and that blood products are ordered for imminent transfusion. Fluid administration with isotonic sodium chloride or lactated Ringer's solution should be continued to treat shock from blood loss until the bleeding and patient's hemodynamics are stabilized.

Endovascular techniques to repair or embolize the bleeding vessel are less invasive than median sternotomy and ligation of the innominate artery, and they require a shorter recovery period. However, median sternotomy and ligation is occasionally needed for definitive treatment.

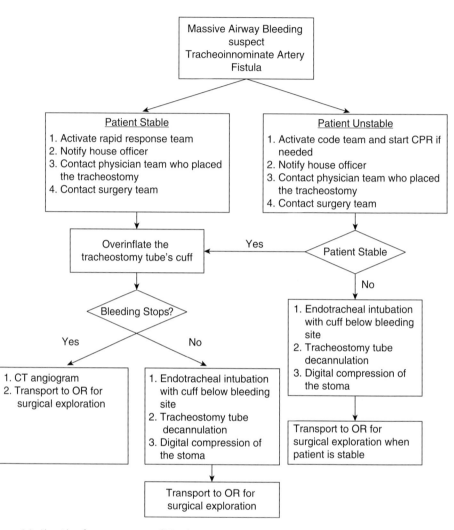

Figure 6.2 Algorithm for management of bleeding

In the case study presented, the otolaryngology surgeon opted for surgical management, but after a discussion with the patient's cardiologist and cardiac surgeon the patient was deemed to be too unstable for sternotomy, given her poor ejection fraction. After an extensive discussion with the family about the risks and benefits, the family opted for a less invasive approach, which turned out to be sufficient for this patient, as her bleeding stopped after embolization of the artery.

Post-management care

Postoperative management should include fluid replacement, including blood transfusions with packed red blood cells, platelets, and fresh frozen plasma. If the patient was on any anticoagulants preoperatively, they should be discontinued for a reasonable duration.

Bedside tracheostomy tube manipulations during bathing or changes in position should be limited. Because the innominate artery and the surrounding tissues can become contaminated with airway secretions, there is a risk for tissue inflammation that could result in wound infection, especially mediastinitis. It is very important to ensure that the patient is treated with broad-spectrum antibiotics and adequate wound care is provided.

Conclusion

Patients with a tracheostomy are at a high risk for complications that can range from temporary cellulitis around the stoma site to long-term tracheal stenosis or tracheomalacia. Certain complications, such as loss of airway from an accidental decannulation or high-volume bleeding from the tracheostomy site, can be life-threatening. These life-threatening complications can lead to devastating neurologic outcomes such as hypoxic/anoxic brain injury or even death, giving rise to medico-legal cases that can result in increased costs to the patient, family members, hospital, and society. Healthcare providers can reduce the number of devastating neurologic outcomes by following standardized protocols and algorithms while caring for these high-risk patients. A survey of 34 Danish intensive care units showed that only 6% of the wards had any type of guideline for accidental decannulation.[6] The situation is likely similar in other countries, but unfortunately very little literature discusses accidental decannulation and none describes the prevalence of guidelines for accidental decannulation. Similarly, healthcare professionals lack awareness about tracheoinnominate fistulae and their management, owing to their infrequency. We have presented algorithms for accidental decannulation and tracheoinnominate fistula bleeds that are being used in a large urban tertiary hospital.

References

1. White AC, Purcell E, Urquhart MB, Joseph B, O'Connor HH. Accidental decannulation following placement of a tracheostomy tube. *Respiratory Care*. Dec 2012;**57**(12):2019–25.

2. Wilkinson K, Martin IC, Freeth H, Kelly K, Mason M. On the right trach? A review of the care received by patients who underwent a tracheostomy: a report. *NCEPOD (National Confidential Enquiry into Patient Outcome and Death) Report*. 2014; 155.

3. Iodice F, Brancaccio G, Lauri A, Di Donato R. Preventive ligation of the innominate artery in patients with neuromuscular disorders. *European Journal of Cardio-Thoracic Surgery: Official Journal of the European Association for Cardio-Thoracic Surgery*. Apr 2007;**31**(4):747–9.

4. Grillo HC, Donahue DM, Mathisen DJ, Wain JC, Wright CD. Postintubation tracheal stenosis. Treatment and results. *The Journal of Thoracic and Cardiovascular Surgery*. Mar 1995;**109**(3):486–92; discussion 492–3.

5. Jones JW, Reynolds M, Hewitt RL, Drapanas T. Tracheoinnominate artery erosion: successful surgical management of a devastating complication. *Annals of Surgery*. Aug 1976;**184**(2):194–204.

6. Mondrup F, Skjelsager K, Madsen KR. Inadequate follow-up after tracheostomy and intensive care. *Danish Medical Journal*. Aug 2012;**59**(8):A4481.

Chapter

7

Subglottic airway emergencies

Seth Manoach and Oren A. Friedman

Case presentation

A 28-year-old man presents to the emergency department in severe respiratory distress. Vital signs are blood pressure: 140/86 mmHg, heart rate: 132 beats per minute, respiratory rate: 38 breaths per minute, and SpO$_2$: 90% on a non-rebreather facemask. The patient sits with his arms behind him and neck extended. He can say only that he has asthma and has been intubated several times, with a recent "emergency neck surgery." The patient has a goatee, a ragged cricothyrotomy scar, and a typical tracheostomy scar. He also exhibits stridor, retractions, and faint wheezing with poor air movement. The emergency physician administers 0.3 mg of subcutaneous epinephrine, nebulized racemic epinephrine, 2 g of magnesium sulfate, and 10 mg of dexamethasone. The patient improves slightly but pulls at his mask. After racemic epinephrine, the emergency team tries 80:20 heliox, but SaO$_2$ levels continue to drop. Anesthesiology and otolaryngology teams are emergency paged, and the patient is moved to the operating room (OR) while seated upright. In the OR, the attending anesthesiologist attempts awake flexible fiberoptic intubation. The patient desaturates to 70% but recovers to 90% after the attempt is aborted. The surgeons prep the patient's neck for tracheostomy while readying a rigid bronchoscope. The anesthesiologist administers 100 mg of ketamine, and the surgeon gently inserts a rigid bronchoscope. The surgeon notes a long area of circumferential subglottic airway narrowing but is able to pass a 6.0 endotracheal tube (ETT). Successive serial dilations are performed through the rigid scope during pauses in ventilation. After serial dilations, a bougie is passed through the scope, the scope is retracted, and a 7.0 ETT is gently rotated over the bougie. The patient is moved to the intensive care unit for stabilization, after which the team plans operative repair of the subglottic defect.

Clinical anatomy

The vocal cords and space between them define the glottis, and the subglottic airway extends inferiorly from the glottis to the inferior margin of the cricoid ring. The glottis and cricoid ring form the narrowest points of the extrathoracic airway. Consequently, they are prone to ETT injury during intubation and subsequent care.[1–6] ETT injury causes 90% of subglottic stenosis (SGS), most often circumferential cricoid narrowing that can progress to airway loss. ETT injury also causes glottic webs that lead to glottic stenosis.[2,4–6]

The anterior external structure of the subglottic airway consists of the thyroid and cricoid cartilages. These are joined by the cricothyroid ligament, membrane, and muscle.

Cases in Emergency Airway Management, ed. Lauren C. Berkow and John C. Sakles. Published by Cambridge University Press. © Cambridge University Press 2015.

The cricoid is the first and only circumferential cartilage of the trachea. The cricothyroid muscle, ligament, and membrane must be incised or punctured when performing a cricothyrotomy or transcricoid catheter ventilation.

The conus elasticus is a fibroelastic membrane that provides conical form and structural integrity to the subglottic airway lumen. The conus originates from the anterior superior cricoid cartilage, forming the lateral cricothyroid membrane. It extends superiorly and fans out, inserting on the inferior anterior aspect of the thyroid cartilage and the posterior aspect of the arytenoid cartilage. Free fibers of the conus give rise to the vocal ligaments.

The posterior aspect of the subglottic airway is supported by the posterior cricoid cartilage, which rises to form a plate connected by the cricoarytenoid ligaments to the inferior arytenoid cartilages. The posterior cricoarytenoid muscles originate from the posterior aspect of the cricoid cartilage and insert on the arytenoids, abducting the vocal cords. These muscles are innervated by the recurrent laryngeal nerve. Unilateral injury to this nerve can cause stridor, and bilateral injury can cause glottic narrowing.

Causes of SGS

Intubation-related injuries are caused by traumatic intubation, oversized tubes, overinflated cuffs, or excessive ETT manipulation.[2,4,5] The cricoid ring is prone to granulation tissue formation and stricture.[6-8] Other causes of SGS include burns, blunt or penetrating trauma, hematomas, and foreign bodies. SGS in children and adults has been caused by objects lodged in the hypopharynx/proximal esophagus posterior to the airway.[9] Esophageal foreign bodies can sometimes cause stridor in children owing to compression of the soft posterior tracheal wall. Foreign body aspiration and airway deformation are more common in children.[1,9]

Uncommon causes of SGS and stridor in children include congenital stenosis and birth injuries (traction of the head on neck causing recurrent laryngeal nerve palsy).[2] Infections can cause reversible SGS. The most common is croup, and others include bacterial tracheitis, retropharyngeal abscess, and fasciitis.[10] Neoplasms can occur in children but increase in frequency with age, smoking, drinking, and human papilloma virus infection.[11] Granulomatosis with polyangiitis, tracheobronchial chondritis, and sarcoidosis also cause SGS.[5] Traumatic and postoperative hematomas can also cause SGS, particularly after cervical discectomy and fusion.[12,13]

Airway physiology and clinical manifestations of SGS

Diaphragmatic contraction creates negative intrathoracic pressure, causing airflow downstream from the mouth and nares toward the lungs. As air encounters the narrow glottis and cricoid ring, flow is deflected, decreases in mass, and increases in velocity. A caudal pressure wave passes through glottic and subglottic tissues, distorting the airway and diminishing its structural support. As airflow velocity rises, intraluminal pressure falls, decreasing transluminal pressure (i.e. luminal pressure minus tissue pressure) and narrowing the airway.[14] At stenotic points, turbulent airflow causes stridor.

Acute insults such as circumferential edema in the pediatric airway, trapped mucus or clot adherent to a partially obstructing intraluminal mass, or webs and strictures inflamed by vomiting or upper respiratory infection may cause rapid loss in luminal area. Because resistance to flow in a tube is proportional to its length and the 4th power of the radius, reduced luminal area causes disproportionate decreases in airflow.[2] This increase in flow velocity, decrease in transluminal pressure, and subglottic airway distortion may precipitate emergent SGS.

Patients with emergent SGS present with dyspnea and stridor that occurs as flow velocity and turbulence increase during forceful inspiration.[11,14] Dyspneic patients with supra- and subglottic airway stenosis typically tripod while extending the head and neck, increasing longitudinal airway tension and reducing the likelihood of airway collapse.[14] If stridor at rest is not caused by a reversible process (e.g. croup, anaphylaxis), one should prepare for emergent intubation, cricothyrotomy, or tracheostomy.[11] Terminal fatigue is often preceded by head drop, neck flexion, and tracheal shortening, which favor airway collapse. As stenosis worsens, biphasic stridor may occur, and finally, as flow diminishes and respiratory arrest approaches, breathing becomes quiet.[14] This sudden disappearance of stridor should prompt a rapid reassessment, as complete airway collapse may be imminent.

General management of emergent SGS and undifferentiated stridor

Truly emergent glottic, subglottic, and extrathoracic tracheal stenoses may be indistinguishable in the absence of direct or collateral history (e.g. a note from a physician or presence of a reliable family member), obvious physical examination findings (e.g. a cricothyrotomy scar), or pre-existing studies. A portable chest X-ray can reveal an alternative diagnosis, such as an anterior mediastinal mass with recurrent laryngeal nerve compression.[15] Soft-tissue films may show subglottic narrowing (e.g. steeple sign) or evidence of epiglottitis (e.g. "thumbprint" epiglottis with supraglottic dilation).[2] Older children and adults may tolerate diagnostic rhinolaryngoscopy or gentle awake video or direct laryngoscopy.[11] Most often, the diagnosis remains uncertain, but all three types of stenoses are approached uniformly:

1. Small children should be left in their parent or guardian's lap while awaiting expert help and equipment.[8] First responders should not use a "blind finger sweep" to attempt to dislodge suspected foreign bodies, as this action may convert a partial to a full obstruction or drive a supraglottic object into the subglottic airway, complicating salvage of the foreign body.[1,16]

2. Interventions such as intravenous placement that increase agitation and respiratory effort should not be initiated until personnel equipped to perform nonsurgical and surgical airway salvage arrive.[1,16,17]

3. An inexperienced or untrained airway manager should initiate airway instrumentation only if the patient rapidly decompensates and death would be imminent without aggressive intervention.[1,16,17]

4. Inexperienced providers may be able to "buy time" using racemic epinephrine, dexamethasone, or heliox.[18] For heliox to provide maximum benefit, patients must be able to tolerate a fraction of inspired oxygen (FiO_2) of 0.2, although heliox at a 70:30 He: O_2 ratio may also be beneficial.[19,20] Airway resistance is a function not only of the structure and dimensions of the airways but also of the density and viscosity of the gases they contain. Helium is less dense and less viscous than nitrogen, and therefore is more likely to maintain laminar rather than turbulent flow through a stenotic airway. Laminar flow increases bulk gas exchange, transiently improves objective respiratory parameters, and may immediately relieve dyspnea.[11] This relief can decrease anxiety and inspiratory effort, reducing the dynamic component of upper airway obstruction.

5. The default method of obtaining airway control in patients with SGS or undifferentiated supraglottic, glottic, and subglottic stridor is to perform a "double setup," ideally in the OR, but often in the field or any place where critically ill and injured patients present. In a double set-up, providers and equipment are ready for transoral/nasal intubation *or* rapid cricothyrotomy, and the patient is prepared for both procedures. Some providers inject local anesthesia in anticipation of surgical salvage.

6. For emergent SGS and other critical upper airway stenosis, one should not ablate spontaneous respiration until the airway is secured by endotracheal intubation, rigid bronchoscopy-supported jet ventilation, cricothyrotomy, or tracheostomy.

7. Patients lose airway tone before diaphragm activity, and supine position favors airway collapse. Therefore, it is recommended that patients be intubated while sitting upright or with the head of the bed elevated.[14]

8. Rigid oral airways can cause trauma, vomiting, laryngospasm, and cough.[11] Nasal airways are more tolerable, as they splint the soft palate off the posterior pharynx, opening the airway.[11]

9. Cricothyrotomy is the emergency surgical airway of choice because data suggest that trained nonsurgical physicians or advanced practice nurses can perform it quickly and safely.[21] The incidence of cricothyrotomy has fallen dramatically since emergency airway managers adopted rapid sequence intubation; therefore, airway providers may be less experienced with surgical cricothyrotomy.[22,23] Seldinger cricothyrotomy kits are often used for percutaneous cricothyrotomy, but evidence suggests that the success rate of these kits when used by inexperienced providers is low compared to that of an open surgical airway technique.[22]

10. Cricothyrotomy is contraindicated in children.[24] In infants, the cricothyroid membrane measures 3 x 3 mm, the hyoid bone overrides the thyroid cartilage, and fat obscures landmarks. Because the cricothyroid membrane is small, many standard jet ventilation catheters (e.g. Cook inner coil 2-mm ID TTJV catheter) are too big, and attempts at surgical cricothyrotomy are likely to ablate the airway. Therefore, a tracheostomy is recommended but should be performed by an otolaryngologist or pediatric surgeon. In a truly emergent situation, nonsurgeons can attempt transtracheal puncture with a fluid-filled syringe and the neck in an extended position. Presence of an air bubble in the syringe confirms tracheal placement, after which an appropriate-sized angio- or Ravussin catheter can be inserted. Ventilation is provided by attaching rigid tubing to a manual jet ventilator, adjusted for age, or to an ENK flow modulator, which is a ventilation catheter with built-in manual oxygen modulator and tubing (Cook Critical Care, Bloomington, IN, USA). Barotrauma and catheter kinking must be identified immediately.[24]

11. In adults or children who need surgical salvage, a supraglottic airway device may be life- and brain-saving. Rescue ventilation with a supraglottic airway device while awaiting experienced help or arranging transfer by highly skilled personnel (e.g. emergency flight crews) may be safer than attempting a difficult high-risk procedure that may fail to provide safe, adequate ventilation.

12. Tracheostomy is preferred to cricothyrotomy in *very* proficient hands because it is a definitive procedure, unlike a cricothyrotomy, which must be revised within a few days. The cricothyroid membrane is often the site of SGS lesions, so tissue defects may complicate the procedure and repeat trauma may worsen long-term prognosis.

Use of topical anesthesia/sedation in patients with SGS

We prefer to use topical anesthesia with 2–4% lidocaine before attempting airway instrumentation. Some literature suggests that lidocaine may cause laryngospasm, which could worsen the airway obstruction.[11] Most patients with upper airway emergencies are agitated and may benefit from topical anesthesia *plus* some sedative agent and much reassurance, but sedation also carries the risk of worsening airway obstruction, so this decision should be made very carefully.

If the airway is managed in the OR, some recommend inducing anesthesia slowly with sevoflurane and/or nitrous oxide to calm the patient while maintaining spontaneous respiration.[1,6,11] Once the patient has reached an appropriate anesthetic plane, the airway manager can gently insert a direct fiberoptic scope or video laryngoscope. The lingual surface and tip should be lubricated with 2% viscous lidocaine, but care should be taken not to soil the optic portion of the device.

For the airway manager without access to volatile anesthetics, ketamine is a reasonable option to facilitate awake intubations of patients with at-risk airways. However, ketamine may precipitate laryngospasm, which the operator must be prepared to manage. With the exception of very few patients who present with malignant tachydysrhythmias, the benefit of intact airway tone, spontaneous respiration, and a dissociated state outweighs the risk of laryngospasm. Glycopyrrolate at 0.2 mg or 0.015 mg/kg can be used as an antisialagogue, if needed. There are no systematic data on benzodiazepines, opiates, or propofol, but all can cause airway collapse.[14]

Management of known emergent SGS

No high-quality randomized controlled data exist to guide management of emergent SGS. A variety of techniques can be used, depending on the preference of the airway manager.

The role of flexible fiberoptic bronchoscopy in SGS

The following points highlight the role of flexible fiberoptic bronchoscopy:

1. When a fiberoptic bronchoscope (FOB) is passed beyond the vocal cords, the scope is contained within the narrowest portion of the airway and is very close to the area of stenosis. In contrast, more distal lesions can be approached slowly and assessed by the scope.[6,11] Therefore, a FOB is more likely to block airflow in patients with SGS than in those with a more distal tracheal lesion.

2. The smallest tube that easily fits over a 5-mm FOB is 6.5 mm, which may be too large to bypass a mass or circumferential cricoid lesion.

3. A very skilled flexible bronchoscopist may be able to assess the caliber of SGS before entering the cords and decide whether or not to proceed.

4. Warming and physically manipulating the ETT may increase flexibility during FOB and increase the likelihood of bypassing a lesion.

5. When SGS is discovered serendipitously during an FOB intubation attempt for undifferentiated stridor, the procedure should be aborted. If an already-stenotic airway is acutely traumatized, the patient may progress to respiratory arrest.[2,6,11]

The role of rigid bronchoscopy in SGS

Rigid bronchoscopy plays a critical role in the management of SGS. This technique requires specific training and may be available only in a specially equipped OR or interventional suite. With rigid bronchoscopy, the operator can use jet ventilation while dilating the airway to facilitate endotracheal intubation. Balloon or Jackson dilators can be passed through a rigid scope and used to increase airway diameter. High-grade and long lesions are more difficult to dilate.[4–8,25] After dilation, the operator can pass a bougie or airway exchange catheter through the scope, then pass an ETT over the catheter. Cautery and large suction catheters can also be passed through a rigid scope. The scope itself can "core" out tissue in patients with a focal obstructing lesion, although this may cause trauma. The rigid bronchoscope can tamponade bleeding and retract a vocal fold to allow visualization of a foreign body impacted against the fold by cough or forceful expiration. Once the airway is secured, additional imaging and/or detailed bronchoscopic examination can be used to guide definitive management.[1,2,5–7]

Standard measures to reduce the risk of patient injury and airway fire should be followed if rigid bronchoscopy is used to facilitate jet ventilation and/or cautery:[5,26]

1. The anesthetist and surgeon must plan, anticipate, and respond in synchrony to unexpected events.[1,6,11]
2. Patients undergoing rigid bronchoscopic jet ventilation with dilation require general anesthesia and neuromuscular blockade to tolerate the procedure and reduce the risk of barotrauma. The procedure is safe once the airway is temporarily secured with a jet ventilation catheter or the tip of the scope itself.
3. Ventilation must be synchronized with balloon dilation and electrocautery.[4,5,11]

Conclusion

The subglottic space contains the narrowest portion of the extrathoracic airway and is subject to stenosis, mostly from intubation trauma and post-intubation injury. Known cases of SGS ideally should be managed by an experienced airway manager in conjunction with an otolaryngologist or cardiothoracic surgeon adept at rigid bronchoscopy and surgical airway salvage. Although potentially useful for management of emergent SGS, a FOB can obstruct the airway. The most important pharmacologic principle is not to ablate airway tone or spontaneous respiration before the airway is secured. Clinicians may need to manage these emergencies without knowing the exact nature of the lesion, and without optimal equipment. These cases must be approached as any other dangerous undifferentiated airway obstruction. If intubation fails, one must shift rapidly to surgical salvage with bougie-assisted cricothyrotomy, or, at times, tracheostomy. Transtracheal catheter ventilation may be successful as an alternative subglottic salvage technique. Primary surgical salvage with local anesthesia and spontaneous ventilation may be the best option in some adults; ketamine is an excellent sedative for these cases. Emergent pediatric SGS is especially dangerous. During surgical salvage, the airway manager must optimize spontaneous breathing with heliox or nebulized epinephrine, or support ventilation using a laryngeal mask.

Acknowledgements

The authors would like to acknowledge Dr. Eugene Shostak, Assistant Professor of Medicine in Cardiothoracic Surgery, and Dr. Joshua I. Levinger, Assistant Professor of Otolaryngology; both at Weil-Cornell Medical College, New York, NY for their helpful comments.

References

1. Sharma HS, Sharma S. Management of laryngeal foreign bodies in children. *Journal of Accident and Emergency Medicine* 1999;**16**(2):150–3.

2. Hammer J. Acquired upper airway obstruction. *Paediatric Respiratory Reviews* 2004;**5**(1):25–33.

3. Campos JH. Fiberoptic bronchoscopy guidelines for the anesthesiologist. *Revista Mexicana de Anestesiología* 2011;**34**(1):264–9.

4. Maunsell R, Avelino MA. Balloon laryngoplasty for acquired subglottic stenosis in children: predictive factors for success. *Brazilian Journal of Otorhinolaryngology* 2014;**80**(5):453–4.

5. Barros Casas D, Fernández-Bussy S, Folch E, Flandes Aldeyturriaga J, Majid A. Patología obstructiva no maligna de la vía aérea central. *Archivos de Bronconeumología* 2014;**50**(8):345–54.

6. Zias N, Chroneou A, Tabba MK, *et al.* Post tracheostomy and post intubation tracheal stenosis: report of 31 cases and review of the literature. *BMC Pulmonary Medicine* 2008;**8**:18. doi: 10.1186/1471-2466-8-18.

7. Grillo HC. Development of tracheal surgery: a historical review. Part 2: treatment of tracheal diseases. *Annals of Thoracic Surgery* 2003;**75**(3):1039–47.

8. Ernst A, Feller-Kopman D, Becker HD, Mehta AC. Central airway obstruction. *American Journal of Respiratory and Critical Care Medicine* 2001;**169**(2):1278–97.

9. Manoach S, Wilkerson RG, Russo CM, Charchaflieh J. Case report: a 12 month-old girl with partial airway obstruction caused by an esophageal coin. *American Society of Critical Care Anesthesiologists Interchange* 2010;**21**(2):13–14.

10. Cheng HC, Dai ZK, Wu JR, Chen IC. Pediatric upper airway emergencies. *Journal of Pediatric Respiratory Disease* 2012;**8**:25–31.

11. Mason RA, Fielder CP. The obstructed airway in head and neck surgery. *Anaesthesia* 1999;**54**(7):625–8.

12. Wells DG, Zelcer J, Wells GR, Sherman GP. A theoretical mechanism for massive supraglottic swelling following carotid endarterectomy. *Australian and New Zealand Journal of Surgery* 1988;**58**(12):979–81.

13. Holdsworth RJ, McCollum PT. Acute laryngeal oedema following carotid endarterectomy. *Journal of Cardiovascular Surgery* 1994;**35**(3):249–51.

14. Hillman DR, Platt PR, Eastwood PR. The upper airway during anaesthesia. *British Journal of Anaesthesia* 2003;**91**(1):31–9.

15. Anders HJ. Compression syndromes caused by substernal goitres. *Postgraduate Medical Journal* 1998;**74**(872):327–9.

16. Berg MD, Schexnayder SM, Chameides L, *et al.* Part 13: pediatric basic life support: 2010 American Heart Association Guidelines for Cardiopulmonary Resuscitation and Emergency Cardiovascular Care. *Circulation* 2010;**122**(suppl 3):S862–75.

17. Berg RA, Hemphill R, Abella BS, *et al.* Part 5: adult basic life support: 2010 American Heart Association Guidelines for Cardiopulmonary Resuscitation and Emergency Cardiovascular Care. *Circulation* 2010;**122**(suppl 3):S685–705.

18. Ho AM, Dion PW, Karmakar MK, Chung DC, Tay BA. Use of heliox in critical upper airway obstruction. Physical and physiologic considerations in choosing the optimal helium:oxygen mix. *Resuscitation* 2002;**52**(3):297–300.

19. Moraa I, Sturman N, McGuire T, van Driel ML. Heliox for croup in children. *Cochrane Database of Systematic Reviews* 2013 Dec 7;12:CD006822. doi: 10.1002/14651858.CD006822.pub4.

20. Bjornson C, Russell K, Vandermeer B, Klassen TP, Johnson DW. Nebulized epinephrine for croup in children. *Cochrane Database of Systematic Reviews* 2013 Oct 10;10:CD006619. doi: 10.1002/14651858.CD006619.pub3.

21. Salvino CK, Dries D, Gamelli R, Murphy-Macabobby M, Marshall W. Emergency cricothyrotomy in trauma victims. *Journal of Trauma* 1993;**34**(4):503–5.

22. Eisenburger P, Laczika K, List M, *et al.* Comparison of conventional surgical versus Seldinger technique emergency cricothyrotomy performed by inexperienced clinicians. *Anesthesiology* 2000;**92**(3):687–90.

23. Chang RS, Hamilton RJ, Carter WA. Declining rate of cricothyrotomy in trauma patients with an emergency medicine residency: implications for skills training. *Academic Emergency Medicine* 1998;**5**(3):247–51.

24. Coté CJ, Hartnick CJ. Pediatric transtracheal and cricothyrotomy airway devices for emergency use: which are appropriate for infants and children? *Paediatric Anaesthesia* 2009;**19**(1):66–76.

25. Myer CM 3rd, O'Connor DM, Cotton RT. Proposed grading system for subglottic stenosis based on endotracheal tube sizes. *Annals of Otology, Rhinology and Laryngology* 1994;**103**(4 Pt 1):319–23.

26. Cortiñas-Díaz J, Manoach S (2013). The role of transtracheal jet ventilation. In Glick DB, Cooper RM, Ovassapian A (eds.), *The Difficult Airway: An Atlas of Tools and Techniques for Clinical Management* (pp. 211–40). New York, NY: Springer Science + Business Media.

Airway management in patients with tracheobronchial traumatic injury

Felipe Urdaneta

Case presentation

A 25-year-old male unrestrained driver was involved in a high-speed motor vehicle accident while intoxicated. Advanced Trauma Life Support (ATLS) guidelines are followed, and an initial survey is performed. Because the patient needs further evaluation and computed tomography (CT) of the head, cervical spine, thorax, and abdomen, the clinical providers determine that airway control and ventilation support are necessary. Rapid sequence intubation using direct laryngoscopy with manual in-line stabilization is performed, leaving the cervical collar in place; two attempts are necessary because the view of the glottic opening is incomplete (Cormack–Lehane grade 3) and bloody secretions are present in the oropharynx. The endotracheal tube (ETT) is placed successfully, and end-tidal CO_2 is confirmed with capnography. The practitioners note the presence of bloody secretions and then blood that requires frequent suctioning after the ETT is secured. Results of his radiologic evaluation reveal multiple rib fractures, bilateral small pulmonary contusions, bilateral pleural effusions, bilateral pneumothoraces (left more prominent than the right), and pneumomediastinum. He also suffered splenic rupture and a closed fracture of the right femur. His cervical spine evaluation does not show any fractures or dislocations. The patient has bilateral thoracostomy tubes placed and is taken to the operating room for exploratory laparotomy, splenectomy, and open reduction external fixation of the femur fracture. Twenty-four hours later, the otolaryngology service is consulted regarding the persistent blood-tinged secretions in the ETT. They perform a flexible bronchoscopic examination that shows a small laceration in the membranous portion of the lower trachea proximal to the location of the ETT cuff, with evidence of recent but not active bleeding. Because there is no evidence of deterioration, difficulty ventilating, or esophageal involvement, the team decides on a conservative, non-surgical approach. Repeat bronchoscopic surveillance performed 24 hours later shows no further signs of bleeding or any other complication. The patient is extubated 2 hours later; no further pulmonary issues or hemoptysis is documented, and the thoracostomy tubes do not show further evidence of air leak.

Introduction

Tracheobronchial traumatic injury (TTI) includes a heterogeneous group of respiratory tract disorders that are anatomically located at any point in the major central airways, from

Cases in Emergency Airway Management, ed. Lauren C. Berkow and John C. Sakles. Published by Cambridge University Press. © Cambridge University Press 2015.

the level of the cricoid cartilage to the bifurcation into the right and left main bronchi. In this chapter we will discuss some pertinent features of airway management in adult patients with TTI, a relatively uncommon and potentially life-threatening condition.

Tracheobronchial traumatic lesions are usually caused by penetrating or blunt trauma, but they have also been described – albeit much less commonly – secondary to iatrogenic causes, such as tracheal and bronchial perforation during tracheal tube placement. Such incidents occur most commonly in the pediatric population or with the use of double-lumen tubes, or during bronchoscopy and tracheal stent placement. They can also occur during procedures performed on nearby organs, such as during cardiac surgery, thyroidectomy, and esophageal surgery; in neonates after vaginal delivery;[1] and after esophageal perforation that results from ingestion of caustic substances.[2] TTI remains a very challenging condition to diagnose and manage. Patients with TTI usually present acutely. They may require emergent and resuscitative efforts, owing to associated injuries, and may need immediate surgery. However, the presentation may be delayed, usually with airway obstruction or stricture months after the initial insult has been described.[3]

The true incidence of TTI is unknown because many patients with TTI die before reaching medical care; consequently, such events go unreported.[4] Improvement in prehospital care and initiation of ATLS have improved overall survival and therefore have increased the rate at which TTI patients actually receive medical care.[5]

Available retrospective reports show that TTI occurs in less than 1% of all trauma cases, with reported figures for TTI between 1 in 1,000 and 1 in 137,000 emergency department for considency visits.[6,7] The incidence of penetrating TTI is approximately 1–2% of all thoracic trauma hospital visits, and 2.8% of blunt traumatic injuries.[8] These figures are just crude estimates because most studies combine all causes of TTI without providing an actual denominator of cervicothoracic injuries in order to estimate an actual incidence of major airway lesions.[9]

In the past, blunt trauma used to be the leading cause of TTI, but recent evidence indicates that penetrating trauma is now the leading cause.[7] Most blunt injuries involve the thoracic trachea and mainstem bronchi, with the right more commonly involved than the left.[10] Most penetrating injuries involve the cervical trachea.

Tracheobronchial anatomy

The adult trachea is approximately 10 to 13 cm in length, with a diameter of 1.8 to 2.3 cm; it is slightly larger and wider in males than in females. The cervical trachea starts at the inferior portion of the larynx at the level of the cricoid cartilage (which corresponds with the 6th cervical vertebra) and ends at the carina, at the level of T4–T5 vertebrae. It contains 18 to 22 cartilaginous rings anteriorly and is membranous posteriorly. Only one cartilage – the cricoid – is complete. The trachea is surrounded by other important structures. The esophagus is located to the left at the level of the neck, and then it is located posteriorly until the level of the carina. The thyroid gland is located anteriorly and the innominate artery crosses the trachea in the midline at the level of the sternal notch; other major vessels of importance include the carotids, located laterally to the trachea and thyroid gland, and brachiocephalic vein, located anteriorly to the innominate artery. The anatomical distribution of the recurrent laryngeal nerve (RLN) is important to describe as it may be involved in both blunt and penetrating traumatic injuries. On the right side it comes off the vagus nerve, wraps around the subclavian artery, and traverses superiorly to enter the larynx between the thyroid and cricoid cartilages. On the left it comes off the vagus beneath the aortic arch and runs in the tracheoesophageal groove.[11] The blood supply is segmental, with the upper half receiving blood from the inferior thyroid artery and the lower half from the bronchial arteries.

Pathophysiology

The tracheobronchial tree is located in the neck and the chest. TTI damage can occur at one or both locations. Damage from TTI varies depending on the mechanism of injury, the anatomic site of the damage, and the severity of respiratory compromise that follows. In general three mechanisms are involved.

Blunt trauma

Blunt trauma occurs most commonly during a motor vehicle accident, when the body has direct impact with the steering wheel, airbags, dashboard (dashboard injury), or seatbelt over the chest. Any impact that produces laryngotracheal distraction and hyperextension of the cervical spine can cause crush injury to the cervical trachea owing to the impact of the semi-rigid trachea against the rigid bony cervical spine. Rapid deceleration and anteroposterior compression forces will increase tracheobronchial pressure and cause shear forces that may lead to damage at levels of the cricoid cartilage and carina, points of tracheobronchial anatomic fixation. Most reports show damage at the level of the cricoid cartilage, 2.5 cm above the carina, or at the takeoff of the right main bronchus.[5,12] Blunt trauma is usually associated with major accompanying injuries (orthopedic, maxillofacial, pulmonary, intra-abdominal, and neurologic), and these injuries may be the primary determinants of overall outcome.

Penetrating trauma

Penetrating injuries are usually caused by stabbing or occur secondary to firearm injury. Less commonly they occur after shrapnel injury. Penetrating injuries usually occur at the cervical trachea, and damage to surrounding structures, such as blood vessels or the esophagus, is very common. Distal tracheal injuries are usually associated with other severe injuries; major vessel involvement is common and usually lethal. Most stabbing injuries occur at the level of the cervical spine and, depending on the severity, may cause lacerations, perforations, transection, or through-and-through injuries. Firearm injury can affect any portion of the central airways; however, most patients seen have lesions at the cervical level. Tissue effects of firearm injury depend on the type of weapon used (low-velocity weapons are less destructive than high-velocity weapons), the caliber of the bullets (larger bullets cause larger area of damage), and the distance at which the weapon was fired (greater distance reduces the velocity at which the projectile reaches the victim and therefore reduces damage). Penetrating lesions of the lower neck and thorax require a thorough evaluation of the vasculature, digestive system, and major airway structures.

Iatrogenic injury

The third leading cause of TTI is iatrogenic. It can result from damage to the tracheal integrity during airway instrumentation (intubation, percutaneous tracheostomy, and bronchoscopy) or from injury to the tracheobronchial tree during procedures in nearby organs. Usually these iatrogenic injuries are detected in the postoperative period.

Diagnosis

The diagnosis of TTI is difficult and requires a high index of suspicion; early diagnosis is critical in order to reduce early complications, mortality, and delayed complications.[5] Major clues that demand additional radiologic evaluation and early bronchoscopy include progressive dyspnea and tachypnea, respiratory distress, cyanosis, voice changes, airway obstruction, hemoptysis, subcutaneous emphysema, large air leak, and persistent lung collapse after tube thoracostomy in patients with blunt or penetrating trauma. TTI should also be ruled out in the presence of injury to nearby structures. Practitioners should evaluate for TTI when patients present with injury to the cervical spine and spinal cord, laryngeal fractures, esophageal injury, vascular injury (carotid arteries and/or jugular veins), rib fractures, injury of intrathoracic great vessels, pulmonary and cardiac injuries, pneumothorax, hemothorax, or pulmonary contusion. Unfortunately, mortality remains high, usually from associated major injuries.[13]

Penetrating TTI is usually apparent. Associated injuries in nearby structures, such as the esophagus, carotid artery, or jugular vein, can be extensive and usually dominate the resuscitative efforts, prognosis, and outcome.

Diagnosis of TTI after blunt trauma is more difficult and may be delayed. It requires a high index of suspicion and radiographic imaging, particularly CT scanning and bronchoscopy. Major head and abdominal injuries, bruising or seatbelt marks on the chest wall, hemoptysis, any degree of respiratory distress, subcutaneous emphysema, and voice changes are clues that the integrity of the respiratory tract might be compromised. Free air in the neck, pneumothorax, and pneumomediastinum should raise immediate concern for potential tracheobronchial damage. Radiologic evaluation with plain films or, more importantly, with CT scanning can identify TTI in most patients. Paratracheal air and pneumomediastinum are usually present with TTI. Bronchoscopy is the most important procedure to locate and assess the extent of TTI.

Airway management

Airway assessment followed by definitive airway protection is a key feature of trauma management (Figure 8.1). Acute management and subsequent surgical repair need to be individualized. Patients with TTIs have a wide range of issues, from minor and localized, to catastrophic and life-threatening. Incorrect management may result in immediate life-threatening consequences or future airway obstruction and/or strictures.

In general, the management plan depends on the clinical circumstances, presence of secondary lesions, and degree of respiratory and hemodynamic instability. Airway providers need to be adept in multiple options and rescue techniques; adequate management requires a stepwise approach and plan dictated by the patient's needs, the clinical circumstances, and the availability of appropriate equipment and experienced, skilled personnel. No single modality or technique is better than others; every option available has potential pitfalls and complications. Patients with TTI may need special considerations with regard to the cervical spine. Cervical spine injury may lead to or exacerbate spinal cord damage, and airway management must be performed with attention to cervical spine immobilization.[14]

If the patient is unstable, airway management may be needed to continue with the evaluation and resuscitative efforts. In these circumstances two options exist for first-line management: (1) oral intubation via direct or indirect laryngoscopy with manual in-line stabilization or (2) an invasive (surgical) approach (tracheostomy or cricothyroidotomy). Controversy exists as to which is the preferred choice. The surgical approach is especially

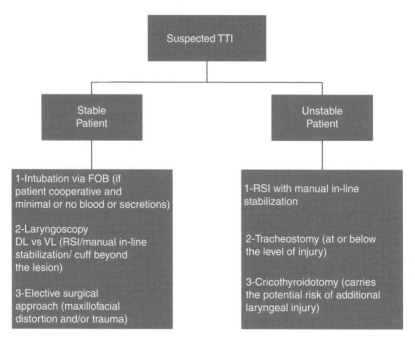

Figure 8.1 Algorithm for management of the patient with suspected transtracheal injury. DL= direct laryngoscopy. VL= video laryngoscopy. RSI = rapid sequence intubation

recommended when the patient has anatomic distortion or has open wounds or fractures from concomitant severe maxillofacial traumatic involvement. In such cases, it is possible to precipitate airway obstruction or convert partial lesions into complete lesions and even transections during attempts at noninvasive or blind tracheal tube placement.[7] In suspected or documented cases of TTI, preparations for definitive surgical airway should be made early in the clinical course. In general, tracheostomy with controlled placement of the tube either at or below the level of the injury is preferred over cricothyroidotomy because it is not uncommon for patients to have laryngeal involvement as well. Intubation over an open neck, chest wound, and surgical field has been described in cases of penetrating injuries.[12,13]

If the patient is stable and cooperative, most authors recommend tracheal tube placement via a flexible fiberoptic bronchoscopy (FOB) approach as the first-line management option. This approach in theory has several advantages over a laryngoscopic approach at intubation: it does not cause movement of the cervical spine, it is usually done with a spontaneously breathing patient, and it allows simultaneous evaluation of the tracheobronchial tree. In practice, however, the FOB approach has many limitations: availability of equipment, experience of personnel using it, and limited view caused by secretions and blood in the oropharynx and central airways. It also requires patient cooperation and time because the technique can be considerably lengthier than conventional laryngoscopy. Most series to date show that conventional laryngoscopic and/or invasive (surgical) options for intubation predominate over the FOB option.[6,7,9,15] Although many studies have shown that video laryngoscopy is superior to direct laryngoscopy for intubation success and decreases cervical spine motion during airway access, to date no published studies or case reports have specifically addressed its use in TTI patients.[16] See Figure 8.1.

Post-intubation care

The most common method for ventilation management is via standard orotracheal tube placement or tube tracheostomy. If there are associated injuries to the central airways, the cuff may be placed under direct bronchoscopic examination beyond the level of the injury. In general, double-lumen tracheal tubes are not used or recommended because their larger caliber and rigidity give them the potential to cause additional damage to the tracheobronchial tree. If lung isolation is needed during surgery, the first approach should be to selectively advance the single-lumen tube into the mainstem bronchus or use bronchial blockers. Placement via the operative field has been reported.[9] Jet ventilation might be used in cases of tracheobronchial injury during reconstructive airway surgery.[17] Depending on the degree of airway compromise and presence of major associated injuries, cardiopulmonary bypass has been used during tracheobronchial reconstruction.[13] However, after major trauma with associated injuries, the added inflammatory effects and need for anticoagulation with extracorporeal circulation may exacerbate damage; therefore cardiopulmonary bypass should be used only in extreme circumstances.

In cases of tracheobronchial reconstructive surgery, the preferred strategy is to extubate the patient after surgery to prevent further damage from mechanical ventilation. However, because of possible RLN involvement and the potential for vocal cord paralysis associated with blunt and penetrating traumatic cases, the clinical provider should take great care during extubation and have a high index of suspicion for abnormal glottic function. Bilateral incomplete damage to the RLN is more dangerous than complete damage. When bilateral damage to the RLN is incomplete, the adductor fibers draw the cords toward each other, the glottic opening is severely compromised, and severe respiratory distress ensues. On the other hand, if bilateral damage is complete, the vocal cord assumes a position midway between abduction and adduction, leaving enough glottic opening to prevent respiratory distress. When patients with associated injuries need prolonged mechanical ventilation, consider performing a surgical airway access/tracheostomy away from the site of surgical repair to prevent contamination, infection, stenosis, or dehiscence of tracheal tissue.

Conclusion

Although TTI occurs infrequently, it is an important condition that is difficult to diagnose and treat. Any portion of the tracheobronchial tree may be involved. Depending on the cause and mechanism of injury, the presentation might be evident or might be masked by other major injuries; presentation might also be delayed. Practitioners should have a high index of suspicion for TTI and use bronchoscopic examination of the trachea to establish the diagnosis and decrease the chance that complications will lead to delayed presentation. Maintaining the airway is a critical aspect of managing patients with trauma, especially those that have damage to the central airways. A stepwise approach to airway management with multidisciplinary care is essential for adequate short- and long-term outcomes of these potentially fatal injuries.

References

1. Kacmarynski DS, Sidman JD, Rimell FL, Hustead VA. Spontaneous tracheal and subglottic tears in neonates. *Laryngoscope* 2002;**112**:1387–93.

2. Chen K-C, Hsiao C-H. Tracheal perforation in esophageal corrosive injury. *Annals of Thoracic Surgery* 2013;**96**:1879.

3. Glazer ES, Meyerson SL. Delayed presentation and treatment of tracheobronchial injuries due to blunt trauma. *Journal of Surgical Education* 2008;**65**:302–8.

4. Blyth A. Thoracic trauma. *BMJ* 2014;**348**: bmj.g1137-bmj.g.

5. Cassada DC, Munyikwa MP, Moniz MP, Dieter RA, Jr., Schuchmann GF, Enderson BL. Acute injuries of the trachea and major bronchi: importance of early diagnosis. *Annals of Thoracic Surgery* 2000;**69**:1563–7.

6. Randall DR, Rudmik LR, Ball CG, Bosch JD. External laryngotracheal trauma. *The Laryngoscope* 2013;**124**:E123–E33.

7. Bhojani RA, Rosenbaum DH, Dikmen E, et al. Contemporary assessment of laryngotracheal trauma. *Journal of Thoracic and Cardiovascular Surgery* 2005;**130**:426–32.

8. Symbas PN, Justicz AG, Ricketts RR. Rupture of the airways from blunt trauma: treatment of complex injuries. *Annals of Thoracic Surgery* 1992;**54**:177–83.

9. Karmy-Jones R, Wood DE. Traumatic injury to the trachea and bronchus. *Thoracic Surgery Clinics* 2007;**17**:35–46.

10. Vantroyen B, De Baetselier. Tracheal rupture after blunt trauma. *European Journal of Trauma and Emergency Surgery* 2008;**34**:410–13.

11. Zervos MD, Prokopakis E, Bizekis C. Benign and malignant disorders of the trachea. In Lalwani AK, ed., *Current Diagnosis and Treatment in Otolaryngology – Head and Neck Surgery*, 3rd edn.: LANGE/McGraw Hill; 2012.

12. Welter S. Repair of tracheobronchial injuries. *Thoracic Surgery Clinics* 2014;**24**:41–50.

13. Lin J, Rajdev P, Mulligan MS. Reconstruction of a complex tracheal injury using an intercostal muscle flap. *Annals of Thoracic Surgery* 2014;**97**:679–81.

14. Crosby ET. Considerations for airway management for cervical spine surgery in adults. *Anesthesiology Clinics* 2007;**25**:511–33, ix.

15. Verschueren DS, Bell RB, Bagheri SC, Dierks EJ, Potter BE. Management of laryngo-tracheal injuries associated with craniomaxillofacial trauma. *Journal of Oral and Maxillofacial Surgery* 2006;**64**:203–14.

16. Hindman BJ, Santoni BG, Puttlitz CM, From RP, Todd MM. Intubation biomechanics: laryngoscope force and cervical spine motion during intubation with Macintosh and Airtraq laryngoscopes. *Anesthesiology* 2014;**121**:260–71.

17. Luyet C, Boudah R, McCartney CJ, Zeldin R, Rizoli S. Low-frequency jet ventilation through a bronchial blocker for tracheal repair after a rare complication of percutaneous dilatational tracheostomy. *Journal of Cardiothoracic and Vascular Anesthesia* 2013;**27**:108–10.

Chapter 9

Airway management of the patient with morbid obesity

Davide Cattano and Ruggero M. Corso

Case presentation

A 62-year-old male patient who is morbidly obese (body mass index [BMI] 45) presents at the emergency department with nausea and acute abdominal pain. He reports 3 days of constipation. He is nauseated but has not vomited. His last meal was the previous night. He reports hypertension (on lisinopril) and diabetes (on metformin). He snores, and his wife confirms that it is loud snoring interrupted by gasping during sleep. Physical examination reveals left lower-, right lower-, and left upper-quadrant tenderness and clinical evidence of colonic obstruction and acute abdomen. A computed tomography (CT) scan and water-soluble contrast enema examination reveal a large colonic perforation and associated collection in the right flank. Vital signs are temperature 39 °C, pulse 115 beats per minute, respiration 30 breaths per minute, and blood pressure 90/42 mmHg. Laboratory data include white blood cell count 6.4 k/cm, neutrophils 87.5%, hemoglobin 11.5 g/dL, and platelets 180,000. After the workup, a diagnosis of bowel perforation and colorectal mass is made, and the patient is scheduled for emergency surgery.

Surgical diagnosis and anesthesia

Colorectal cancer is the third most commonly diagnosed cancer in the world. In 15–30% of cases, patients require emergency surgery for obstruction, perforation, or bleeding.[1,2] Emergency surgery for colorectal cancer is a common occurrence in anesthetic practice and is associated with a poor outcome.[3] Although a high BMI is not an independent predictor of mortality after emergency surgery,[4] morbid obesity has several other implications that will be discussed in detail later in the chapter. The patient described above is exhibiting systemic inflammatory response syndrome that could precipitate into septic shock, which would complicate the clinical picture. The NPO (nil per os) status and the anesthetic technique will need to be addressed in order to proceed safely with appropriate maintenance of perfusion once the airway is secured. The airway manager should be aware of challenging problems in morbidly obese patients.[5]

Cases in Emergency Airway Management, ed. Lauren C. Berkow and John C. Sakles. Published by Cambridge University Press. © Cambridge University Press 2015.

Morbid obesity

Anatomic and physiologic changes

Obesity leads to a set of physiologic alterations, and those that involve the respiratory system are particularly important for the airway manager. The accumulation of fat around the chest wall, diaphragm, and into pharyngeal tissues decreases pharyngeal area and leads to reduced chest wall compliance, thereby defining an actual restrictive lung disease.[6] The reduction in lung volume causes a significant decrease in oxygen reserve by reducing the period of safety apnea, and contributes to decreased ventilation of the lung bases with subsequent ventilation–perfusion mismatch and hypoxemia. These conditions are made worse by the supine position and general anesthesia. Obese patients also have increased oxygen consumption and carbon dioxide production owing to the metabolic activity of excess body tissue and the increased work of breathing.[7]

The airway manager must therefore be aware that: (1) in case of a difficult airway, these patients desaturate very quickly; (2) alveolar hypoventilation may also increase the risk of postoperative pulmonary complications; (3) decreased compliance of the respiratory system leads to increased breathing effort during spontaneous ventilation, with subsequent rapid fatigue of respiratory muscles; and (4) the resulting increase in O_2 consumption and alveolar–arterial oxygen gradient requires careful planning of tracheal extubation.

Morbid obesity and obstructive sleep apnea

Obstructive sleep apnea (OSA) is a condition that affects the general population and has been implicated as a comorbid factor in various clinical conditions. The signs, symptoms, and consequences of OSA are a direct result of the derangements caused by the repetitive collapse of the upper airway. They include sleep fragmentation, hypoxemia, hypercapnia, marked variations in intrathoracic pressures, and increased sympathetic activity. Obesity is a classic risk factor for OSA, with prevalence as high as 70% in bariatric surgery, presumably owing to the accumulation of fat tissue at the neck level.[8] However, despite its frequency, most patients do not have a formal diagnosis and therefore do not receive therapy. Moreover, chronic, untreated OSA is an independent risk factor for increased all-cause mortality in the general population. The characteristic collapsibility of the upper airway and associated comorbidities also place OSA surgical patients at increased risk for complications during the perioperative period.[9]

Given the high prevalence of undiagnosed OSA among obese patients, many authors suggest using polysomnography to diagnose OSA in all obese patients undergoing bariatric surgery. However, costs and limitations associated with the availability of sleep centers make this approach somewhat unrealistic. A different strategy involves using some bedside screening tests. Although all of these screening tools appear to improve the likelihood of identifying OSA preoperatively, the quickest and simplest to use seems to be the STOP questionnaire.[10] This questionnaire has also been modified to include questions about additional risk factors for OSA such as BMI (B), age (A), neck circumference (N), and gender (G); the modified tool is called the STOP-BANG questionnaire. Patients with STOP-BANG scores of 0–2 may be considered to have a low risk of OSA, 3–4 an intermediate risk, and 5–8 a high risk. STOP-BANG scores that indicate a high risk of OSA have been associated with a heightened risk of postoperative complications in patients undergoing elective surgery, confirming its value to predict OSA severity and triage patients in the perioperative period.[11]

Evaluation and predictive factors of difficult airway

The term "difficult airway" encompasses a spectrum of difficulty ranging from mask ventilation to the surgical airway. The United Kingdom Fourth National Audit Project (NAP4) reviewed major complications of airway management and reported a significant increase in risk in obese patients. However, laryngoscopy typically is not considered more difficult in morbidly obese patients (see *Direct laryngoscopy and intubation* below). In the NAP4 review study, complications occurred in all phases of anesthesia, including tracheal extubation in seven cases.[12,13]

Airway strategies

Mask ventilation

Obesity has been identified as an independent predictor of difficult mask ventilation in several studies. More importantly, obesity is an independent risk factor for impossible mask ventilation.[14] Recently, in a retrospective database-based study, a BMI of 30 or more was identified as an independent predictor of difficult mask ventilation combined with difficult laryngoscopy. Hence, obesity is associated with potential difficult mask ventilation. Limited protruding mandible, neck circumference, and the Mallampati class may be good predictors of difficult mask ventilation in these patients.

Supraglottic airway devices

Supraglottic airway devices (SGAs) are commonly used in both elective and rescue airway management, but how safe are these devices in the obese patient? Obesity is an independent predictor for failed use of a laryngeal mask airway (LMA),[15] but second-generation SGAs, which provide higher leak pressures, have been shown to provide effective ventilation in morbidly obese patients.[16] However, one should not underestimate the problem of gastric content aspiration, as 8 of the 23 cases of gastric content aspiration reported in NAP4 occurred in obese patients. In cases of difficult and impossible mask ventilation, when laryngoscopy has also been proven difficult if not impossible by routine means, a SGA is an effective management tool to provide rescue ventilation.

Direct laryngoscopy and intubation

Are obese patients more difficult to intubate than nonobese patients? In the literature, we find studies in favor of, but also against this hypothesis. Certainly the BMI alone is not a risk factor for difficult intubation. Additionally, ultrasound quantification of anterior soft-tissue thickness failed to predict difficult laryngoscopy in obese patients. However, a combination of features in the obese patient, such as Mallampati Class 3 and larger neck circumference, increases the risk of difficult laryngoscopy and difficult tracheal intubation.[17]

Optimizing preoxygenation, positioning

The correct positioning of the patient is, perhaps, the most important element to ensure the success of airway control. The 25-degree head-up and reverse Trendelenburg positions increase the duration of apnea without arterial desaturation and allow more time for tracheal intubation. The "ramped" position can also facilitate direct laryngoscopy (see

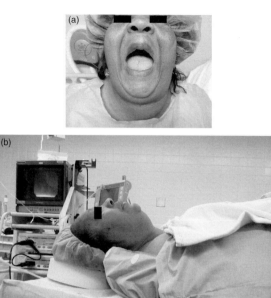

Figure 9.1 Obese patient in the ramped position. (a) Mallampati class and neck circumference in morbid obese patient. (b) Positioning to improve airway management (laryngoscopy and bag-mask ventilation) and ventilation/oxygenation. (Note on the background the presence of a flexible fiberoptic bronchoscope and tower, as well as a video laryngoscope.) Morbid obesity is not a predictor of difficult laryngoscopy per se; however, morbid obesity increases the factorial contribution of known risk factors such as the neck circumference and Mallampati class. Other aspects of airway management, such as bag-mask ventilation, oxygenation, and, for instance, the surgical airway, may be affected by obesity. Proper positioning is essential for best airway access as well as to improve ventilation/oxygenation

Figure 9.1). This is achieved by aligning the sternal notch horizontally with the external auditory meatus using folded blankets or commercially available pillows under the upper body, shoulders, and head.[18] It is also important to provide optimal preoxygenation to avoid hypoxemia after induction of general anesthesia. In obese patients any form of positive airway pressure support (PAP), supplemental nasopharyngeal oxygen insufflation, and noninvasive ventilation during spontaneous ventilation can be beneficial before induction of general anesthesia.

Airway management plans

The key to safely managing the airway in the obese patient lies in the ability to predict difficulty and in creating a strategy that includes multiple exit routes if needed.

Plan A: rapid sequence intubation (RSI), direct laryngoscopy/video laryngoscopy, backup SGAs

RSI

RSI historically has been used to minimize the risk of aspiration in surgical patients with a "full stomach." The traditional components of the technique include oxygen administration, rapid injection of an anesthetic agent followed immediately by succinylcholine, application of cricoid pressure, and avoidance of positive-pressure ventilation before tracheal intubation with a cuffed endotracheal tube. Currently, it is the gold standard for anesthesia induction in patients with full stomachs. However, some aspects of the RSI technique may be deleterious in obese patients. The application of cricoid pressure can worsen the laryngoscopic view by altering the airway anatomy. The lack of test for ability to mask ventilate the patient before administering a muscle relaxant, as required for classical RSI, may precipitate a "cannot intubate, cannot oxygenate" scenario. A recent meta-analysis showed that there is no evidence to support or refute the use of RSI.[19] The RSI is considered standard of care in patients at high risk of aspiration; however, it should be avoided if a difficult airway is predicted.

Dosing of medications for airway management

In RSI, a potent sedative-hypnotic is administered with the goal of inducing unconsciousness. Particularly important in the obese patient is the right dosing, which depends on the type of drug. Etomidate is lipophilic and theoretically should be administered according to total body weight. In contrast, more evidence supports dosing ketamine according to lean body mass. Midazolam is the benzodiazepine most used by airway managers because of its favorable pharmacokinetic profile. Based on its properties, a single intravenous dose should be increased in proportion to total body weight. In anesthetic practice, propofol is the induction agent of choice for obese patients. It is a highly lipophilic drug that has fast onset and offset because of its rapid redistribution to the inactive tissues, such as muscle and fat. According to the evidence, the dose of propofol for both induction and maintenance of general anesthesia in obese patients should be based on total body weight. Although opiates are lipophilic, the pharmacokinetics of these drugs are difficult to predict in obesity. It is a common practice of the authors to administer the first bolus based on ideal body weight and adjust subsequent doses according to individual patient response. When RSI is used, succinylcholine, dosed at 1 mg/kg of total body weight, provides excellent conditions for tracheal intubation. Rocuronium is an acceptable alternative when succinylcholine is contraindicated, and should be administered at a dose of 1.2 mg/kg of ideal body weight for RSI.

Direct laryngoscopy versus video laryngoscopy

With proper preparation, direct laryngoscopy is often easy for an experienced airway manager. The use of a gum-elastic bougie or an intubating malleable stylet should be considered when suboptimal glottic views are obtained. Recently, video laryngoscopy has become popular in clinical practice. Several studies have shown that video laryngoscopy improves intubation conditions in morbidly obese patients.[20] However, practitioners should remember that, although video laryngoscopes improve glottis visualization, they often prolong tracheal intubation times and do not necessarily translate into easier intubation. Today, no single video laryngoscope has shown superiority for use in the obese patient, and research to identify predictive factors of difficult video laryngoscopy is just beginning. Nevertheless, video laryngoscopes do provide better glottis visualization in obese patients and should be readily available.

Use of SGAs as intubating adjuncts

In the anesthetized patient, fiberoptic intubation may be made very difficult due to collapse of the upper airway tissues. SGAs can act as conduits to maintain an open airway and provide access to the laryngeal inlet.[21] Several techniques have been described. An endotracheal tube may be "railroaded" over a bronchoscope through the SGA, or an Aintree intubating catheter (Cook Critical Care, Bloomington, IN, USA) may be advanced over the bronchoscope into the trachea through the SGA. The fiberscope and SGA are then removed, leaving the intubating catheter *in situ* to act as a "railroading" device for the endotracheal tube. Several case reports have described the use of this technique in morbidly obese patients; however, additional research is needed on the efficacy and safety of this technique in this patient population.[22]

Plan B: awake fiberoptic intubation

An awake fiberoptic intubation (AFOI) is recommended for use in obese patients with a predicted difficult airway. Critical to the success of the technique are topical anesthesia with lidocaine and sedation. Among drugs used for sedation, remifentanil target-controlled infusion appears to provide better conditions for AFOI than propofol target-controlled infusion in normal-weight patients. However, evidence regarding the best sedation technique for AFOI in obese patients is lacking. Awake tracheal intubation with video laryngoscopy has emerged as a new approach that can be used instead of AFOI.

Surgical airway

Emergency cricothyroidotomy is, in a cannot intubate, cannot ventilate scenario, the rescue technique of choice. It can be particularly challenging in the obese patient because anatomical landmarks may not be identifiable. However, the use of ultrasound guidance can allow the airway manager to identify the cricothyroid membrane accurately in patients with a large neck circumference and impalpable landmarks. Ultrasound-guided bougie-assisted cricothyroidotomy is a new approach that could be beneficial in obese patients.[23]

Postoperative management

Safe extubation

It has long been known that many airway-related complications occur at the time of tracheal extubation, resulting in significant morbidity and mortality.[12] To standardize tracheal extubation and minimize patient risk, the Difficult Airway Society guidelines suggest a stepwise approach.[24] Individuals who are obese or have OSA are regarded as high-risk patients for whom awake tracheal extubation is suggested. We refer the reader to Chapter 17 for more details.

Postoperative PAP

Morbidly obese patients are at high risk of atelectasis under general anesthesia. Potential solutions to improve postoperative lung function include the application of continuous PAP (CPAP) and use of respiratory physical therapy in the recovery room. Patients have shown improved postoperative oxygenation and better maintenance of spirometry lung function with both interventions.[25] OSA patients should maintain their preoperative airway support system if possible (CPAP, biphasic PAP). The Boussignac CPAP mask could be used as an effective and safe alternative device in cases where CPAP systems are contraindicated. In summary, morbidly obese patients are at high risk of hypoxemia postoperatively. Incentive spirometry and CPAP administered early after tracheal extubation can reduce postoperative pulmonary complications.

References

1. Quinten C, Martinelli F, Coens C, *et al*. A global analysis of multitrial data investigating quality of life and symptoms as prognostic factors for survival in different tumor sites. *Cancer* 2013;**120**:302–11.

2. Rabeneck L, Paszat LF, Li C. Risk factors for obstruction, perforation, or emergency admission at presentation in patients with colorectal cancer: a population-based study. *Am J Gastroenterol* 2006;**101**:1098–103.

3. McArdle CS, Hole DJ. Emergency presentation of colorectal cancer is associated with poor 5-year survival. *Br J Surg* 2004;**91**:605–9.

4. Ferrada P, Anand RJ, Malhotra A, Aboutanos M. Obesity does not increase mortality after emergency surgery. *J Obes* 2014;**2014**:492127.

5. El-Solh AA. Clinical approach to the critically ill, morbidly obese patient. *Am J Respir Crit Care Med* 2004;**169**:557–61.

6. Salome CM, King GG, Berend N. Physiology of obesity and effects on lung function. *J Appl Physiol* 2010;**108**:206–11.

7. Dargin J, Medzon R. Emergency department management of the airway in obese adults. *Ann Emerg Med* 2010;**56**:95–104.

8. Lopez PP, Stefan B, Schulman CI, *et al*. Prevalence of sleep apnea in morbidly obese patients who presented for weight loss surgery evaluation: more evidence for routine screening for obstructive sleep apnea before weight loss surgery. *Am Surg* 2008;**74**:834–8.

9. Kaw R, Chung F, Pasupuleti V, Mehta J, Gay PC, Hernandez AV. Meta-analysis of the association between obstructive sleep apnoea and postoperative outcome. *Br J Anaesth* 2012;**109**:897–906.

10. Chung F, Yegneswaran B, Liao P, *et al*. STOP questionnaire: a tool to screen patients for obstructive sleep apnea. *Anesthesiology* 2008;**108**:812–21.

11. Corso R, Petrini F, Buccioli M, *et al*. Clinical utility of preoperative screening with STOP-BANG questionnaire in elective surgery. *Minerva Anesthesiol* 2014;**80**:877–84.

12. Cook TM, Woodall N, Frerk C; Fourth National Audit Project. Major complications of airway management in the UK: results of the Fourth National Audit Project of the Royal College of Anaesthetists and the Difficult Airway Society. Part 1: anaesthesia. *Br J Anaesth* 2011;**106**:617–31.

13. Cook TM, Woodall N, Harper J, Benger J; Fourth National Audit Project. Major complications of airway management in the UK: results of the Fourth National Audit Project of the Royal College of Anaesthetists and the Difficult Airway Society. Part 2: intensive care and emergency departments. *Br J Anaesth* 2011;**106**:632–42.

14. Kheterpal S, Martin L, Shanks AM, Tremper KK. Prediction and outcomes of impossible mask ventilation: a review of 50,000 anesthetics. *Anesthesiology* 2009;**110**:891–7.

15. Ramachandran SK, Mathis MR, Tremper KK, Shanks AM, Kheterpal S. Predictors and clinical outcomes from failed Laryngeal Mask Airway Unique™: a study of 15,795 patients. *Anesthesiology* 2012;**116**:1217–26.

16. Nicholson A, Cook TM, Smith AF, Lewis SR, Reed SS. Supraglottic airway devices versus tracheal intubation for airway management during general anaesthesia in obese patients. *Cochrane Database Syst Rev* 2013;**9**:CD010105.

17. Brodsky JB, Lemmens HJ, Brock-Utne JG, Vierra M, Saidman LJ. Morbid obesity and tracheal intubation. *Anesth Analg* 2002;**94**:732–6.

18. Cattano D, Melnikov V, Khalil Y, Sridhar S, Hagberg CA. An evaluation of the rapid airway management positioner in obese patients undergoing gastric bypass or laparoscopic gastric banding surgery. *Obes Surg* 2010;**20**:1436–41.

19. Neilipovitz DT, Crosby ET. No evidence for decreased incidence of aspiration after rapid sequence induction. *Can J Anaesth* 2007;**54**:748–64.

20. Cattano D, Corso RM, Altamirano AV, *et al*. Clinical evaluation of the C-MAC

D-Blade videolaryngoscope in severely obese patients: a pilot study. *Br J Anaesth* 2012;**109**:647–8.

21. Wong DT, Yang JJ, Mak HY, Jagannathan N. Use of intubation introducers through a supraglottic airway to facilitate tracheal intubation: a brief review. *Can J Anaesth* 2012;**59**:704–15.

22. Berkow LC, Schwartz JM, Kan K, Corridore M, Heitmiller ES. Use of the laryngeal mask airway–Aintree intubating catheter fiberoptic bronchoscope technique for difficult intubation. *J Clin Anesth* 2011;**23**:534–9.

23. Curtis K, Ahern M, Dawson M, Mallin M. Ultrasound-guided, Bougie-assisted cricothyroidotomy: a description of a novel technique in cadaveric models. *Acad Emerg Med* 2012;**19**:876–9.

24. Popat M, Mitchell V, Dravid R, Patel A, Schampillai C, Higgs A. Difficult Airway Society guidelines for the management of tracheal extubation. *Anaesthesia* 2012;**67**: 318–40.

25. Neligan PJ, Malhotra G, Fraser M, *et al.* Continuous positive airway pressure via the Boussignac system immediately after extubation improves lung function in morbidly obese patients with obstructive sleep apnea undergoing laparoscopic bariatric surgery. *Anesthesiology* 2009;**110**:878–84.

Adult and pediatric epiglottitis

Calvin A. Brown III

Case presentation

A 42-year-old man presents to the emergency department (ED) with 4 days of clear rhinorrhea, mild nonproductive cough, and minor sore throat. However, in the past 36 hours he has developed severe throat pain, difficulty swallowing, and a muffled voice. He has started to drool at home and is having difficulty drinking liquids. He does not report dyspnea, chest pain, recent travel, or sick contacts. He has a history of hypertension and diabetes for which he takes atenolol and metformin.

On examination he appears unwell and is diaphoretic. Vital signs show an oral temperature of 100.9 °F, heart rate of 117 beats per minute, blood pressure of 141/83 mmHg, respiratory rate of 24 breaths per minute, and oxygen saturation of 96% on room air. Brief oral inspection shows mild erythema of the pharyngeal arches without obvious swelling or exudates. He has had a tonsillectomy. Palpation of the anterior neck reveals tenderness over the larynx and bilateral anterior cervical lymphadenopathy. His pulmonary examination is clear. Cardiac examination reveals a regular tachycardic heart rate without obvious pathologic murmurs or gallops.

The nurse places an 18-gauge peripheral intravenous (IV) line in the right arm, and nasal cannula oxygen is applied with an oxygen saturation of 98%. He is placed on telemetry, and isotonic fluid resuscitation is started at 150 cc/hour.

What is the differential diagnosis, diagnostic workup, and management decision tree? Does this patient need to be intubated?

Overview of epiglottitis

Epiglottitis is most often a focal bacterial cellulitis of the supraglottic structures, including the arytenoids, inter-arytenoid notch, vallecula, and lingual tonsils, as well as the epiglottis. Thus, it is often, more accurately, described as supraglottitis. Infection can occur from direct invasion or hematogenous spread after bacteremia. The epiglottic epithelium and supporting soft tissues are loosely attached on the superior (lingual) surface of the epiglottis, allowing a potential space for inflammatory fluid and edema to collect. Inflammation and vascular congestion result in distention and distortion of the epiglottis and other supraglottic structures. As the infection progresses, the glottic inlet narrows and swollen supraglottic tissue obstructs the tracheal aperture, resulting in asphyxia and death. The airway manager's chief

Cases in Emergency Airway Management, ed. Lauren C. Berkow and John C. Sakles. Published by Cambridge University Press. © Cambridge University Press 2015.

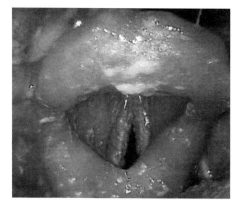

Figure 10.1 Fungal epiglottitis. Courtesy of Michael F. Murphy, MD. Zone Chief of Anesthesiology, Alberta Province, Canada.

concern is the sudden and sometimes unpredictable airway occlusion that can occur, especially in children. The diagnosis must be made quickly so that medical treatment and airway management can be initiated before the airway becomes obstructed. Accurate identification, appropriate preparation, and skill with rescue surgical techniques are paramount to avoid patient morbidity and mortality. Complete airway occlusion may occur rapidly, but cardinal signs of severe airway obstruction (stridor, drooling, tachypnea, cyanosis, retractions, and dyspnea) may become evident only as the airway is on the verge of total obliteration.[1]

Epiglottitis occurs across all age groups, although it is discussed, classically, in the context of pediatric airway emergencies. Epiglottitis is most often caused by a bacterial infection, although it can result from viruses and fungi on occasion (Figure 10.1). Noninfectious causes include caustic and thermal injury. Historically, *Haemophilus influenzae* type b caused most cases of epiglottitis; however, the incidence of pediatric bacterial epiglottitis has dropped significantly since the development of the *H. influenzae* vaccine in 1985. Despite this, *H. influenzae* type b is the most commonly isolated bacterial organism in both children and adults.[2] Although it is unusual, *H. influenzae* epiglottitis infection still occurs in immunized individuals.[3,4] Contemporary pediatric microbiology has become much more varied and includes *Staphylococcus aureus*, group A beta hemolytic strep, and *Streptococcus pneumoniae*.[5] The current incidence of pediatric epiglottitis is estimated to be 0.6 to 0.8 cases per 100,000 and occurs more often in older children, most commonly between the ages of 6 and 12.[6] The incidence of epiglottitis is twice as high in adults (> 18 years) and is currently estimated at 1.6 cases per 100,000.

The clinical presentation varies by age group. Pediatric epiglottitis typically begins with an abrupt onset of fever and marked sore throat followed quickly by change in phonation, drooling, difficulty breathing, stridor, and anxiety as a result of worsening airway obstruction. Cough is typically absent. The child may present in a "sniffing" position with both his/her jaw and head protruded forward in an effort to maintain airway patency.[7] The degree of obstructive symptoms is related to patient age. Young children (< 2 years of age), with smaller-caliber airways, will exhibit more significant airway obstruction, whereas older children and young adults require more swelling before obstruction is clinically evident. Older pediatric patients are more often misdiagnosed as having croup and streptococcal or viral pharyngitis. Young children may appear toxic and have altered levels of alertness. Overall, pediatric patients with fever, drooling, or stridor should be considered to have epiglottitis until proven otherwise.

In adults, epiglottitis does not have a seasonal trend or "season," as is observed with other infectious diseases, such as influenza. The onset is often insidious with what may appear, at first, to be an ordinary upper respiratory illness. The initial symptoms may last for several days before the onset of severe sore throat, dysphagia, and altered phonation.[8] Although fever is nearly universal in pediatric epiglottitis cases, it is present in only 50% of adult patients.[8] Additionally, epiglottitis should be considered in adult patients who have a benign pharyngeal examination yet report severe throat pain. Rapid-onset symptoms are more common in adult patients who have chronic illnesses, in particular diabetes, which put them at risk for serious infections. In adults, rapid-onset symptoms may predict the need for airway management. The differential diagnosis includes retropharyngeal abscess, peritonsillar abscess, streptococcal and mononucleosis-associated pharyngitis, anaphylaxis, Ludwig's angina, tumors, laryngeal trauma, and caustic and thermal supraglottic exposure.

General management principles

When epiglottitis is suspected, the first decision is whether the airway needs to be managed emergently. Patients who have severe respiratory distress, refractory hypoxia (despite supplemental oxygen), or rapidly developing obstructive symptoms have an immediate need for airway management, and emergency intubation trumps all other treatment and diagnostic considerations at that moment.

If time allows for a workup, a structured, efficient diagnostic path should start immediately with the goal of accurately confirming the diagnosis. However, in children, one should avoid unnecessary airway manipulation, which can cause patient agitation, increased airway turbulence, and swelling and may precipitate laryngospasm. The diagnostic pathway differs slightly for adults and children. In children specifically, confirmatory testing may not be necessary when classic or severe symptoms are present. In this instance, stable pediatric patients should have blow-by supplemental oxygen as needed, but otherwise, they should be left in a comfortable, calm position until anesthesia and otolaryngology specialists can perform definitive airway evaluation and intubation in a controlled setting, optimally in the operating room (OR). It is critical to avoid airway evaluation that causes pharyngeal manipulation because it can precipitate immediate airway obstruction with rare reports of cardiac arrest.[9] Children with mild or atypical symptoms can undergo a gentle oral examination. Alternatively, a lateral soft-tissue plain radiograph can aid in the diagnosis. A thickened epiglottic shadow (> 8 mm), also known as the "thumb print" sign, along with lack of air in the vallecula confirms the diagnosis. A provider with expertise in emergency airway management must remain with the patient at all times during any diagnostic testing or airway evaluation in case acute respiratory distress or obstruction occurs. Antibiotics against *H. influenzae* and other common pathogens are indicated as soon as possible. However, the benefit of early IV antibiotics should be weighed very carefully against the risk of agitation and airway obstruction that can occur during peripheral IV placement. In general, antibiotics are reserved until after the patient is intubated.

The practitioner should attempt to visualize the airway of adults with suspected epiglottitis. In contrast to children, adults are amenable to an oral and laryngeal evaluation without the same risk of acute obstruction. Laryngoscopy is the confirmatory test of choice, but soft-tissue lateral X-rays have high sensitivity and can be ordered to aid in the workup.[8,10] Adult patients do not typically require intubation; however, dyspnea, drooling, hypoxia, stridor, and inability to phonate indicate significant obstruction and increase

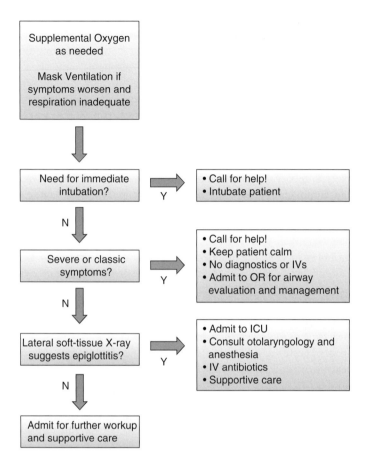

Figure 10.2 Management algorithm for suspected pediatric epiglottitis. IV, peripheral intravenous line

the likelihood of intubation.[8,10] As with children, adult patients with severe respiratory distress, hypoxia, or rapidly progressive symptoms require emergent intubation.

Pediatric airway management principles

In pediatric patients with suspected epiglottitis, the initial management is dependent on patient acuity and respiratory distress (Figure 10.2). Whereas adult patients usually do not require intubation, most treatment algorithms promote placement of a definitive airway for all pediatric patients with proven epiglottitis, especially young children or toddlers (< 6 years), because a large registry of data suggested that it reduces mortality compared to that with careful observation.[11] Small case series data have since suggested that some patients can be managed successfully in an intensive care unit (ICU) setting after a fiberoptic evaluation of the airway has been performed.[12,13] Older children (> 6 years) and those with a reassuring fiberoptic examination are more likely to matriculate from an observation protocol. In all cases where epiglottitis is diagnosed or deemed likely based on clinical grounds, the practitioner should call for help (often otolaryngology, anesthesia, or both). If the patient is stable, then only supportive measures are indicated (oxygen) and no attempt should be made to examine the oral cavity, pharynx, or larynx. Agitated children produce increased respiratory effort and turbulent airflow that can accelerate supraglottic swelling and airway obstruction. In general, the patient should be left alone until he/she can be moved to a stable environment, such as the OR. At all times, an expert airway manager as well as basic and difficult airway devices should be kept in the patient's room. Patients with respiratory failure, rapidly progressive symptoms, or sudden obstruction should undergo immediate rescue mask ventilation. Appropriately configured self-inflating (e.g. Ambu) bags, with excellent mask seal, can generate 50–100 cm H_2O ventilation pressure and, in general, can produce enough force to overcome soft-tissue obstruction. However, pediatric Ambu bags are often configured with positive-pressure relief valves sometimes called "pop-off" valves. These safety devices are designed to prevent accidental barotrauma secondary to vigorous ventilation. In the case of airway obstruction, this extra force may be needed and pressure release valves should be either detached or disarmed to ventilate effectively. Oral and nasal adjuncts may be needed but often are unnecessary in children. Effective bag-mask ventilation (BMV) can buy time to construct a plan for either awake laryngoscopy or rapid sequence intubation with a double setup for a percutaneous or open surgical airway.

If rescue ventilation fails (a rare event in epiglottitis), then immediate recourse to a surgical airway is required. In patients less than 5 years of age, needle cricothyrotomy is the preferred method. For patients 5 to 10 years old, either a needle cricothyrotomy or a Melker (Seldinger-style) surgical airway can be performed. For children over the age of 10, standard surgical techniques can be used. There are no published data that definitively support the most effective mode of ventilation after a needle cricothyrotomy. Transtracheal jet ventilation is an option but it can be complicated by barotrauma.[14] In the absence of proven benefit, if equipment and familiarity with setting up a transtracheal jet ventilation circuit are lacking, it is recommended that practitioners attach an Ambu bag to the end of the needle adapter and mask ventilate by hand.

Adult airway management principles

Adult patients with suspected airway obstruction from epiglottitis who are apneic or in extremis need to be intubated immediately. They should undergo rapid sequence intubation (sedation with paralysis) under the "forced to act" principle of difficult emergency airway management.[15] The practitioner should *always* proceed with a double setup for a rescue surgical cricothyrotomy in case the first laryngoscopy and intubation attempt fail. Thankfully, such failure is rare. In general, adult patients will be stable enough to undergo an awake evaluation of the airway. Depending on patient acuity, provider skill, and specialist support, this can happen in the ED, OR, or ICU. The initial diagnostic and therapeutic maneuvers are identical (Figure 10.3) to that of children. If the patient is not in crisis, fiberoptic laryngoscopy is the preferred approach, and in preparing the patient for examination, the table is also set for awake intubation if it is deemed necessary. Successful awake fiberoptic laryngoscopy is predicated on two principles: dense topical anesthesia and judicious use of sedation. If time permits, a drying agent such as glycopyrrolate (0.01 mg/kg IV) should be administered 15 to 20 minutes before topicalization. Glycopyrrolate dries the mucosal surfaces, allowing a more robust and complete anesthetic block. A nasal approach is used most often. With this approach, a vasoconstrictor (oxymetazoline or phenylephrine) should be administered in each nostril to prolong topical anesthesia and reduce the incidence

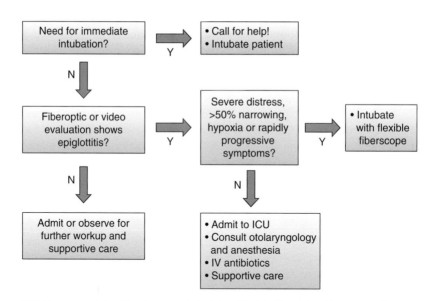

Figure 10.3 Management algorithm for suspected adult epiglottitis. IV, peripheral intravenous line

of epistaxis. After administration of glycopyrrolate and phenylephrine, topicalization can proceed with both nebulization and atomization of aqueous lidocaine. The practitioner should nebulize 2–3 mL of a 4% aqueous lidocaine solution for 10 minutes followed by atomization in the nasal passage. A small endotracheal tube (ETT; 6.5 mm) should be placed in the nasal passage and inserted just beyond the bony turbinate so that the tip is in the posterior nasopharynx. Before insertion, the distal four inches of the tube should be coated with lidocaine jelly to further contribute to topical anesthesia. Lidocaine jelly should not be applied inside the nose (as is done during nasogastric tube placement) because the ETT will have to travel through a wall of lidocaine, potentially creating a plug of jelly in the ETT lumen and soiling the end of the scope during insertion. Topical anesthesia may need to be augmented with token doses of sedation to facilitate the procedure. The benefit from sedation should be balanced carefully against the risk of sudden airway collapse and obstruction that occur when protected airway reflexes and stenting upper airway tone is reduced. If necessary, very small doses of midazolam (1 mg IV) or fentanyl (50 mcg IV) can be used.

Once the ETT is in place, an assistant can hold the proximal end of the tracheal tube while the operator inserts the flexible video or fiberoptic bronchoscope through it. If properly placed, the bronchoscope will exit the ETT in the distal nasopharynx and, with very little manipulation, the larynx should come into view. The advantage of placing an ETT in the nostril before proceeding with laryngoscopy is that it allows for intubation over the scope, at that moment, without needing to retract the scope and start the procedure over again.

Awake laryngoscopy can also be performed with either a conventional laryngoscope or a video laryngoscope. However, these techniques may be less practical because the patient often can't tolerate laying supine for a laryngoscopic attempt. In addition, compression of the base of the tongue and epiglottis by the laryngoscope blade may precipitate laryngospasm. If a laryngoscope is used, the GlideScope or C-MAC D-blade would be optimal, as each has a hyper-curved blade and can be used to visualize the glottis with very little manipulation while the patient is sitting upright.

The following equipment should be at the bedside before any awake evaluation is performed: Ambu bag, oral and nasal airways, a direct or video laryngoscope, and equipment to perform an open surgical cricothyrotomy. If the airway suddenly becomes obstructed, immediate rescue mask ventilation with an oral and nasal airway should be attempted. Given the level of the obstruction (just above the glottic opening) placement of an extraglottic device such as a laryngeal mask airway, laryngeal tube, or combitube will not be helpful if BMV is ineffective. However, laryngospasm and other forms of soft-tissue obstruction can often be overcome by using a pristine two-handed, two-person BMV technique and airway and nasal adjuncts. If BMV fails, one (and only one) immediate attempt at laryngoscopy is reasonable while preparations are made for an immediate surgical airway. In this setting, a video laryngoscope is preferred to a conventional laryngoscope because it provides better glottic exposure and intubation success.[16,17]

Once the airway is visualized, the decision to intubate is multifactorial and will depend on the appearance of the glottic opening, progression of symptoms, patient distress, and vital signs. An approach that calls for mandatory intubation of all adult patients with epiglottitis and one that uses a selective approach based on laryngoscopic findings have both been advocated. However, most experts agree that selective intubation in adults is the best approach. Patients with more than a 50% glottic obliteration, an epiglottic abscess, or a compromised immune system should be intubated during the fiberoptic procedure.[18,19] In general, it is safer to err on the side of intubation because an ETT that is placed but removed shortly thereafter provides a better patient outcome than continued observation of a high-risk dynamic airway obstruction that results in sudden occlusion and hypoxic injury.

Post-intubation management

Post-intubation management of the patient with epiglottitis should include a strategy for ongoing sedation and pain control to keep the patient comfortable while ventilated. In addition, extra precautions should be taken to prevent accidental extubation, as it could be a terminal event. Hand restraints may be required. A surgical airway kit should always be kept at the patient's bedside in case of extubation. IV antibiotics that cover common bacterial agents for epiglottitis should be started as soon as possible. Second- and third-generation cephalosporins are good initial agents. If methicillin-resistant *Staphylococcus aureus* is a concern, vancomycin should be added. The role of glucocorticoids in acute epiglottitis is controversial and not currently recommended. Intubation for 2–3 days is often required. Extubation can be entertained with resolution of supraglottic edema and the presence of a cuff leak around the ETT.

References

1. Glynn, F. and J.E. Fenton, Diagnosis and management of supraglottitis (epiglottitis). *Curr Infect Dis Rep*, 2008. **10**(3):200–4.

2. Frantz, T.D. *et al.*, Acute epiglottitis in adults. Analysis of 129 cases. *JAMA*, 1994. **272**(17):1358–60.

3. Shah, R.K. *et al.*, Epiglottitis in the *Hemophilus influenzae* type B vaccine era: changing trends. *Laryngoscope*, 2004. **114**(3):557–60.

4. Gonzalez Valdepena, H. *et al.*, Epiglottitis and *Haemophilus influenzae* immunization: the Pittsburgh experience – a five-year review. *Pediatrics*, 1995. **96**(3 Pt 1):424–7.

5. Somenek, M. *et al.*, Membranous laryngitis in a child. *Int J Pediatr Otorhinolaryngol*, 2010. **74**(6):704–6.

6. Tanner, K. *et al.*, *Haemophilus influenzae* type b epiglottitis as a cause of acute upper airways obstruction in children. *BMJ*, 2002. **325**(7372):1099–100.

7. Stroud, R.H. and N.R. Friedman, An update on inflammatory disorders of the pediatric airway: epiglottitis, croup, and tracheitis. *Am J Otolaryngol*, 2001. **22**(4):268–75.

8. Ng, H.L. *et al.*, Acute epiglottitis in adults: a retrospective review of 106 patients in Hong Kong. *Emerg Med J*, 2008. **25**(5):253–5.

9. Oropharyngeal examination for suspected epiglottitis. *Am J Dis Child*, 1988. **142**(12):1261–7.

10. Solomon, P. *et al.*, Adult epiglottitis: the Toronto Hospital experience. *J Otolaryngol*, 1998. **27**(6):332–6.

11. Cantrell, R.W. *et al.*, Acute epiglottitis: intubation versus tracheostomy. *Laryngoscope*, 1978. **88**(6):994–1005.

12. Andreassen, U.K. *et al.*, Acute epiglottitis – 25 years experience with nasotracheal intubation, current management policy and future trends. *J Laryngol Otol*, 1992. **106**(12):1072–5.

13. Damm, M. *et al.*, Airway endoscopy in the interdisciplinary management of acute epiglottitis. *Int J Pediatr Otorhinolaryngol*, 1996. **38**(1):41–51.

14. Craft, T.M. *et al.*, Two cases of barotrauma associated with transtracheal jet ventilation. *Br J Anaesth*, 1990. **64**(4):524–7.

15. Walls, R.M., The emergency airway algorithms. In *Manual of Emergency Airway Management*, 3rd edn., eds. R.M. Walls, M.F. Murphy, and R.C. Luten. 2008, Philadelphia, PN: Lippincott, Williams & Wilkins / Wolters Kluwer Health, pp. 8–22.

16. Brown, C.A., 3rd *et al.*, Improved glottic exposure with the video Macintosh laryngoscope in adult emergency department tracheal intubations. *Ann Emerg Med*, 2010. **56**(2):83–8.

17. Sakles, J.C. *et al.*, A comparison of the C-MAC video laryngoscope to the Macintosh direct laryngoscope for intubation in the emergency department. *Ann Emerg Med*, 2012. **60**(6):739–48.

18. Berger, G. *et al.*, The rising incidence of adult acute epiglottitis and epiglottic abscess. *Am J Otolaryngol*, 2003. **24**(6): p. 374–83.

19. Mayo-Smith, M.F. *et al.*, Acute epiglottitis. An 18-year experience in Rhode Island. *Chest*, 1995. **108**(6):1640–7.

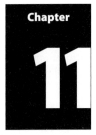

Chapter 11

Management of foreign body aspiration in pediatric and adult patients

Neal Patrick Moehrle and Narasimhan Jagannathan

Case presentation

A 3-year-old boy has a sudden choking episode at home while playing. His mother witnesses her child "turning blue," upon which she taps vigorously on his back. With this maneuver, the child appears to have some improvement. He is then rushed to the emergency department (ED). On arrival to the ED, the child has a respiratory rate of 40 breaths per minute, heart rate of 140 beats per minute, and oxygen saturation of 92% on room air. His breath sounds are markedly decreased over the right lung fields. A chest X-ray is then ordered and appears normal.

Introduction

Aspiration of a foreign body is a potentially life-threatening medical emergency. It has significantly high rates of morbidity, especially with delayed diagnosis and treatment, and is a leading cause of accidental death in children. This chapter will focus on the various techniques that can be used for airway management in adult and pediatric foreign body aspiration (FBA).

A medical review of FBA

Epidemiology

Although FBA can occur at any age, it predominantly affects the pediatric population. Approximately 80% of all cases occur in pediatric patients, and most of those are in children under the age of 3 years.[1] Several reasons explain the increased risk of FBA in children. Because they lack posterior molars, children are often unable to chew their food completely.[2] Large food boli that do not enter the esophagus may obstruct the glottic opening, and smaller food particles may enter the trachea and become lodged in the distal airways. Furthermore, many children are orally fixated and use their mouths as a means to explore their surroundings.[2] Putting foreign objects in their mouths puts them at increased risk for accidentally aspirating the object.

In adults, the incidence of FBA tends to increase with age.[1] Common risk factors include difficulty swallowing and an impaired cough reflex, both of which become more prevalent later in life. These impairments may also result from neurologic disorders, such as those

Cases in Emergency Airway Management, ed. Lauren C. Berkow and John C. Sakles. Published by Cambridge University Press. © Cambridge University Press 2015.

caused by cerebrovascular accidents, or may be associated with medications like antic-holinergics and sedatives.[1] Aspiration of dental supplies and teeth has been shown to be a complication associated with various dental procedures in adults.[3]

The incidence of FBA is higher among boys than girls, occurring in a ratio of approximately 1.5:1.[4] A similar gender bias has been reported in the adult population, although some studies have found no difference between men and women.[5]

Pathogenesis

Any object small enough to fit through the glottic opening can be aspirated. Most cases involve the aspiration of organic materials such as nuts (especially peanuts), seeds, and other food particles.[3,4] In addition to physically obstructing the airway, organic materials often induce inflammation in the bronchi and bronchioles; this inflammatory reaction can then lead to the formation of granulation tissue, airway stenosis, and further respiratory complications.[4] Less commonly, a patient will inhale a pin, dental appliance, glass, or other miscellaneous inorganic materials. Inorganic materials are less likely to induce an inflammatory response, but the presence of sharp edges can cause additional damage to the airway.

Where a foreign body lodges in the respiratory tract depends on its size. Objects larger than the diameter of the trachea tend to obstruct the upper airway near the larynx or oropharynx, a potentially fatal scenario that results in rapid oxygen deprivation and death if not treated quickly. Smaller objects commonly obstruct the distal airways. Notably, the right side is more often involved than the left.[2,4,5] This difference can be explained in part by the right mainstem bronchus being more vertically orientated than the left.[2]

Failure to remove a foreign body in a timely fashion can result in several complications, including chronic cough, bronchitis, recurrent pneumonia, bronchiectasis, pneumomedias-tinum, or pneumothorax.[1,2] Because the sequelae arising from delayed treatment can lead to complications, early diagnosis and removal of the object are imperative.

Clinical manifestations

Aside from a choking episode, the signs and symptoms of FBA are often nonspecific and subtle. In both adults and children, the most frequent symptom is a "penetration syndrome," characterized by acute onset of choking and coughing, with or without vomiting.[1,5] A recent history of penetration syndrome significantly aids in the diagnosis of FBA, but unfortunately it is reported in only about half of all cases.[1]

In the absence of choking, FBA may present with nonspecific signs such as coughing, wheezing, shortness of breath, or fever.[1] Physical examination may show decreased breath sounds on the affected side. If the aspiration is complicated by pneumonia, evidence of consolidation may also be present, including dullness of breath sounds, bronchial breath sounds, and increased tactile fremitus. In children, the presence of stridor and cyanosis are highly specific for FBA.[4] In adults, the nonspecific findings are often misattributed to other respiratory conditions, such as chronic obstructive pulmonary disease (COPD), atypical asthma, or pneumonia.[1] This presentation in adults makes the diagnosis of FBA difficult. Often, clinicians require a high index of clinical suspicion, which can delay diagnosis and treatment and increase the risk for additional complications.

Patients with suspected FBA routinely undergo chest radiography to aid in the diagnosis. Ideally, the radiograph will help clinicians to visualize the foreign object, but visualization depends on the type of material that is aspirated. Radiopaque objects like coins, pins, and other metals can usually be picked up by X-ray. However, organic materials, which represent a majority of cases, are typically radiolucent and thus cannot be visualized by X-ray. Nevertheless, plain films of patients with FBA show abnormalities in approximately 75% of cases.[2] Air trapping is the most common radiographic finding in pediatric patients and is best seen by examining both inspiratory and expiratory films.[2,5] In contrast, the presence of atelectasis is the predominant feature on X-rays in the adult population.[5] In patients who develop pneumonia, radiographs may show pulmonary infiltrates in the parenchyma surrounding the obstruction.

Chest X-rays may be falsely normal in up to 25% of patients.[2] If FBA is still suspected in these patients, the superior sensitivity and specificity of computed tomography (CT) may improve detection of foreign bodies missed by standard radiography. The higher resolution of CT enables clinicians to visualize the aspirated object with greater frequency than that with plain films. In addition, presence of atelectasis, air trapping, and other abnormal findings may be more evident. The use of CT is limited because it is more costly than standard radiography and exposes the patient to more radiation; therefore, for the initial examination, X-ray is usually the imaging modality of choice.

Management of FBA

Bronchoscopy is the gold standard for diagnosis of FBA. The bronchoscope not only allows the operator to identify and localize the foreign body, but also provides a means by which the object can be removed from the respiratory tract. Since the late 1890s, when rigid bronchoscopes were first used for this purpose, mortality associated with FBA has decreased significantly, with a reported drop from 24% to 2% by 1936.[3] Rigid bronchoscopy became the primary method of treatment until the 1960s, when the development of the flexible bronchoscope provided a possible alternative to the prototype. Once the benefits of flexible bronchoscopy became clearer, this alternative method became an increasingly popular tool for the initial evaluation of FBA. These two methods of bronchoscopy will be discussed here for both pediatric and adult airway management scenarios.

Initial airway management for partial obstructions in adults and children

In patients with suspected FBA, maintaining adequate oxygenation and ventilation should be the primary goal. Some patients with a partial obstruction may present with normal oxygen saturation and unhindered breathing, whereas others may require assistance. Supplemental oxygen or, in some cases, bag-mask ventilation should be provided.[1] The latter is a skill that requires minimal training for most clinicians, but it delivers oxygen less efficiently than other alternatives. Bag-mask ventilation also has the potential to cause gastric insufflation, which may lead to regurgitation of gastric contents. Additionally, administration of oxygen with too much force via bag-mask (high peak inspiratory pressures) could potentially dislodge a foreign body and worsen the obstruction, or convert a partial obstruction into a complete airway obstruction. In any case, the patient's lungs should be properly oxygenated until he or she can be taken to the operating room for bronchoscopy.

Treatment of partial airway obstruction in children and infants

Before the advent of flexible bronchoscopy, the rigid open-tube bronchoscope was primarily used for diagnosis and removal of an inhaled foreign body. Even today, rigid bronchoscopy remains the procedure chosen by most physicians to remove an object from a pediatric airway. Flexible bronchoscopy, however, offers several benefits, including the ability to assess the size and magnitude of obstruction, especially if the foreign body is located in the distal airways. When choosing which type of bronchoscope to use, it is important to consider the likelihood that FBA is the correct diagnosis.

When the history and clinical manifestations strongly suggest that the patient has inhaled a foreign body, rigid bronchoscopy should be used to confirm the diagnosis and subsequently to remove the object.[6] If the diagnosis is less certain, however, many clinicians turn to the flexible fiberoptic bronchoscope for their initial diagnostic tool.[4,6] If an inhaled foreign body is excluded as a cause of the patient's symptoms, then general anesthesia and an unnecessary rigid bronchoscopic procedure can be avoided, thereby reducing treatment costs and sparing the patient from possible complications. If flexible bronchoscopy confirms the presence of a foreign body, a rigid bronchoscope can then be used to extract it.[6] The initial visualization of the object with a flexible bronchoscope may provide helpful information for the operator, such as the size of the foreign body and the type of rigid bronchoscope and forceps needed for subsequent removal. This two-step process has been shown to decrease the negative finding rate of rigid bronchoscopy without increasing the length of hospital stay.[6]

As clinicians have become more comfortable with the flexible bronchoscope, it has become useful not only for the diagnosis of FBA in children, but also for object retrieval. A retrospective review of over 1,000 children found that foreign bodies were successfully and safely removed by flexible bronchoscopy in 91.3% of patients.[7] Several advantages warrant the use of flexible over rigid bronchoscopy for diagnosis and treatment of FBA. In contrast to the general anesthesia required for rigid bronchoscopy, a combination of local anesthesia and mild sedation is usually sufficient for flexible bronchoscopy.[4] This regimen reduces procedure cost and shortens the hospital stay.[6] Additionally, because the flexible broncho-scope has a smaller diameter and greater flexibility than the rigid bronchoscope, it is better able to access foreign bodies located in more distal airways or in the upper lobe bronchi.[3,7] These advantages are highlighted in Table 11.1.

Nevertheless, use of the flexible bronchoscope in children has some limitations. Its feasibility often depends on the patient's ability to cooperate and lie still during the procedure. Excessive movement makes foreign body removal more difficult and increases the patient's risk of complications, such as tissue trauma and bleeding. This drawback

Table 11.1 Advantages and disadvantages of flexible bronchoscopy compared to rigid bronchoscopy

Advantages	Disadvantages
• Can be performed under local anesthesia and/or sedation • Improved access to distal airways • Reduced cost	• Less control of ventilation • Dependent on patient cooperation

partly explains why the shift to flexible bronchoscopy as a treatment modality for FBA has been slower in the pediatric population than in the adult population, as children tend to be less cooperative than adults.

Although rigid bronchoscopy remains the primary therapy for FBA in children, flexible bronchoscopy is a safe and efficacious method for managing the pediatric airway.[7] The decision to use rigid or flexible bronchoscopy ultimately depends on the operator's expertise with each device.

Treatment of partial airway obstruction in adults and adolescents

The management of FBA in adults and adolescents is slightly different than that in young children and infants. Regardless of the degree of clinical suspicion, flexible bronchoscopy is often used as the initial diagnostic tool. If a foreign body is detected in the respiratory tract, the operator can attempt to remove it with the flexible bronchoscope and avoid rigid bronchoscopy altogether.[3] In a case series of 426 patients, foreign bodies were successfully removed by flexible bronchoscopy in 86% of the cases (366 of 426 patients).[3] With relatively high success rates and advantages over rigid bronchoscopy, flexible bronchoscopy has become the first-line therapeutic procedure for FBA in adults and older children. Rigid bronchoscopy, once the only means by which a foreign body could be extracted from an airway, is now mainly performed in this age group only when flexible bronchoscopy fails.

Anesthetic and airway management during flexible bronchoscopy in adult and pediatric patients

Pharmacologic management

In adults, a combination of topical anesthetic and mild sedation is often sufficient for flexible bronchoscopy. For example, a lidocaine 4% spray will anesthetize the airway while midazolam or fentanyl is introduced intravenously for sedation. In patients who are not able to tolerate an awake procedure, general anesthesia with an artificial airway may be necessary.

Supraglottic airway vs. endotracheal tube ventilation

During flexible bronchoscopy, a patient's airway can be managed with either a supraglottic airway (SGA) or an endotracheal tube (ETT). Compared to bag-mask ventilation, these methods provide more direct access to the trachea, and insertion of an ETT provides a more secure airway that ventilates the lungs more effectively. Nevertheless, bronchoscopy through an ETT is restricted to smaller-diameter bronchoscopes and for evaluation of foreign bodies located more distally in the tracheobronchial tree.[8] Compared with tracheal intubation, SGAs may provide better visualization of the supraglottic larynx and allow the use of larger-diameter flexible bronchoscopes.[8] Regardless of which management option is chosen, it is important to have a deep plane of anesthesia to minimize reflex activation of the airway (coughing, bearing down, laryngospasm, bronchospasm), which can also lead to foreign body dislodgement. Topical anesthesia and/or titrated doses of opioids may help accomplish this.

Anesthetic and airway management during rigid bronchoscopy in children

Pharmacologic management

General anesthesia is primarily induced by inhalation or intravenous anesthesia, although the former is more widely practiced.[4] Spontaneous ventilation is often maintained while anesthesia is being induced.[4,9]

In children, sevoflurane is the pharmacologic agent of choice for mask induction and maintenance of anesthesia. Sevoflurane is preferred because it poses a lower risk for cardiac arrhythmias than halothane, which is still used in many developing countries.[4] Intravenous anesthetics (i.e. propofol and remifentanil) are becoming increasingly popular for anesthesia maintenance because they provide a more constant level of anesthesia that is not dependent on native ventilation.[4] With intravenous administration, air leakage around the rigid bronchoscope will not affect anesthetic depth, as it can when volatile agents are used alone. Additionally, the risk of atmospheric contamination of volatile gases is lower. Nevertheless, both inhaled and intravenous methods are effective means by which anesthesia can be delivered to children undergoing rigid bronchoscopy.

Controlled vs. spontaneous ventilation

Maintaining adequate ventilation and control of the airway is essential during removal of a foreign body with a rigid bronchoscope. For many clinicians, choosing whether to have the patient on controlled or spontaneous ventilation is a difficult decision, as both methods have advantages and disadvantages. For example, compared with positive-pressure ventilation, spontaneous ventilation is less likely to advance the foreign body more distally, which would make removal of the object more challenging.[9] Under controlled ventilation, the patient experiences brief periods of apnea as the operator maneuvers through the airway; in contrast, ventilation is uninterrupted if the patient is allowed to breathe spontaneously. Spontaneous ventilation, however, is associated with higher risk of patient movement and reflex activation of the airway (coughing, bearing down, laryngospasm, and bronchospasm), which can make foreign body removal more arduous and can potentially lead to additional complications.[9] These complications can often be managed by increasing the depth of anesthesia with an intravenous agent, such as propofol, or neuromuscular blocking drugs. Topicalization of the tracheobronchial tree with local anesthesia will also help blunt airway reflexes.[4] In addition to its lower risk of patient movement and airway reactivity, controlled ventilation may decrease atelectasis and hypercarbia, thus improving oxygenation.[9] The advantages and limitations of controlled and spontaneous ventilation are compared in Table 11.2.

To date, research to determine whether controlled or spontaneous ventilation is more beneficial during foreign body removal has been inconclusive. Although controlled ventilation is associated with shorter operative times, the incidence of oxygen desaturation is not significantly different between the two, according to a recent meta-analysis.[10] In most cases, preserving spontaneous ventilation initially may be the safest method to prevent dislodgement of the foreign body. The anesthesiologist can later convert to controlled ventilation if necessary.[4] More research must be conducted to definitively determine which mode of ventilation is better for both the bronchoscopist and patient.

Table 11.2 Comparison of controlled and spontaneous ventilation for rigid bronchoscopy

Controlled ventilation		Spontaneous ventilation	
Advantages	**Disadvantages**	**Advantages**	**Disadvantages**
• Decreases atelectasis • Associated with shorter operative times • Less potential for hypercarbia • Rapid airway control in case of full stomach	• Increased risk of foreign body dislodgement with positive-pressure ventilation • Intermittent apnea during removal	• Decreased risk of foreign body dislodgement • Better V/Q matching, less air trapping • Easier to ventilate through bronchoscope • Airway is preserved and ventilation maintained during manipulation of foreign body	• Increased risk of reflex activation of the airway (laryngospasm, coughing), hypercarbia, and patient movement • Prolonged emergence from anesthesia

V/Q, ventilation/perfusion

Technique for foreign body removal

Removal of a foreign body from a pediatric or adult airway requires precision and dexterity. Bronchoscopy enables the clinician to locate and visualize the object, but various types of forceps and other instruments are used for retrieval. Forceps selection is typically based on the shape and nature of the foreign body. Once the bronchoscopist has established a secure grasp on the object, the forceps, object, and bronchoscope are removed simultaneously.[3] This practice allows for constant visualization of the object as it moves up the respiratory tract.

Inadvertent release of the foreign body during removal is a potentially life-threatening complication, as objects in the proximal airway may cause complete obstruction. In this situation, it may be best to push the object more distally into one of the main bronchi – preferentially the bronchus where it originated – in order to preserve at least partial ventilation.[4] The bronchoscopist can then re-grasp the foreign body and make a second attempt at removal.

To facilitate removal and reduce the risk of accidentally dropping the object, the clinician should relax the vocal cords with topical lidocaine or a muscle relaxant.[4,9] The bronchoscope, forceps, and foreign body can then pass through the trachea and larynx more easily. After the object is successfully removed, a second bronchoscopy is usually performed to check for remnants of the foreign body that may have separated during the extraction and to assess for any airway damage.

Management of a complete airway obstruction by a foreign body

Although less common than partial obstructions of the tracheobronchial tree, complete obstruction of the larynx and trachea by a foreign body is associated with high mortality rates. Progression to respiratory failure, coma, and death occurs so rapidly that many patients never reach the hospital. This situation requires immediate attention and stabilization of the patient's airway. Signs of a complete obstruction include the inability to speak or cough, choking, and respiratory distress. Recognition of these signs is imperative so that first aid can be administered as soon as possible according to the age-specific Basic Life Support (BLS) guidelines (i.e. Heimlich maneuver developed by the American Heart Association). These maneuvers should not be performed for a partial obstruction, as they can cause progression to a complete obstruction.

If initial first aid is unsuccessful, direct laryngoscopy should be used to locate the foreign body in the upper airway. The object should be safely removed with Magill forceps if it is easily accessible.[1] If immediate removal of the foreign body by direct laryngoscopy is not feasible, or if respiratory status is rapidly deteriorating, clinicians should stabilize the airway first with bag-mask ventilation or an SGA before attempting to remove the object. When indicated, a cricothyrotomy should be performed expeditiously to minimize the risk of hypoxic brain damage.[1] Once ventilation is restored, the foreign body can be removed by rigid or flexible bronchoscopy as described in the preceding sections.

Algorithm for the management of FBA

As technology for bronchoscopy has become more advanced, algorithms for the management of FBA have changed. Figure 11.1 illustrates a possible algorithm that can be used for airway management of patients with partial and complete obstructions.

Post-management care

Barring any major intraoperative complications, pulmonary status should improve after bronchoscopy; most patients are discharged from the hospital within 2 days of the

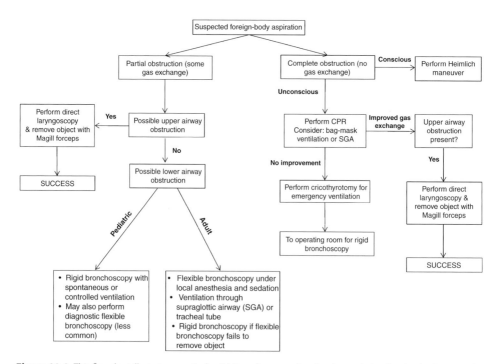

Figure 11.1 This flowchart illustrates practical guidelines for managing the airway during foreign body removal in pediatric and adult patients whose airways are completely or partially obstructed

procedure, and approximately 60% of patients are stable enough to go home the same day.[4] Several factors can prolong recovery time, including magnitude of airway inflammation, prolonged duration of bronchoscopy, and the occurrence of intra- and postoperative complications.[2]

The severity of complications positively correlates with recovery time. The occurrence of pneumothorax, acute pulmonary edema, pneumonia, and subglottic edema in children has been shown to extend hospitalization to more than one week.[2] If pneumonia is suspected, a culture should be obtained during bronchoscopy so that targeted antibiotic therapy can be administered. Serious complications from rigid and flexible bronchoscopy are relatively uncommon, occurring in less than 1% of cases.[3,4] Fortunately, most complications from bronchoscopy are less serious. For example, laryngeal edema and minor bleeding only marginally affect the length of recovery.[2] Given its high success rate and low incidence of complications, bronchoscopy is an effective and safe procedure for the management of FBA in adults and children.

Discussion of the case presentation

An otolaryngologist called to the ED decides that he will first perform a diagnostic flexible bronchoscopy, based on the lack of convincing evidence suggesting FBA. Flexible bronchoscopy reveals a large red object resembling a Lego® piece lodged in the child's right mainstem bronchus. Because the object is large, and the child is uncooperative and distressed, the otolaryngologist decides to proceed with rigid bronchoscopy under general anesthesia for the removal of the foreign body.

Anesthesia is induced with sevoflurane via mask and titrated doses of fentanyl before the rigid bronchoscope is placed. The rigid bronchoscope is then inserted into the trachea, and anesthesia is maintained with intravenous propofol. Oxygenation is possible through the rigid bronchoscope while spontaneous ventilation is maintained. When the otolaryngologist attempts to extract the foreign body with laryngeal forceps, the child coughs vigorously, leading to foreign body dislodgement and a sudden inability to ventilate the lungs. Oxygen saturation falls precipitously to 60%. Succinylcholine is administered intravenously with immediate placement of the rigid bronchoscope, which reveals that the foreign body is lodged in the lower trachea above the carina. The otolaryngologist then uses the rigid bronchoscope to advance the foreign body into the right mainstem bronchus to permit one lung oxygenation and ventilation. After oxygen saturations improve, the foreign body is successfully extracted under controlled ventilation through the rigid bronchoscope. The remaining procedure is completed without complications, and the patient has an uneventful recovery.

References

1. Boyd, M. et al., Tracheobronchial foreign body aspiration in adults. South Med J, 2009. 102(2):171–4.

2. Tan, H.K. et al., Airway foreign bodies (FB): a 10-year review. Int J Pediatr Otorhinolaryngol, 2000. 56(2):91–9.

3. Rafanan, A.L. and A.C. Mehta, Adult airway foreign body removal. What's new? Clin Chest Med, 2001. 22(2):319–30.

4. Fidkowski, C.W. et al., The anesthetic considerations of tracheobronchial foreign bodies in children: a literature review of 12,979 cases. Anesth Analg, 2010. 111(4):1016–25.

5. Baharloo, F. et al., Tracheobronchial foreign bodies: presentation and management in children and adults. Chest, 1999. 115(5):1357–62.

6. Martinot, A. et al., Indications for flexible versus rigid bronchoscopy in children with

suspected foreign-body aspiration. *Am J Respir Crit Care Med*, 1997. **155**(5):1676–9.

7. Tang, L.F. *et al.*, Airway foreign body removal by flexible bronchoscopy: experience with 1,027 children during 2000–2008. *World J Pediatr*, 2009. **5**(3):191–5.

8. Baker, P.A. *et al.*, A prospective randomized trial comparing supraglottic airways for flexible bronchoscopy in children. *Paediatr Anaesth*, 2010. **20**(9):831–8.

9. Farrell, P.T., Rigid bronchoscopy for foreign body removal: anaesthesia and ventilation. *Paediatr Anaesth*, 2004. **14**(1):84–9.

10. Liu, Y. *et al.*, Controlled ventilation or spontaneous respiration in anesthesia for tracheobronchial foreign body removal: a meta-analysis. *Paediatr Anaesth*, 2014. **24**(10):1023–30.

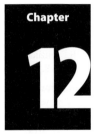

Management of anterior mediastinal mass

Basem Abdelmalak

Case presentation

A 29-year-old man has been having symptoms related to an upper respiratory infection (URI) for the last few days, and now presents to the emergency department (ED) with shortness of breath and respiratory distress that he has attributed to URI-induced exacerbation of his bronchial asthma. His history revealed complaints of fatigue, weight loss, dysphagia, cough, and shortness of breath exacerbated by lying flat. He also reported noting progressive swelling of the neck and face in the last couple of weeks before his presentation.

In the ED, after his initial assessment, the patient receives supplemental oxygen via facemask, as well as nebulized albuterol treatment, but shows minimal improvement. A chest X-ray reveals a large mediastinal mass, which is further confirmed with computed tomography (CT) imaging. The mass is compressing the trachea and compromising the lumen, leaving only 15% of its original diameter. The mass is large enough to compress the right atrium at the superior vena cava insertion site. Immediate management includes repositioning the patient into different positions: sitting, lateral, and even prone. The position that best improves breathing and ventilation for the patient is sitting up and leaning forward. Moreover, his supplemental oxygen is replaced with heliox, which improves oxygen saturation and reduces work of breathing. The patient is then admitted to the hospital and scheduled to have a transtracheal needle biopsy for tissue diagnosis and insertion of a silicone Y stent to support the trachea and relieve his tracheal compression symptoms prior to definitive treatment.

Introduction

The presence of an anterior mediastinal mass (AMM) constitutes a major airway management challenge. It has been described as one of the most concerning encounters in anesthesia practice.[1] Although it may sound like an extreme exaggeration, this description has some truth to it. AMM can predispose patients to severe respiratory or cardiovascular complications, and the risk becomes even more pronounced during sedation or anesthesia. These complications may include airway obstruction, compression of the cardiac chambers, and compression of the great vessels, especially the pulmonary artery.[2] Each of these complications, either alone or in combination, can cause death. Moreover, compression of the superior vena cava (SVC) along with the right atrium is not uncommon. Because this compression reduces venous return, it further compromises hemodynamic status. It also

Cases in Emergency Airway Management, ed. Lauren C. Berkow and John C. Sakles. Published by Cambridge University Press. © Cambridge University Press 2015.

causes facial plethora/swelling. The constellation of these signs and symptoms is often referred to as SVC syndrome. The SVC-syndrome-associated head and neck swelling may further complicate airway management because swelling/congestion of the mucosal lining of the oropharynx narrows the airway to such an extent that visualization of the vocal cords during laryngoscopy becomes very difficult. In addition, the airway becomes more prone to bleeding upon very minor trauma. Thus, the swelling converts what is essentially a lower airway challenge into both an upper and lower airway dilemma.

Airway management strategies

In the ED

It is important to note that not all mediastinal masses are the same. The physiologic and anatomic impact on the airway/cardiovascular system will depend on many factors. In fact some authors, for example Blank and de Souza,[3] have proposed a clinical risk assessment score for anticipating airway/hemodynamic complications of mediastinal masses:

- low risk: no to mild symptoms with no airway compression;
- moderate risk: mild to moderate postural symptoms and < 50% tracheal compression;
- high risk: severe symptoms and > 50% tracheal compression.

The airway management of low-risk and some moderate-risk patients (those without any other indication of anticipated airway management difficulty) can successfully proceed in the usual fashion if they require emergent and/or elective intubation. On the other hand, high-risk patients, including those with larger AMMs (causing > 50% reduction in airway diameter as seen on a CT scan, Figure 12.1), should be managed very cautiously. These patients are better managed in the operating room, where all needed specialists are available, and specialized equipment, such as a rigid bronchoscope, are set up and immediately ready for use. However, other initial management strategies can prove to be very helpful, such as changing the patient to a lateral, prone, or sitting-up-and-leaning-forward position. Such positioning can take advantage of gravity forces and may pull the mass away from the airway to relieve compression.

The airway stenosis caused by tumor compression and the added airway edema and bronchospasm caused by the AMM result in a turbulent airflow pattern and increased work of breathing. Heliox, a mixture of oxygen (30%) and helium (70%), decreases gas density and improves laminar flow through a stenosed airway.[4] Using interventions such as repositioning and heliox can relieve symptoms[5] and buy time until operating room personnel and clinicians have mobilized and constructed an airway management plan.

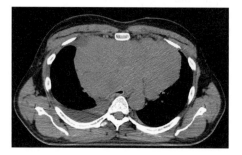

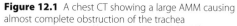
Figure 12.1 A chest CT showing a large AMM causing almost complete obstruction of the trachea

In the operating room

Many cautious anesthetic approaches have been described to minimize the physiologic impact these masses can have when a patient is under anesthesia. It has been highly recommended that practitioners preserve spontaneous ventilation during airway management of patients with AMM,[6] avoid use of muscle relaxants, and maintain negative intrapleural pressure.[7] Classic teaching states that when muscle tone is eliminated and/or negative intrathoracic pressure is lost owing to the use of positive-pressure ventilation, the AMM may collapse upon the trachea, causing severe tracheal stenosis/occlusion regardless of whether an endotracheal tube is present. Although the physiologic explanation for this scenario may not be easily understood, or accepted by many, such occurrences have been confirmed in the published literature (mainly as case reports owing to the difficulty in conducting a trial for this relatively infrequent and high-risk clinical presentation). The reader is referred to the thorough review by Blank and de Souza[3] for more details on this concept. A rigid bronchoscope (even when the surgical plan does not include it) and expertise in using it can be helpful to establish (stent) the airway if for any reason the mass occludes the airway.

Many techniques have been described for spontaneous ventilation anesthesia, starting with awake intubation performed while the patient is positioned in the least symptomatic position. Awake intubation can be accomplished with any available airway device; however, a flexible fiberoptic/videoscope is commonly used because it is versatile, causes minimal airway trauma, and is better tolerated than rigid devices. During awake intubation, patients can be sedated with various regimens such as small, titrated doses of fentanyl and/or midazolam; small, titrated doses of intravenous (IV) ketamine; and small doses of propofol infusion. Remifentanil infusion has also been used, but this drug has respiratory depressant effects and increases the risk of chest wall rigidity in the presence of an already compromised lower airway. Respiratory sparing agents such as dexmedetomidine have also been used successfully when administered as an infusion.[8] Dexmedetomidine is a selective α2 agonist with sedative, analgesic, amnestic,[9] and antisialagogue properties. It maintains spontaneous respiration with minimal respiratory depression. Patients sedated with dexmedetomidine are easy to arouse, which can be very helpful during awake fiberoptic-assisted intubation.[8] However, this advantage may not hold at higher doses (non-FDA approved usage). Alternatively, in select patients without SVC syndrome, a titrated inhalational anesthetic mask induction that maintains spontaneous ventilation may work just as well in experienced hands.

It has been suggested that cardiopulmonary bypass capabilities should be on stand-by with femoral vessel cannulation before induction is initiated in the management of high-risk AMM patients.[6,10] However, having bypass equipment on stand-by may not always ensure a favorable outcome.[7] Even if the cardiopulmonary bypass team is immediately available, achieving adequate oxygenation after complete airway obstruction may take 5–10 minutes,[11] during which the patient is at risk for hypoxic neurologic injury. Hence, it is important to use an anesthetic plan that lessens the chance of needing such a very invasive intervention.

Index case management

In the case described above, after the patient was initially stabilized in the ED by positioning in the least symptomatic position, bronchodilator therapy, and heliox administration, he was transferred to the operating room for airway management. The anesthesiologist, interventional pulmonologist, and thoracic surgeon discussed the proposed interventions, sequence of events, airway management, and primary and contingency management plans. The patient was premedicated with 1 mg of IV midazolam. Then he was sedated with dexmedetomidine IV infusion.[12] After topicalization of the patient's airway, the anesthesiologist performed an awake fiberoptic intubation using a size 5.0 mm ID microlaryngeal tube (MLT). The dexmedetomidine infusion was gradually increased toward anesthetic levels (up to seven times the maximum recommended dose for sedation, approximately 7.0 mcg/kg/h). Small amounts of sevoflurane 0.7% were also added to ensure amnesia. A rigid bronchoscope was inserted to the level of the vocal cords, the MLT was removed, and then positioning of the rigid bronchoscope was completed. A flexible bronchoscope was introduced through the rigid bronchoscope, and a transtracheal biopsy was obtained. The mass proved to be a lymphoma. The rigid bronchoscope was also used as a conduit for the Y-stent placement. Stenting of the airway with the silicone Y stent provides temporary relief for airway obstruction and alleviates symptoms until definitive treatment is contemplated and implemented.

Conclusion

AMM continues to be an airway management challenge. Patients with mild risk and some with moderate risk can be managed via routine airway management techniques. In high-risk patients (symptomatic, > 50% airway stenosis), airway managers should exercise extreme caution, create a management plan in advance, and communicate clearly with all involved clinicians. Placing the patient in the least symptomatic position and administering heliox have been found to be very helpful as initial measures. Maintaining spontaneous ventilation throughout airway management is still recommended for managing such challenging clinical scenarios.

References

1. Fabbro M, Patel PA, Ramakrishna H, et al. CASE 5–2014 challenging perioperative management of a massive anterior mediastinal mass in a symptomatic adult. J Cardiothorac Vasc Anesth. 2014;28(3):819–25.

2. Bittar D. Respiratory obstruction associated with induction of general anesthesia in a patient with mediastinal Hodgkin's disease. Anesth Analg. 1975;54(3):399–403.

3. Blank RS, de Souza DG. Anesthetic management of patients with an anterior mediastinal mass: continuing professional development. Can J Anaesth. 2011;58(9):853–9.

4. Doyle D. Use of heliox in managing stridor: an ENT perspective. In Abdelmalak BDD, editor, Anesthesia for Otolaryngologic Surgery, Cambridge: Cambridge University Press, 2013, pp. 101–4.

5. Galway U, Doyle DJ, Gildea T. Anesthesia for endoscopic palliative management of a patient with a large anterior mediastinal mass. J Clin Anesth. 2009;21(2):150–1.

6. Goh MH, Liu XY, Goh YS. Anterior mediastinal masses: an anaesthetic challenge. Anaesthesia. 1999;54(7):670–4.

7. Slinger P, Karsli C. Management of the patient with a large anterior mediastinal mass: recurring myths. Curr Opin Anaesthesiol. 2007;20(1):1–3.

8. Abdelmalak B, Makary L, Hoban J, Doyle DJ. Dexmedetomidine as sole sedative for awake intubation in management of the critical airway. J Clin Anesth. 2007;19(5):370–3.

9. Ebert TJ, Hall JE, Barney JA, Uhrich TD, Colinco MD. The effects of increasing plasma concentrations of dexmedetomidine in humans. Anesthesiology. 2000;93(2):382–94.

10. Azizkhan RG, Dudgeon DL, Buck JR, *et al.* Life-threatening airway obstruction as a complication to the management of mediastinal masses in children. *J Pediatr Surg.* 1985;**20**(6):816–22.

11. Tempe DK, Arya R, Dubey S, *et al.* Mediastinal mass resection: femorofemoral cardiopulmonary bypass before induction of anesthesia in the management of airway obstruction. *J Cardiothorac Vasc Anesth.* 2001;**15**(2):233–6.

12. Abdelmalak B, Marcanthony N, Abdelmalak J, *et al.* Dexmedetomidine for anesthetic management of anterior mediastinal mass. *J Anesth.* 2010;**24**(4):607–10.

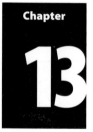

Chapter 13

The asthmatic crisis

Sal J. Suau and Peter M. C. DeBlieux

Case presentation

It is a busy day in the emergency department (ED) when emergency medical services bring a 42-year-old man with a history of asthma, who is complaining of shortness of breath and chest tightness. EMS reports that the patient is conscious, pale, and diaphoretic, with a heart rate (HR) of 115 beats per minute; a blood pressure (BP) of 101/60 mmHg; a respiratory rate (RR) of 29 breaths per minute; and pulse oxygen saturation (SpO_2) of 91% on room air. They treated the patient en route with albuterol–ipratropium bromide nebulizer, but it provided minimal improvement. The patient is speaking in two–three-word sentences and reports being "short of breath." His family reports that the patient has a history of asthma, hypertension, and diabetes; they also report a few days of generalized malaise, cough, and "not looking so well today prior to calling 911." The patient denies any allergies and affirms "running out" of all his medications about 1 week ago. He also confirms being intubated 4 years ago for shortness of breath.

Introduction

Asthma is an inflammatory disease of the airways that often requires emergent medical evaluation and treatment. It accounts for more than 2 million visits to EDs, and approximately 4,000 deaths annually in the United States.[1] It is characterized by increased bronchial hyper-responsiveness, increased vascular permeability, smooth muscle spasm, and the release of inflammatory mediators. This pathophysiology translates into recurrent episodes of wheezing, difficulty breathing, chest tightness, and coughing.[2] Asthma exacerbations are variable and can be triggered by a plethora of environmental agents, infectious precipitants, emotional or exercise states, and diverse exposure to ingested or inhaled agents.[3] Regardless of the inciting etiology, it is paramount that risk stratification and treatment modalities be initiated immediately and expeditiously to decrease clinical deterioration, morbidity, and mortality.

Risk stratification of the severely asthmatic patient requires several steps and can be a difficult feat when an undifferentiated asthmatic presents to your ED. First, the practitioner should take a detailed history and determine whether the patient has had previous endotracheal intubations (ETI), prior intensive care unit (ICU) admissions, ≥ 2 non-ICU hospitalizations in the past year, ≥ 3 ED visits in the past month, chronic use of oral corticosteroids, history of noncompliance, lives in poverty without access to adequate

Cases in Emergency Airway Management, ed. Lauren C. Berkow and John C. Sakles. Published by Cambridge University Press. © Cambridge University Press 2015.

Box 13.1 Important risk factors in the asthma patient

- Previous endotracheal intubations
- Previous ICU admissions
- ≥ 2 non-ICU hospitalizations in the past 1 year
- ≥ 3 ED visits in the past month
- Chronic use of oral corticosteroids
- Medication noncompliance
- Living in poverty with no access to healthcare
- Using ≥ 2 SABA pressurized metered dose inhalers monthly

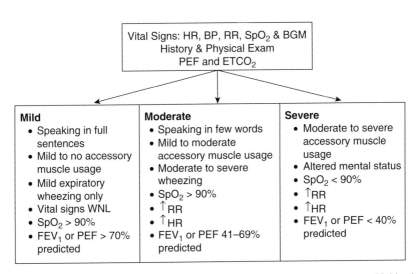

Figure 13.1 Asthma exacerbation severity stratification pathway. BGM, blood glucose monitor; BP, blood pressure; FEV_1, forced expiratory volume in 1 second; HR, heart rate; PEF, peak expiratory flow; RR, respiratory rate; WNL, within normal limits

healthcare, and uses ≥ 2 short-acting β2-agonist (SABA) pressurized metered dose inhalers monthly (Box 13.1).[4]

Second, asthma exacerbation severity can also be assessed with objective physical findings such as vital signs, including oxygen saturation, heart rate, and respiratory rate; degree of wheezing and air movement; use of accessory muscles; degree of difficulty with speech; peak expiratory flow (PEF); and/or end-tidal carbon dioxide ($ETCO_2$) monitoring.[4] These historical and physical findings can aid a physician during evaluation and information gathering. It is imperative to understand that the absence of severity markers does not exclude the presence of a life-threatening disease process. A helpful algorithm to aid in differentiating between mild, moderate, and severe exacerbation is found in Figure 13.1.

The final step during primary assessment of the asthmatic patient is the essential consideration that wheezing and respiratory distress can also be found in multiple other disease entities. An adequate differential diagnosis must be formulated to prevent the creation of an anchoring bias, a predetermined diagnosis which would prevent a clinician

Box 13.2 Differential diagnosis of wheezing

Adults	Children
• Upper respiratory tract infection	• Upper respiratory tract infection
• Pneumonia	• Croup
• Chronic obstructive pulmonary disease	• Tracheomalacia
• Congestive heart failure (CHF)	• Bronchiolitis
• Chronic bronchitis	• Pneumonia
• Gastroesophageal reflux disease	• Foreign body
• Acute coronary syndrome (ACS)	
• Pulmonary embolism	
• Foreign body	
• Pneumothorax	
• Cystic fibrosis	
• Vocal cord dysfunction	

from maintaining a broad differential diagnosis. Box 13.2 illustrates a differential diagnosis of wheezing in adults and children.

After the initial assessment is complete, therapeutic interventions must be initiated promptly. The current cornerstone in the treatment of all asthma exacerbations begins by administering SABA combined with ipratropium bromide via a pressurized metered dose inhaler with a holding chamber or an oxygen-driven nebulizer; oral or parenteral steroids; and intravenous (IV) or nebulized magnesium sulfate. Upon completion of these initial interventions, any additional treatment is based on the patient's clinical status. Figure 13.2 illustrates a suggested treatment algorithm for patients with severe asthma.

Airway management scenario and discussion #1

The patient has been given multiple rounds of nebulized SABA and ipratropium bromide combinations. He has also been given IV methylprednisolone, IV magnesium sulfate, 20 mL/kg of IV fluids, and 5 L of oxygen by nasal cannula. His condition continues to deteriorate. He then receives 0.5 mL of 1:1,000 L-epinephrine intramuscularly. Despite these aggressive treatments, his vital signs reveal a HR of 121 beats per minute, RR of 33 breaths per minute, BP of 115/71 mmHg, and SpO$_2$ of 88%. It is evident that this patient has a severe exacerbation that is refractory to first-line therapy. He demonstrates accessory muscle utilization, a paradoxical pulse greater than 25 mmHg, persistent tachycardia, tachypnea > 30 breaths per minute, limited speech, and hypoxia. If it were attained, his peak expiratory flow rate or forced expiratory volume in 1 second (FEV$_1$) would be < 50% predicted volume.

Airway management of decompensating asthmatic patients who are not responding to first-line therapy warrants early recognition and appropriate modification to prevent mortality. Evidence translated from patients who have chronic obstructive pulmonary disease and are in acute respiratory failure has suggested that noninvasive positive-pressure ventilation (NPPV) is an effective treatment alternative.[6] This treatment modality is best provided via full facial mask. It is postulated that NPPV is a direct bronchodilator.[7] NPPV

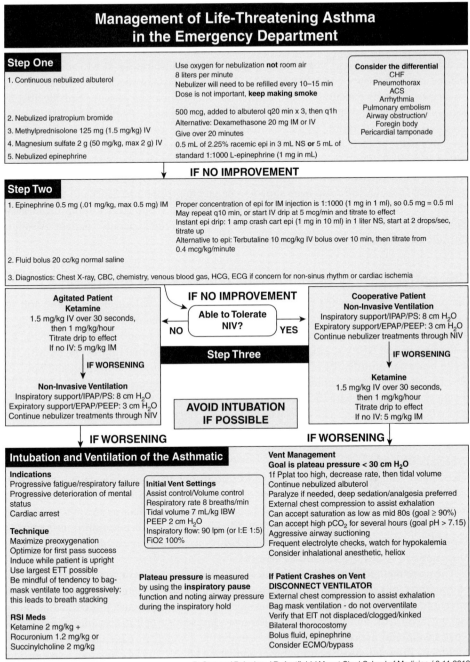

Figure 13.2 Management algorithm in severe to life-threatening asthma (with authorization from the authors with accreditation to emupdates.com)[5] IBW, ideal body weight; CBC, complete blood count; HCG, human chorionic gonadotropin; ECG, electrocardiogram

also recruits alveoli secondary to external positive end-expiratory pressure (PEEP) offsetting intrinsic PEEP.[8] Alveolar recruitment improves ventilation–perfusion mismatch by preventing airway closure and reducing the work of breathing.[9] NPPV can be used for short periods of time as deemed clinically necessary and carries a lower risk of nosocomial pneumonia than ETI does.[10] Figure 13.2 suggests starting inspiratory (IPAP) and expiratory positive airway pressure (EPAP) at 8 cm H_2O and 3 cm H_2O, respectively. The authors of this chapter strongly encourage that the practitioner remain at the patient's bedside directly monitoring the work of breathing and serially increasing both IPAP and EPAP to higher pressures within a 30 minute trial to optimize the patient's comfort and work of breathing. A recent Cochrane review indicated that patients with acute asthma exacerbation who were treated with NPPV had decreased hospital admission rates, decreased length of ICU stay, and an overall reduced hospital stay,[11] although there was no clear benefit for reduced ETI or mortality. Lastly, NPPV has been shown to be safe in pregnant patients and the pediatric population.[6] Relative contraindications include facial or esophageal trauma or surgery, deformities of the upper airway, copious secretions, or an uncooperative patient. Absolute contraindications are cardiac or respiratory arrest.[12]

Alternative airway management scenario and discussion #2

The patient initially benefits from NPPV with continuous nebulizer treatment, but he continues to tire and becomes agitated. He is administered a bolus of 0.5 up to 1.5 mg/kg of IV ketamine over 30 to 60 seconds, followed by an infusion of 1 mg/kg/h while receiving his IV fluid bolus and NPPV treatment. His vital signs show a minimal improvement, with HR of 125 beats per minute, RR of 31 breaths per minute, BP of 121/78 mmHg, and SpO_2 of 89%. Despite these improvements, his mentation begins to deteriorate.

The decision to intubate should not be taken lightly, as manipulation of the airway in an asthmatic patient can cause laryngospasm, worsen bronchospasm, and increase morbidity. It is estimated that the mortality rate of ICU patients who are intubated for severe asthma is 10–20%.[13] Some studies have advocated that the severe asthmatic patient can be adequately managed without resorting to intubation.[14,15] Despite attempting to refrain from intubating a decompensating asthmatic, once first- and second-line therapies have failed, the practitioner must seriously consider ETI. The clinical decision regarding when to intubate a decompensating asthmatic patient can be aided by clinical signs such as an $SpO_2 < 90\%$ with maximal supplemental oxygen, bradypnea leading to hypercapnia and respiratory acidosis, altered level of consciousness, or physical exhaustion.[16] The only absolute indications for intubation are respiratory or cardiac arrest.[17]

The usual method for intubating a patient in asthmatic crisis is maximal preoxygenation followed by rapid sequence intubation. Ketamine and propofol are both valid options for induction agents. Ketamine creates a catecholamine release that causes bronchodilation by relaxing bronchial smooth muscles.[18] Because this release of catecholamines can cause hypertension and arrhythmias, ketamine should be avoided in patients with active dysrhythmias. Propofol also has some bronchodilating effects, but it can cause hypotension; therefore, patient selection for this drug also should be considered carefully.

Succinylcholine and rocuronium are the two main choices of muscle relaxant for rapid sequence intubation in the ED. It is essential that their respective benefits and possible side effects be understood before selecting an agent. Traditionally, rocuronium has been considered to have a slower time of onset than succinylcholine. However, onset is slower

Table 13.1 Side effects of succinylcholine

Side effect	Remarks
Bradycardia	Occurs especially in small children after repeat doses
Hyperkalemia	May increase potassium ~ 0.4 mmol/L in normal patients, but may lead to life-threatening elevations in amyotrophic lateral sclerosis, multiple sclerosis, muscular dystrophies, inherited myopathies, denervating injuries, burns, and crush injuries
Fasciculations	Increase: • oxygen consumption that may cause myalgia • intragastric pressure, likely by increasing lower esophageal sphincter tone • intracranial pressure • intraocular pressure
Malignant hyperthermia	Rare

only if rocuronium is used at lower doses of 0.6 to 0.9 mg/kg IV. If a dose of 1.2 mg/kg IV is used, no difference exists in the time of onset of "ideal intubating conditions," although the higher dose will lengthen the duration of paralysis.[19] The duration of paralysis with rocuronium is also dose-dependent; time to paralysis recovery is reported to occur as early as 30 minutes with a dose of 0.6 mg/kg IV, but it will be double or even triple after a 1.2 mg/kg dose.[19] Table 13.1 provides the common side effects encountered with succinylcholine. The most troubling, but rare, side effect of rocuronium is anaphylaxis. Regardless of the agent used for paralysis, understanding respective mechanisms of action and side effects is essential.

Initial ventilator settings should be optimized to prevent hyperinflation and auto-PEEP in asthmatic patients. Hyperinflation pathophysiology could result in hypotension and barotrauma.[20] This goal is achieved by reducing both respiratory rate and tidal volume. These maneuvers shorten the inspiratory time and lengthen the time for exhalation, resulting in permissive hypercapnia. Permitting hypercapnia in this patient population is safer than causing hyperinflation while attempting to reach a normal partial pressure of CO_2 (PCO_2).[13] While intubated, the patient will require inhalational therapy to reverse the reactive airway disease process. Metered dose inhalers can be used instead of nebulizers, as they may decrease nosocomial pneumonia rates.[17] Deep sedation should be used in an attempt to minimize neuromuscular blockade. Prolonged paralysis has been associated with increases in pneumonia rates and ICU length of stay.[21]

As a final note, practitioners should be diligent in documenting the intubation procedure. A detailed medical record will greatly aid the clinician who attempts extubation when the pathophysiologic state has been reversed. The practitioner should document the Cormack–Lehane score, the laryngoscope blade used, any airway adjuvants utilized, the number of intubation attempts made, a description of any complications, and any confirmation modalities used in the airway management.

Alternative adjuvants: devices and resources

Ketamine is a potent dissociative analgesic that can be used as a rescue agent in patients who have severe asthma and are refractory to first-line treatment options. It is characterized by an onset of action within 60 seconds, peak tissue distribution within 7–11 minutes, and hepatic excretion half-life of 2–3 hours.[22] Ketamine holds several properties that can aid the severely asthmatic patient. First, it has been postulated to block the activation of NMDA (N-methyl-D-aspartic acid) receptors in the lung parenchyma, which are responsible for stimulating the unwanted pulmonary edema and bronchoconstriction found during severe asthmatic crisis.[23] Second, in the lung, ketamine has been found to downregulate production of nitric oxide that is responsible for bronchospasm.[24] Third, ketamine has been found to block the recruitment of macrophages, interfere with cytokine production, and decrease interleukin-4 concentrations. These mechanisms are responsible for unwanted inflammatory changes, airway hyper-reactivity, and bronchoconstriction in the acutely severe asthmatic patient.[25] All of these properties, along with the previously discussed upregulation of catecholamine levels and the anticholinergic effects on bronchial smooth muscle, argue strongly for ketamine as an advantageous adjuvant agent in the management of the decompensating asthmatic patient. Lastly, it is important to emphasize that ketamine, like all analgesic, amnestic, anesthetic, and muscle relaxants, should be administered in a monitored environment where SpO_2, $ETCO_2$, BP, HR, and appropriate nursing staffing is continuously available.

Heliox is a compound mixture of 80% helium and 20% oxygen. It can also be considered as an adjuvant in the early management of asthma before oxygen saturation requirements become the deciding parameter. Helium is a chemically inert, odorless, tasteless, noncombustible gas that has a lower molecular density than oxygen and air.[26] This lower density can serve as a better transport modality than traditional room air or 100% oxygen-driven nebulizers for the penetration of bronchodilating, anticholinergic, and anti-inflammatory agents. It has been shown that heliox-driven bronchodilation brings about more rapid and greater improvement in FEV_1, FVC (forced vital capacity), and FEFmax (maximal expiratory flow rate) than the traditional nebulizer methods.[27] Therefore, in asthmatic patients with an $FEV_1 \leq 50\%$, heliox-driven nebulization treatments lead to better spirometry measurements than do air-driven nebulization treatments.[26] Currently, evidence is insufficient to support routine delivery of heliox via NPPV or in intubated asthmatic patients.

Inhaled anesthetics such as sevoflurane can also be used as adjuvant agents in the post-intubation period. It is a potent bronchodilator and can decrease airway responsiveness. Logistically, sevoflurane may be a difficult treatment modality because it requires an anesthesia circuit and appropriate monitoring. It may also cause myocardial depression and therefore must be used with caution in patients who are hypotensive or unstable.

The last resort in a clinically decompensating asthmatic patient would be the initiation of extracorporeal membrane oxygenation (ECMO). This technology is considered in those patients who cannot be maintained on mechanical ventilation with adequate oxygenation. ECMO requires a dedicated support staff and equipment.

Post-management care and follow-up

Weaning and extubation criteria have not been adequately studied in the acutely asthmatic patient.[13] Asthma exacerbations that require ETI typically are slow to resolve and require aggressive therapy for more than 24 hours before weaning and extubation can be considered. Before assessing the patient for possible extubation, the practitioner must confirm that the asthmatic pathophysiologic state that warranted intubation has resolved. First, all sedation and muscle relaxants must be discontinued and prophylactic antiemetic treatment provided. The head of the bed should be raised to > 45 degrees. Adequate time must be allowed for the patient to be able to follow simple commands such as opening his eyes, tracking with his eyes, grasping with both hands, and protruding the tongue on command with no evidence of bronchospasm or hemodynamic decompensation. Once appropriate time has elapsed, the cuff leak test should be performed. This test is used to evaluate for any laryngeal edema that might have occurred during the ETI and throughout the treatment.[28] When no mucosal swelling is evident, the third step is the assessment of oxygenation and ventilation. Adequate oxygenation and ventilation can be assessed with a spontaneous breathing trial on reduced pressure support of 5 cm H_2O. If the patient is able to maintain the following parameters with no bronchospasm, an attempt at extubation can be considered:[29]

- SpO_2 > 92% (PaO_2 > 70) on fraction of inspired oxygen (FiO_2) less than 40% and PEEP is less than 5 cm H_2O;
- tidal volume > 5 mL/kg;
- mean arterial pressure (MAP) > 60 mmHg with no aid of vasopressor agents;
- RR < 30 and > 6 breaths per minute;
- HR < 100 and > 60 beats per minute.

If the patient remains stable with no evidence of bronchospasm for approximately 30 minutes, one can move forward with the negative inspiratory force test. A value greater than −30 cm H_2O (normal, −90 to −120 cm H_2O) indicates that the strength of the diaphragm and other inspiratory muscles is adequate to attempt extubation. A final assessment modality to predict a successful extubation is the rapid shallow breathing index. This index relies on the idea that patients on a ventilator who cannot tolerate independent breathing tend to breathe with high frequency and shallow tidal volumes. Therefore, a score of less than ~100 is considered by most an adequate indication of weaning readiness.[30] Upon successful completion of all these steps, extubation may be undertaken. Safe extubation of a patient requires equipment such as suction, oral airway, supplemental oxygen, and equipment that may be needed if reintubation is required. A non-rebreathing mask and NPPV should be at the bedside because extubation may elicit laryngeal edema, bronchospasm, and post-extubation stridor that require nebulized epinephrine and further treatment. In short, extubation should always be approached in a logical and cautious manner. Every step should be meticulously anticipated and cautiously executed in order to prevent re-exacerbation or other complications.

The final component of post-asthmatic crisis care is a detailed asthma care plan, which includes explicit discharge instructions, necessary medications and education on how to use them, education in self-assessment, a future action plan for managing recurrence of airflow obstruction, and an explicit follow-up appointment. Asthma care plans have been associated with improved outcomes and medication compliance.[31] It is recommended that patients follow up with an asthma-specialized clinician within 1 week of discharge. These final moments before the patient returns home after an asthmatic crisis are the ideal opportunity for clinicians to provide appropriate care plans that will assist patients with future exacerbations, encourage partnership with primary care physicians, and promote ongoing discussions of home asthma care.

References

1. Moorman JE, Rudd RA, Johnson CA. National surveillance for asthma – United States, 1980–2004. *MMWR Surveill Summ* 2007;**56**:1–54.

2. Sellers WFS. Inhaled and intravenous treatment in acute severe and life-threatening asthma. *Br J Anaesth* 2013;**110**(2):183–90.

3. Murata A, Ling PM. Asthma diagnosis and management. *Emerg Med Clin North Am* 2012;**30**:203–22.

4. National Asthma Education and Prevention Program. Expert panel report III: guidelines for the diagnosis and management of asthma. Bethesda (MD): National Heart, Lung, and Blood Institute; 2007 (NIH publication no. 08–4051).

5. When the patient can't breathe, and you can't think: the emergency department life-threatening asthma flowsheet. *Emergency Medicine Updates* 2011, Dec 14. See http://emupdates.com/192011/12/14/when-the-patient-cant-breathe-and-you-cant-think-the-emergency-departement-life-threatening-asthma-flowsheet/.

6. Carson KV, Usmani ZA, Smith BJ. Noninvasive ventilation in acute severe asthma: current evidence and future perspectives. *Curr Opin Pulm Med* 2014;**20**:118–23.

7. Buda AJ, Pinsky MR, Ingels NB Jr, *et al.* Effect of intrathoracic pressure on left ventricular performance. *N Engl J Med* 1979;**301**:453–9.

8. Broux R, Foidart G, Mendes P, *et al.* Use of PEEP in management of life-threatening status asthmaticus: a method for the recovery of appropriate ventilation–perfusion ratio. *Appl Cardiopulm Pathophysiol* 1991;**4**:79–83.

9. Soroksky S, Stav D, Shpirer I. A pilot prospective, randomized, placebo-controlled trial of bilevel positive airway pressure in acute asthmatic attack. *Chest* 2003;**123**:1018–25.

10. Nourdine K, Combes P, Carton MJ, *et al.* Does noninvasive ventilation reduce the ICU nosocomial infection risk? A prospective clinical survey. *Intens Care Med* 1999;**25**:567–73.

11. Lim WJ, Mohammed Akram R, Carson KV, *et al.* Noninvasive positive pressure ventilation for treatment of respiratory failure due to severe acute exacerbations of asthma. *Cochrane Database Syst Rev* 2012;**12**:CD004360.

12. Yeow ME, Santanilla JI. Noninvasive positive pressure ventilation in the emergency department. *Emerg Med Clin North Am* 2008;**26**:835–47.

13. Brenner B, Corbridge T, Kazzi A. Intubation and mechanical ventilation of the patient in respiratory failure. *J Emerg Med* 2009;**37**(2S):S23–S34.

14. Braman SS, Kaemmerlen JT. Intensive care of status asthmaticus. A 10-year experience. *JAMA* 1990;**264**:366–8.

15. Mountain RD, Sahn SA. Acid–base disturbances in acute asthma. *Chest* 1990;**98**:651–5.

16. Murase K, Tomii K, Chin K, *et al.* The use of non-invasive ventilation for life-threatening asthma attacks: changes in the need for intubation. *Respirology* 2010;**15**:714–20.

17. Schauer SG, Cuenca PJ, Johnson JJ, Ramirez S. Management of acute asthma in the emergency department. *Emerg Med Pract* 2013;**15**(6):1–28.

18. Brown RH, Wagner EM. Mechanisms of bronchoprotection by anesthetic induction agents: propofol versus ketamine. *Anesthesiology* 1999;**90**:822–8.

19. Perry JJ, Lee JS, Sillberg VA, *et al.* Rocuronium versus succinylcholine for rapid sequence induction intubation. *Cochrane Database Syst Rev* 2008;(2): CD002788.

20. Lougheed MD, Fisher T, O'Donnell DE. Dynamic hyperinflation during bronchoconstriction in asthma: implications for symptom perception. *Chest* 2006;**130**:1072–81.

21. Adnet F, Racine SX, Lapostolle F, *et al.* Full reversal of hypercapnic coma by noninvasive positive pressure ventilation. *Am J Emerg Med* 2001;**19**:244–6.

22. Stevenson C. Ketamine: a review. *Update Anaesth* 2005;**20**:25–9.

23. Sato T, Hirota K, Matsuki A, Zsigmond EK, Rabito SF. The role of the N-methyl-D-aspartic acid receptor in the relaxant effect of ketamine on tracheal smooth muscle. *Anesth Analg* 1998;**87**:1383–8.

24. Zhu MM, Qian YN, Zhu W, *et al.* Protective effects of ketamine on allergen-induced airway inflammatory injury and high airway reactivity in asthma: experiment with rats. *Zhonghua Yi Xue Za Zhi* 2007;**87**:1308–13.

25. Goyal S, Agrawal A. Ketamine in status asthmaticus: a review. *Indian J Crit Care Med* 2013;**17**(3):154–61.

26. El-Khatib MF, Jamaleddine G. Effect of heliox- and air-driven nebulized bronchodilator therapy on lung function in patients with asthma. *Lung* 2014;**192**:377–83.

27. Bag R, Bandi V, Fromm RE Jr, Guntupalli K. The effect of heliox-driven bronchodilator aerosol therapy on pulmonary function tests in patients with asthma. *J Asthma* 2002;**39**(7):659–65.

28. Zhou T, Zhang HP, Chen WW, *et al.* Cuff-leak test for predicting postextubation airway complications: a systematic review. *J Evid Based Med* 2011;**4**(4):242–54.

29. Salam A, Tilluckdharry L, Amoateng-Adjepong Y, Manthous CA. Neurologic status, cough, secretions and extubation outcomes. *Intens Care Med* 2004;**30**:1334–9.

30. Meade M, Guyatt G, Cook D, *et al.* Predicting success in weaning from mechanical ventilation. *Chest* 2001;**120**(6 Suppl):400–24S.

31. McCarty K, Rogers J. Inpatient Asthma Education Program. *Pediatr Nursing* 2012;**38**(5):257–263.

Airway management
of the pregnant patient

Mohammed A. Abdel-Rahim, Lori Ann Suffredini,
and Jean-Pierre P. Ouanes

Case presentation

A 32-year-old female (height 155 cm, weight 120 kg) with severe pre-eclampsia at 35 weeks' gestation presents for an emergent cesarean delivery because of severe, unrelenting fetal bradycardia. An epidural catheter was placed prior to her rapid decrease in platelet count from 120,000/mm^3 to 50,000/mm^3 over the course of 6 hours. Airway examination reveals a Mallampati Class 3, mouth opening > 3 cm, thyromental distance > 5 cm, and a short thick neck. On transport to the operating room she is administered 30 mL of sodium citrate. Upon transfer to the operating room table, the epidural catheter is noted to be completely out of the patient's back. The anesthesiologist calls for a neonatal team, difficult airway cart, and medical personnel skilled at surgical airway procedures. Fetal intrauterine resuscitation attempts fail to resolve the fetal bradycardia. The patient is instructed to take three large vital capacity volume breaths of 100% oxygen before rapid sequence intubation with cricoid pressure. The first attempt at direct laryngoscopy with a Macintosh three laryngoscope blade yields a grade 3 Cormack–Lehane view and a failed endotracheal intubation. A second attempt by an attending anesthesiologist with the same laryngoscope blade and a gum-elastic bougie also fails. By this time, saturation is declining rapidly (the lowest SpO$_2$ is 85%); however, two-person bag-mask ventilation with an oral airway provides successful ventilation, and the oxygen saturation returns to 100%. A third attempt with video laryngoscopy results in successful endotracheal intubation. A nuchal cord times three is noted on delivery of a 1,600 g female with APGAR scores of three at 1 minute, five at 5 minutes, and nine at 10 minutes. At the conclusion of the surgery, the mother is hemodynamically stable and successfully extubated without any further events.

Introduction

Despite advances in airway equipment, airway-related events remain one of the top 10 causes of maternal deaths. Between 3% and 12% of all maternal deaths are due to anesthesia, with failed intubation and aspiration being the leading causes. The incidence of failed intubation in the obstetric population has been reported as 1:300–1:250 and is approximately 10 times more than that in the general surgical population (1:3,000–1:2,000). The main risk factors are emergency procedures, obesity, and hypertensive disorders of pregnancy, all of which were present in the case described above.[1–3]

Cases in Emergency Airway Management, ed. Lauren C. Berkow and John C. Sakles. Published by Cambridge University Press. © Cambridge University Press 2015.

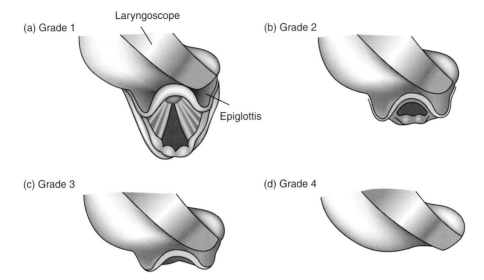

Figure 14.1 Cormack–Lehane classification: (a) grade 1 view, (b) grade 2 view, (c) grade 3 view, (d) grade 4 view

In 1984, Cormack and Lehane classified the causes of difficult intubation into four grades based on laryngoscopy view (Figure 14.1).[4] Their frequency analysis of failed intubations in obstetrics revealed that the grade 3 view was the most common one encountered during failed intubations. They concluded that the grade 3 view is fairly rare but unpredictable because assessing the size and mobility of the tongue is difficult. Additionally, obstetric anesthesiologists are not prepared for such cases because use of general anesthesia in obstetrics is limited. Consequently, Cormack and Lehane recommend drills and simulations in routine anesthesia.[4] Below, we review the airway changes that occur in pregnancy and discuss airway assessment and management.

Airway changes in pregnancy

Throughout pregnancy, a woman's body undergoes multiple anatomic and physiologic changes, some of which directly affect airway management during general anesthesia. For example, increases in progesterone levels throughout the course of pregnancy result in generalized edema and increased total body water. In addition, capillary engorgement of airway mucosa causes airway edema, increased tissue friability, nasal hyperemia, and increased secretions.[5] Thus, to facilitate intubation and prevent trauma, practitioners should use smaller endotracheal tubes and make fewer intubation attempts.

When the parturient is supine, enlarged breasts may interfere with insertion of the laryngoscope. Short laryngoscope handles can be an advantage in this situation. Placing the patient in the left uterine tilt position to avoid vena cava compression syndrome is necessary but may increase the difficulty of intubation. Maternal, fetal, and placental metabolic requirements result in a 60% increase in oxygen consumption during pregnancy.[6] Functional residual capacity is reduced by 0.6 L, or 20%, by term gestation, secondary to the gravid uterus and elevation of the diaphragm.[7] The net result is that PaO$_2$ (the partial pressure of oxygen in arterial blood) can decrease rapidly, at twice the rate of nonpregnant women.[8] Preoxygenation of pregnant patients with 100% oxygen prior to induction is mandatory and will allow approximately 3 minutes of apnea before hypoxemia ensues, comparable to that of an obese adult.[8]

Airway assessment

Due to the nature of obstetric anesthesiology, patients are often managed in an urgent or emergent setting; thus, the airway cannot always be assessed before the patient needs airway manipulation. However, practitioners should take the time to examine the obstetric patient's airway whenever possible to try to predict whether an airway might be challenging with regard to mask ventilation or intubation. By conducting this examination, the practitioner might prevent a potential airway disaster by anticipating difficulty, having additional help or equipment available, or avoiding airway manipulation altogether.[9]

Airway assessment of the parturient should begin with an assessment of the patient's body habitus. Obesity, as defined by a body mass index $> 30 \, kg/m^2$, is associated with an increased risk of difficult mask ventilation and difficult intubation.[10]

The airway manager should perform several assessments of the patient's airway. The Mallampati class should be noted; a class ≥ 3 is associated with difficulty in securing the endotracheal tube. It is imperative to perform frequent airway assessments, as the Mallampati class might worsen significantly during the course of labor itself[11] and is even more pronounced in patients with pre-eclampsia.

Thyromental distance should also be measured. A length $\geq$ three fingerbreadths is desirable because it indicates ease of alignment of the oral, pharyngeal, and laryngeal axes. The degree of mouth opening should be at least three fingerbreadths as well to accommodate the laryngoscope and allow for reasonable alignment of the three axes. Length of the incisors and inter-incisor distance should also be observed; qualitatively long incisors lead to a sharper angle between the oral and pharyngeal axes, and an inter-incisor distance $< 3 \, cm$ indicates that one might encounter difficulty in inserting the Macintosh blade. The patient should be asked to protrude the mandibular teeth anterior to the maxillary teeth; the ability to do this correlates with ease of obtaining a good view with laryngoscopy. The length, thickness, and range of motion of the neck should also be assessed. A short, thick neck reduces the ability to align the airway axes. Decreased ability to flex or extend the neck decreases the chance that the patient will be able to attain "sniffing position," which eases intubation by allowing for proper alignment of the oral, pharyngeal, and laryngeal axes. The presence or absence of teeth should be noted; patients who are edentulous are more difficult to bag-mask ventilate, although the absence of teeth can make intubation somewhat easier.[8]

No single assessment of the airway has been shown to predict difficulty in securing the airway; however, when several assessments are taken together, the sensitivity and specificity of predicting a difficult airway are improved. Multiple studies have shown various sensitivities and specificities in predicting a difficult airway when different airway assessments are combined.[8] The important point to take from these analyses is that performing one aspect of the airway examination will not identify whether an airway will be difficult to secure; one must take into account as many pieces of information as can be obtained. The more indicators of difficult intubation that are present, the greater one's index of suspicion should be. One should then prepare by bringing in extra help, obtaining specialized airway equipment, or planning to avoid airway manipulation altogether.

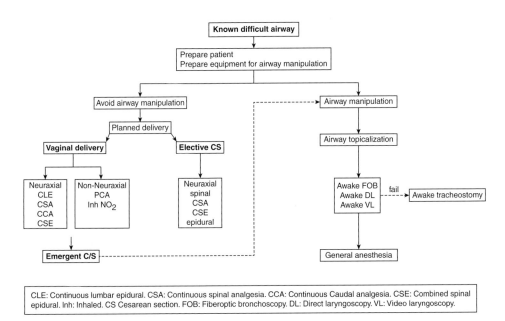

CLE: Continuous lumbar epidural. CSA: Continuous spinal analgesia. CCA: Continuous Caudal analgesia. CSE: Combined spinal epidural. Inh: Inhaled. CS Cesarean section. FOB: Fiberoptic bronchoscopy. DL: Direct laryngoscopy. VL: Video laryngoscopy.

Figure 14.2 Algorithm for known difficult airway in an obstetric patient

Management of the anticipated difficult airway

The parturient with an anticipated difficult airway, such as the one presented in this case, requires careful planning and preparation, with appropriate airway equipment and a backup plan to definitively secure the airway. The clinician should consider the likely course of delivery and suggest a management strategy that best suits the clinical situation and patient comorbidities and complements the provider's skill set. The algorithm shown in Figure 14.2 illustrates a strategy for managing a parturient with a known difficult airway.

Algorithm details

Proposed mode of delivery: vaginal

When the proposed delivery plan is spontaneous vaginal delivery, the anesthesiologist may consider an early continuous lumbar epidural (CLE), combined spinal epidural (CSE), or continuous spinal catheter to provide labor analgesia. These techniques have the added benefit of being usable as the primary surgical anesthetic if an emergency cesarean section becomes necessary. All plans that include avoidance of airway manipulation must be coupled with a backup plan to definitively secure the airway. Advanced airway equipment should be prepared in the operating room in case the epidural fails to provide adequate anesthesia during surgery. Some partially functional epidurals can be supplemented with opioids, ketamine, or infiltration of the surgical field with local anesthesia. These adjuncts may be enough to compensate for a less-than-optimal neuraxial block or, by improving patient comfort, provide time for the practitioner to secure the backup airway plan before inducing general anesthesia.

Proposed mode of delivery: cesarean section

In the case of a planned cesarean section, the options are to place a neuraxial block with spinal anesthesia, CSE, or CLE and avoid airway instrumentation. Alternatively, the airway can be secured before the start of the cesarean section. Securing the airway in an awake patient allows for maintenance of maternal pharyngeal tone and spontaneous ventilations.

A key to successful awake airway instrumentation is patient preparation and topical anesthesia of the upper airway. Benumof described this process in detail in his article on management of the difficult adult airway.[12] Preparation includes asking the patient for cooperation, standard monitoring of the patient, and using topical anesthesia as the primary anesthetic. In addition to applying the topical anesthesia to the mucosa, two nerve blocks may be helpful. Benumof argued that the nerve blocks are necessary to eliminate the gag reflex and hemodynamic response to laryngoscopy, but others have suggested that meticulous topical anesthesia provides adequate intubation conditions. Regional and topical anesthesia of the airway for awake intubation are described in detail elsewhere in this book.

Once the airway has adequate topical anesthesia, it can be secured by advancing the endotracheal tube over a fiberoptic bronchoscope and delivering it into the proper tracheal position. A number of reports describe successful intubation in a difficult airway with topicalization and use of video laryngoscopes.[13] As a backup plan, skilled surgeons can perform tracheostomies in awake patients under local anesthesia.

Management of the unanticipated failed intubation

For more than two decades, anesthesiologists and other airway managers have expressed the need for guidelines and training specific to managing the obstetric airway. As such, a new algorithm (Figure 14.3) was developed specifically to address six scenarios unique to general anesthesia in obstetrics.[14] The algorithm and scenarios are simulated and discussed in detail by Balki et al.[14] These scenarios are "can and cannot ventilate" in three situations specific to obstetrics anesthesia: maternal emergency, fetal emergency, and elective cesarean section.

Algorithm details

Light pressure should be applied to the cricoid cartilage when the patient is awake to prevent coughing, retching, and esophageal rupture. After the patient loses consciousness, a clinical provider applies firm downward force (enough pressure to compress 20 mL of an air-filled syringe to 10 mL) and maintains pressure until endotracheal tube placement is confirmed and the cuff is inflated. Cricoid pressure along with strict adherence to American Society of Anesthesiologists (ASA) NPO (nil per os) guidelines and preoperative administration of antacids is the standard of care in any case with a high risk of aspiration. However, the value of cricoid pressure is questionable, as the application of downward force on the cricoid cartilage has been found to push the esophagus out of midline instead of compressing it.[15] Avoidance of general anesthesia remains the best way to prevent aspiration and has been the main contributor to a decrease in aspiration-related mortality.

The Canadian Airway Focus Group recommends making only two intubation attempts.[16] Other algorithms differ on this point. In an article on failed intubations developed from 17 years of experience at a British teaching maternity unit, Hawthorne et al. allow for a third and fourth attempt *only* if the cords are visible with a Cormack–Lehane grade 3 or better.[3]

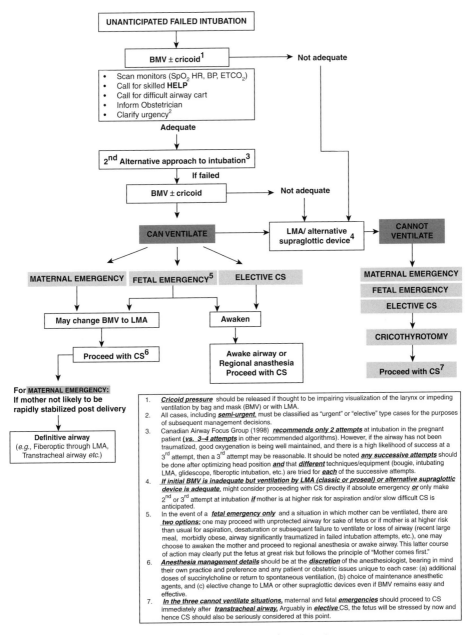

Figure 14.3 Algorithm for unanticipated failed intubation in an obstetric patient

The laryngeal mask airway (LMA) is the rescue device of choice when a patient cannot be intubated and cannot be ventilated. Cricoid pressure should be released if it is impairing the placement of an LMA. The LMA can become wedged in the hypopharynx if cricoid pressure prevents further advancement to its correct position, with the tip at the C5 level fully occupying the hypopharynx, seated behind the arytenoids and cricoid cartilage.[17]

It is crucial that the airway manager communicates and verifies the *urgency* of the case with the surgeon whenever any airway issue is recognized and to differentiate between true emergencies and patients who can tolerate waiting for alternative approaches to general anesthesia. The scenario at the beginning of this chapter described a true fetal emergency that left no time for alternative approaches. However, some argue that if the maternal aspiration risk is unacceptably high, the anesthesiologist should avoid putting the mother at risk and follow the rule "mother comes first." This approach would place the fetus at grave risk while the anesthesiologist/airway manager secures an airway via an awake fiberoptic intubation or achieves anesthesia via the neuraxial route. The decision is an ethical issue that is larger than the scope of this chapter.[14] An alternative technique would be to perform the cesarean section under local anesthetic and intravenous ketamine, as mentioned earlier.

This chapter described a clinical scenario specific to anesthesiology and the operating room. However, many of the principles of emergency airway management in the parturient can be applied in other clinical settings.

References

1. B. K. Ross. ASA closed claims in obstetrics: lessons learned. *Anesthesiol Clin North Am* 2003;**21**:183–97.

2. G. Lyons. Failed intubation. Six years' experience in a teaching maternity unit. *Anaesthesia* 1985;**40**:759–62.

3. L. Hawthorne, R. Wilson, G. Lyons, M. Dresner. Failed intubation revisited: 17-yr experience in a teaching maternity unit. *Br J Anaesth* 1996;**76**:680–4.

4. R. S. Cormack and J. Lehane. Difficult tracheal intubations in obstetrics. *Anaesthesia* 1984;**39**:1105–11.

5. R. Jouppila, P. Jouppila, A. Hollmén. Laryngeal oedema as an obstetric anaesthesia complication: case reports. *Acta Anaesthesiol Scand* 1980;**24**:97–8.

6. L. Spätling, F. Fallenstein, A. Huch. The variability of cardiopulmonary adaptation to pregnancy at rest and during exercise. *Br J Obstet Gynaecol* 1992;**99**(Suppl 8):1–40.

7. J. A. Milne. The respiratory response to pregnancy. *Postgrad Med J* 1979;**55**:318–24.

8. J. A. Thomas and C. A. Hagberg. The difficult airway: risks, prophylaxis, and management. In Chestnut D. H., Polley L. S., Tsen L. C., Wong C. A., eds., *Chestnut's Obstetric Anesthesia: Principles and Practice*, 4th edn., Philadelphia, PN: Mosby Elsevier, 2009, pp. 651–76.

9. U. Munnur, B. de Boisblanc, M. S. Suresh. Airway problems in pregnancy. *Crit Care Med* 2005;**33**:S259–68.

10. S. Kheterpal, R. Han, K. K. Tremper, *et al.* Incidence and predictors of difficult and impossible mask ventilation. *Anesthesiology* 2006;**105**:885–91.

11. B. S. Kodali, S. Chandrasekhar, L. N. Bulich, *et al.* Airway changes during labor and delivery. *Anesthesiology* 2008;**108**:357–62.

12. J. L. Benumof. Management of the difficult adult airway. With special emphasis on awake tracheal intubation. *Anesthesiology* 1991;**75**:1087–110.

13. E. Gaszynska, T. Gaszynski. The King Vision videolaryngoscope for awake intubation: series of cases and literature review. *Ther Clin Risk Manag* 2014;**10**:475–8.

14. M. Balki, M. E. Cooke, S. Dunington, *et al.* Unanticipated difficult airway in obstetric patients: development of a new algorithm for formative assessment in high-fidelity simulation. *Anesthesiology* 2012;**117**:883–97.

15. K. J. Smith, J. Dobranowski, G. Yip, *et al.* Cricoid pressure displaces the esophagus: an observational study using magnetic resonance imaging. *Anesthesiology* 2003;**99**:60–4.

16. E. T. Crosby, R. M. Cooper, M. J. Douglas, *et al.* The unanticipated difficult airway with recommendations for management. *Can J Anaesth* 1998;**45**:757–76.

17. R. F. Reardon and M. Martel. The intubating laryngeal mask airway: suggestions for use in the emergency department. *Acad Emerg Med* 2001;**8**:833–8.

Management of patients with laryngospasm

15

Kenneth H. Butler

Case presentation

A 22-year-old man is brought to the emergency department by ambulance after he experienced the acute onset of audible stridor. He is accompanied by his significant other, who states this difficulty in speaking began while they were arguing. The partner states that, at the onset, the patient could not breathe well. An audible sound then followed. The patient has no history of direct laryngeal trauma or chemical inhalation. His past medical history is non-contributory. He is not taking any medication, and his family history is unremarkable.

On physical examination, you hear inspiratory stridor. The patient appears distressed and anxious, with his hands around his neck. He is mildly tachycardic but hemodynamically stable, non-dyspneic, and afebrile. Pulse oximetry shows a saturation of 95% on room air with good wave form. Examination of the neck shows that the trachea is midline. You find no edema, palpable mass, or crepitance, and the patient does not show evidence of pain. The oral examination reveals no obstruction or pooling of secretions, no edema, and no exudates, but mild erythema is present. The pulmonary examination indicates adequate air exchange with no abnormal breath sounds.

Clinical definition

Laryngospasm is the spasmodic closure of the glottic aperture. It can be complete or partial. It is a relatively uncommon condition, and it is potentially life-threatening. True laryngospasm is complete closure of the larynx caused by external stimulation. The false cords are tightly occluded, the intra-pharyngeal part of the epiglottis moves posteriorly, and ventral movements of both arytenoid cartilages effectively seal the larynx. In partial spasm, the vocal cords are pressed firmly against each other, leaving a small lumen at the posterior commissure, which allows minimal ventilation.[1,2] The associated morbidity varies from cardiac arrest to oxygen desaturation.

Paradoxical vocal fold motion (PVFM) describes inappropriate motion of the true vocal folds. The term refers to a clinical phenomenon rather than one specific or strictly defined clinical diagnosis. PVFM is most commonly observed as inappropriate adduction of the vocal folds on inspiration. Its emergency department presentation is usually wheezing, stridor, or apparent upper airway obstruction.[3] In this setting, it is indistinguishable from laryngospasm, and the clinical approach to both is the same; therefore, the two conditions are discussed interchangeably in this chapter.

Cases in Emergency Airway Management, ed. Lauren C. Berkow and John C. Sakles. Published by Cambridge University Press. © Cambridge University Press 2015.

PVFM has unintentionally become a catch-all term for functional laryngeal disorders. It is also called laryngeal dyskinesia, vocal cord dysfunction, paradoxical vocal cord motion, inspiratory adduction, periodic occurrence of laryngeal obstruction, Munchausen's stridor, episodic paroxysmal laryngospasm, psychogenic stridor, functional stridor, hysterical croup, emotional laryngeal wheezing, factitious asthma, pseudoasthma, and irritable larynx syndrome.[3]

Anatomic findings

In the normal larynx, the true vocal folds abduct, or open, during inspiration and partially adduct, or close, during expiration. In addition to inspiration, abduction can also be induced by sniffing and panting. Normal adduction of the true vocal folds occurs with phonation, coughing, throat clearing, and swallowing and during a Valsalva maneuver. Adduction of 10–40% is normal during expiration. Normal cough mechanics involve vocal fold adduction for 0.2 seconds following the end of the inspiratory phase.[3,4]

PVFM can be seen during inspiration, expiration, or both.[5] The false vocal folds and supraglottic tissue may also dynamically constrict the airway. It is imperative to visualize full abduction during laryngoscopy to rule out other causes of laryngeal obstruction.[3]

Causes of PVFM

Many comorbidities have been associated with PVFM. Because PVFM is a descriptive term rather than a specific diagnosis, the etiology is often multifactorial. Occasionally, no specific inciting agent can be clearly identified.[3]

Asthma

PVFM is often misdiagnosed as asthma; in fact, the two conditions can be seen concomitantly.[6] In Forrest et al.'s study of asthmatic patients who were referred for a suspected diagnosis of PVFM, the diagnosis was confirmed by laryngoscopy in 75% of cases.[7]

Exercise

Exercise accounts for approximately 14% of PVFM diagnoses.[8] This type of PVFM occurs predominantly in young female athletes who present with dyspnea and sometimes stridor triggered by exercise. In Marcinow et al.'s series of 831 patients with PVFM, 46 were elite athletes and, of those, 70% were female and 46% had noisy breathing during exercise. Elite athletes with PVFM were less likely to have a history of reflux, psychiatric diagnosis, dysphonia, cough, or dysphagia than non-athletes with PVFM.[9]

Intraoperative prevention of laryngospasm

Several strategies have been proposed to reduce the incidence of laryngospasm during general anesthesia. Based on a meta-analysis of data from 19 studies, Luce and colleagues concluded that the use of the laryngeal mask airway during pediatric anesthesia significantly reduced the incidence of several postoperative adverse events, including laryngospasm, compared with tracheal intubation.[10]

Similarly, based on another meta-analysis, Mihara and associates reported that lidocaine reduced the likelihood of laryngospasm in children in whom general anesthesia was induced. Both intravenous and topical routes of administration were found to be effective. The timing of intravenous lidocaine administration was observed to be important in terms of its protective effects. The authors suggest that the drug be given within 5 minutes before tracheal intubation.[11]

Endotracheal extubation

The post-intubation onset of acute dyspnea and stridor is much more likely to be caused by laryngospasm than by PVFM.[12] Laryngospasm is usually a brief episode of vocal fold adduction, often seen during emergence from general anesthesia. PVFM can occur shortly after extubation of patients who have been intubated in the emergency department. The two can be differentiated from other pulmonary causes of respiratory distress with flexible laryngoscopy.[13]

Ketamine

Laryngospasm is rare in patients who have received ketamine, reportedly occurring in 0.3% of cases.[14] In a meta-analysis, Green and colleagues showed that low intramuscular doses of ketamine (< 3.0 mg/kg) were associated with significantly fewer adverse airway and respiratory events than other induction agents.[15] In fact, none of the children in the lower-dose group experienced either laryngospasm or apnea.

Irritants that can trigger PVFM

Some patients attribute PVFM to inhalational exposure to an irritant such as ammonia, soldering fumes, cleaning chemicals, aerosolized machining fluids, construction dust, or smoke.[16] The onset of PVFM symptoms typically occurs within 24 hours after the exposure. Patients might feel that ongoing problems with PVFM are related to a previous inhalational irritant exposure. An acute exposure might cause temporary laryngeal irritation, but it is unclear how a previous remote exposure would cause ongoing episodes of PVFM.

Laryngopharyngeal reflux

Reflux of gastric contents into the larynx and pharynx, known as laryngopharyngeal reflux (LPR), is associated with PVFM. However, it is unclear whether the two have a causal relationship.

Psychosocial disorders and stress

PVFM has been associated with a variety of psychosocial disorders. It is very rarely considered a form of malingering[7]; it would be difficult to produce the condition intentionally for secondary gain. In a prospective cohort of 45 patients with PVFM, 18 were found to have conversion disorder and 11 had no psychopathology.[17] In a series of military personnel with PVFM, 52% reported symptoms related to high stress and anxiety, and 39% reported symptoms during exertion.[18]

Clinical presentation of PVFM

In terms of gender-related incidence, PVFM has a female predominance.[7] It affects people of all ages, from children to the elderly.

The hallmark of PVFM is inspiratory stridor accompanied by respiratory distress. Often, the diagnosis is suspected after multiple visits to the emergency department for these episodes (lasting several minutes to hours) or during evaluation for severe asthma. In addition to dyspnea, patients might complain of throat tightness, a choking sensation, dysphonia, and cough. The onset of symptoms can be spontaneous or associated with triggers such as exercise, irritant exposure, or anxiety.

Stridorous sounds can be inspiratory, expiratory, or both. They are usually loudest over the anterior neck and less audible through the chest wall, where the sound is attenuated by transmission through the airways and the pulmonary parenchyma. Typically, albuterol has minimal to no beneficial effect.[19]

Some patients experience dysphonia, often associated with vocal fold hyperfunction (e.g. excessive false vocal fold adduction and anterior–superior laryngeal compression during phonation).[8]

The severity of respiratory distress and anxiety of patients with PVFM occasionally leads clinicians to perform endotracheal intubation or tracheostomy to restore airway patency before diagnostic tests are completed. Immediately afterward, wheezing and stridor typically cease, suggesting that the airflow limitation was caused by an upper airway process instead of asthma.[3]

Evaluation and diagnosis

Laryngoscopy is the gold standard for the diagnosis. Pulmonary function tests and imaging can be performed prior to laryngoscopy, depending on the clinical presentation and degree of clinical suspicion for the diagnosis.[3] Visualization of the larynx with a flexible fiberoptic nasopharyngeal scope is imperative to confirm abnormal adduction of the true vocal folds and exclude other laryngeal pathology. Full visualization of the vocal folds with complete abduction is also necessary to rule out supraglottic or subglottic obstruction and bilateral vocal fold immobility. In some patients, PVFM is apparent on laryngoscopy even when the patient is asymptomatic.[8] Others have findings of PVFM on laryngoscopy only after provocation.[3]

If the patient can tolerate the procedure, local topical 4% lidocaine could be all that is necessary for insertion of the scope through the nares. For patients who require sedation, ketamine is the optimal choice because it has analgesic, sedational, and amnesic properties and maintains the patient's respiratory drive. An additional safety factor is that ketamine does not induce dose-dependent apnea.

PVFM is diagnosed when laryngoscopy reveals abnormal adduction of the true folds (solely during inspiration, throughout the respiratory cycle, or, rarely, solely during expiration). The glottic aperture might be obliterated, except for a posterior diamond-shaped passage. Adduction or bunching of the false vocal folds might be observed.[20] Although these findings are normally seen only during an acute episode, they can often be reproduced on examination when the patient is asked to mimic what happens during an attack.[3]

Imaging is used predominantly to exclude other causes of dyspnea. Chest radiographs are often obtained to exclude an intrathoracic cause of dyspnea. If the trachea cannot be examined during laryngoscopy, high-resolution computed tomography of the upper airways can be used to exclude subglottic stenosis, tracheal and extratracheal (e.g. thyroid) masses, and tracheomalacia.[3]

Treatment

Various treatment strategies have been used, although none has been studied in a controlled fashion. The treatment of PVFM can sometimes be guided by medical management of the possible underlying cause, such as extubation, exposure to an irritant, or laryngopharyngeal reflux.[7] Because the underlying cause is rarely known, such treatments are empiric rather than evidence-based.[3]

The following acute management strategies can be useful[3]:

- Reassurance and supportive care until the episode resolves spontaneously. Asking patients to pant can sometimes abort an episode; panting activates the posterior cricoarytenoid muscle, causing abduction of the true vocal folds.[21]
- Continuous positive airway pressure (CPAP).[20,22] The persistent positive airflow from the CPAP device signals the brain to keep the vocal cords apart.
- Inhalation of a helium–oxygen mixture (heliox). In a case series, four of five PVFM patients experienced improvement in symptoms, including anxiety, with heliox inhalation during acute episodes.[23,24]
- Gentle chest compression after extubation. In a study of children undergoing elective tonsillectomy, Al-Metwalli and colleagues found that gentle chest compression accompanied by the delivery of 100% O_2 via tight-fitting mask is a simple and effective technique for responding to post-extubation laryngospasm.[25] The technique involves placing the extended palm of the free hand on the middle of the child's chest, with the fingers directed caudally, and applying a compression force no more than half that used for cardiopulmonary resuscitation, at a rate of 20 to 25 per minute. None of the children in the study experienced gastric distension as a result of this procedure.
- The vast majority of patients with PVFM do not require endotracheal intubation or tracheostomy. These procedures should be reserved for patients at risk for airway obstruction from causes other than PVFM.[22]

In some cases of laryngospasm, airway management alone will not be enough to stabilize the patient and resolve the symptoms. Intravenous medications are often indicated. Succinylcholine is the gold standard for treatment of persistent laryngospasm. It can be administered at a dose of 0.25 to 0.50 mg/kg, perhaps in combination with small doses of propofol or another anesthetic.[26] In a study of children (3 to 10 years of age) undergoing minor surgical procedures, Afshan and colleagues found that a small dose of propofol (0.8 mg/kg) was effective at relieving laryngeal spasm in patients who did not respond fully to gentle positive-pressure ventilation.[27]

Case resolution

After explaining the procedure to the patient and obtaining his consent, you decide to inspect the larynx and vocal cords using a flexible fiberoptic scope. With the patient in a seated upright position, you administer 4% liquid lidocaine and phenylephrine hydrochloride to achieve topical anesthesia and vasoconstriction of the nasal mucosa.

Through the scope, you see that the nasal cavity is normal. Visualization of the oropharynx, hypopharynx, vallecular, and tongue reveals no abnormalities. Turning to the larynx, you see that the patient's epiglottis is crisp without edema. The glottis has no evidence of edema or a foreign body, and there is no evidence of inappropriate adduction during inspiration or expiration that would be consistent with PVFM.

You reassure the patient by telling him that you have experienced similar episodes during times of anxiety and stress. After documenting your diagnosis of psychogenic PVFM, you discharge the young man to his home, with instructions to follow up with his primary care physician.

Summary and recommendations

PVFM is often mistaken for asthma because it is episodic, it can be brought on by exertion, and its stridor might sound similar to wheezing. Indeed, some patients have both asthma and PVFM. Flow-volume curves might show flattening of the inspiratory loop consistent with extrathoracic airway obstruction. Between episodes, spirometry readings are often normal. The diagnosis is confirmed by flexible laryngoscopy with visualization of abnormal adduction of the vocal folds and exclusion of other causes of glottic and subglottic obstruction. In some patients, the glottic aperture is obliterated during inspiration, except for a posterior diamond-shaped passage.

In patients with an acute episode of PVFM, an initial approach that includes a combination of reassurance and panting maneuvers is recommended. If these measures are not effective, CPAP might be helpful, and inhalation of heliox may be considered.

The symptoms of PVFM and laryngospasm are often indistinguishable. Laryngospasm is more common in the perioperative environment but its overall incidence is much lower. It is also more likely than PVFM to require airway management.

References

1. D. Hampson-Evans, P. Morgan, M. Farrar. Pediatric laryngospasm. *Paediatr Anaesth* 2008; **18**: 303–7.

2. E. Sumner, D. J. Hatch (eds.). *Paediatric Anesthesia*, 2nd edition. London: Arnold; 1999.

3. J. Shapiro, J. Dowdall, C. Thompson. Paradoxical vocal fold motion. Updated May 22, 2014. www.UpToDate.com. (Accessed November 21, 2014.)

4. F. D. McCool. Global physiology and pathophysiology of cough: ACCP evidence-based clinical practice guidelines. *Chest* 2006; **129**(suppl 1): 48S–53S.

5. K. B. Newman, U. G. Mason 3rd, K. B. Schmaling. Clinical features of vocal cord dysfunction. *Am J Respir Crit Care Med* 1995; **152**: 1382–6.

6. K. Yelken, A. Yilmaz, M. Guven, A. Eyibilen, I. Aladag. Paradoxical vocal fold motion dysfunction in asthma patients. *Respirology* 2009; **14**: 29–33.

7. L. A. Forrest, T. Husein, O. Husein. Paradoxical vocal cord motion: classification and treatment. *Laryngoscope* 2012; **122**: 844–53.

8. T. Chiang, A. M. Marcinow, B. W. deSilva, B. N. Ence, S. E. Lindsey, L. A. Forrest. Exercise-induced paradoxical vocal fold motion disorder: diagnosis and management. *Laryngoscope* 2013; **123**: 727–31.

9. A. M. Marcinow, J. Thompson, T. Chiang, *et al*. Paradoxical vocal fold motion disorder in the elite athlete: experience at a large division I university. *Laryngoscope* 2014; **124**: 1425–30.

10. V. Luce, H. Harkouk, C. Brasher, *et al*. Supraglottic airway devices vs. tracheal intubation in children: a quantitative meta-analysis of respiratory complications. *Pediatr Anesth* 2014; **24**: 1088–98.

11. T. Mihara, K. Uchimoto, S. Morita, *et al*. The efficacy of lidocaine to prevent laryngospasm in children: a systematic review and meta-analysis. *Anaesthesia* 2014; **69**: 1388–96.

12. B. Larsen, L. J. Caruso, D. B. Villariet. Paradoxical vocal cord motion: an often misdiagnosed cause of postoperative stridor. *J Clin Anesth* 2004; **16**: 230–4.

13. G. A. Arndt, B. R. Voth. Paradoxical vocal cord motion in the recovery room: a masquerader of pulmonary dysfunction. *Can J Anaesth* 1996; **43**: 1249–51.

14. S. M. Green, M. G. Roback, R. M. Kennedy, B. Krauss. Clinical practice guideline for emergency department ketamine dissociative sedation: 2011 update. *Ann Emerg Med* 2011; **57**: 449–61.

15. S. M. Green, M. G. Roback, B. Krauss. Laryngospasm during emergency department ketamine sedation. *Pediatr Emerg Care* 2010; **26**: 798–802.

16. J. J. Perkner, K. P. Fennelly, R. Balkissoon, *et al.* Irritant-associated vocal cord dysfunction. *J Occup Environ Med* 1998; **40**: 136–43.

17. O. F. Husein, T. N. Husein, R. Gardner, *et al.* Formal psychological testing in patients with paradoxical vocal fold dysfunction. *Laryngoscope* 2008; **118**: 740–7.

18. M. J. Morris, R. T. Oleszewski, J. B. Sterner, *et al.* Vocal cord dysfunction related to combat deployment. *Mil Med* 2013; **178**: 1208–12.

19. S. M. Neustein, L. M. Taitt-Wynter, M. A. Rosenblatt. Treating stridor with opioids: a challenging case of paradoxical vocal cord movement. *J Clin Anesth* 2010; **22**: 130–1.

20. J. Goldman, M. Muers. Vocal cord dysfunction and wheezing [editorial]. *Thorax* 1991; **46**: 401–4.

21. A. E. Pitchenik. Functional laryngeal obstruction relieved by panting. *Chest* 1991; **100**: 1465–7.

22. J. M. Heiser, M. L. Kahn, T. A. Schmidt. Functional airway obstruction presenting as stridor: a case report and literature review. *J Emerg Med* 1990; **8**: 285–9.

23. M. Weir. Vocal cord dysfunction mimics asthma and may respond to heliox. *Clin Pediatr (Phila)* 2002; **41**: 37–41.

24. M. J. Morris, P. F. Allan, P. J. Perkins. Vocal cord dysfunction. *Clin Pulm Med* 2006; **13**: 73–86.

25. R. R. Al-Metwalli, H. A. Mowafi, S. A. Ismail. Gentle chest compression relieves extubation laryngospasm in children. *J Anesth* 2010; **24**: 854–7.

26. J. Butterworth, D. C. Mackey, J. Wasnick (eds.). *Morgan and Mikhail's Clinical Anesthesiology*, 5th edition. New York: McGraw-Hill; 2013: pp. 309–41.

27. G. Afshan, U. Chohan, M. Qamar-Ul-Hoda, *et al.* Is there a role of a small dose of propofol in the treatment of laryngeal spasm? *Paediatr Anaesth* 2002; **12**: 625–8.

Airway compression by expanding hematoma

16

Michael Seltz Kristensen and Wendy H. L. Teoh

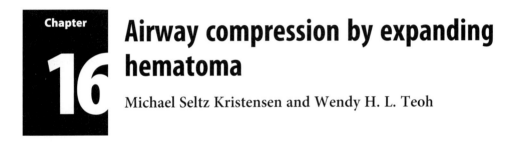

Case presentation

A 68-year-old woman, previously healthy apart from arterial hypertension and mild gastro-intestinal disturbances, height 168 cm, weight 78 kg, went to see an otolaryngolist because she experienced increased sensation of tension by her necklace and later slight discomfort while swallowing. A fine-needle aspiration from a lump in the neck revealed thyroid follicular neoplasia. The patient underwent uneventful general anesthesia and intubation following direct laryngoscopy that revealed a grade 1 Cormack–Lehane view. A right-sided thyroid carcinoma was encountered that had invaded the right internal jugular vein and regional lymph nodes. The internal jugular vein was ligated and lymph nodes with invasion were removed. The tumor did not directly invade the trachea but it was very close. The patient was extubated uneventfully. Three hours later the patient was seen by an attending otolaryngologist. Endoscopy showed edema of the left arytenoid region, right vocal cord palsy, and reduced movement of the left vocal cord. There was moderate swelling on the neck above the right clavicle. The patient had a neck circumference of 46 cm but no stridor. A surgical knife was placed by the patient's side with the instruction, "In case of acute respiratory distress, cut the sutures in the skin and pre-tracheal layer and call the on-call doctor." Four hours postoperatively the patient had "light stridor," and during the next 24 hours, she experienced intermittent dyspnea. Twenty-four hours postoperatively, stridor was diminished, but the patient had audible respiration and a slightly affected voice. The swelling on the neck was unchanged and flexible endoscopy showed the same as the day before; the drainage tube was removed. Forty hours postoperatively, the patient had audible respiration. Both inspection of the external neck and flexible laryngoscopy revealed that the patient was slightly less affected than the previous day. Fifty hours postoperatively, the patient had swelling at the level of the surgical wound and felt oppression. Sixty-eight hours postoperatively, swelling was present around the surgical wound, under the chin, and up the right cheek. The patient had increasing dyspnea, sensation of having a lump in the throat, and increasing pain. Oxygen saturation was 98% on room air. Ultrasound examination revealed a large accumulation of fluid. A needle aspiration was attempted without success. Flexible nasoendoscopy revealed a large, right-sided swelling in the piriform sinus extending to the vallecular and covering the aryepiglottic fold and false cords on the right side. The surgeon decided to operate, and in the meantime an inhalation with epinephrine was initiated.

Cases in Emergency Airway Management, ed. Lauren C. Berkow and John C. Sakles. Published by Cambridge University Press. © Cambridge University Press 2015.

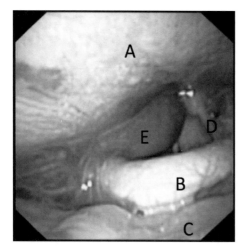

Figure 16.1 The image obtained during advancement of the flexible videoscope from the oral cavity toward the vocal cords. A = Posterior pharyngeal wall. B = Tip of the epiglottis. C = Tongue. D = Left aryepiglottic fold. E = In-bulging from external compression by the expanding hematoma

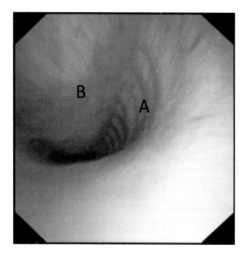

Figure 16.2 The image obtained during advancement of the flexible videoscope in the trachea. A = Tracheal rings. B = In-bulging of the posterior tracheal wall caused by the external expanding hematoma

The pre-anesthetic examination revealed a sitting patient in respiratory distress with a Mallampati Class 2 and mouth opening approximately 3.5 cm. The practitioner decided to perform awake intubation. The patient was placed in semi-sitting position, given glycopyrrolate 200 mcg, nasal oxygen at 4 L/min, and marginal sedation with 0.5 mg of midazolam. Lidocaine 10% spray was administered to the tongue and oral, pharyngeal, and laryngeal structures before a flexible videoscope was introduced orally via a Berman airway. The videoscope was advanced until the tip was 5 cm above the carina, and then the endotracheal tube was railroaded over it. During the flexible endoscopy it was noted that not only was there swelling and in-bulging above the vocal cords (Figure 16.1) but the upper half of the tracheal lumen was narrowed (Figure 16.2) owing to external compression of the posterior, soft part of the trachea.

A large amount of coagulated blood was present at the site of surgery and extended deep into the thoracic cavity along the trachea. After the coagulated blood was removed, the patient was kept intubated and transferred to the intensive care unit. The patient's trachea was extubated the following day.

Pertinent review of the medical problem/condition and relevant literature review

Airway obstruction from an expanding hematoma can arise after trauma to the airway[1] or adjacent structures, or after surgery.[2] The obstruction can arise at any level in the respiratory tract from the oral cavity,[1] pharynx, and larynx to the level of the distal trachea. Surgery of the neck, including cervical exploration for thyroid or parathyroid disease and anterior cervical spine surgery,[3] carries an inherent risk of postoperative hematomas that can cause airway obstruction. It is difficult to identify reliable predictors regarding which patients who undergo cervical exploration will develop postoperative hematoma.[4] Additionally, the time from surgery until onset of symptoms varies widely, with 43% presenting within 6 hours, approximately 19% presenting beyond 24 hours,[4] and life-threatening hematomas occurring up to a week post-surgery.[5] Approximately 1 in 200 patients develop a hematoma that requires surgical intervention after thyroid/parathyroid surgery.

Airway compromise can develop by two mechanisms. The first mechanism consists of the hematoma itself acting as a mass in the airway or compressing the airway from the outside, thereby diminishing the cross-sectional area of the airway. In the second mechanism, pressure exerted on the vessels by the hematoma impairs venous and lymphatic drainage, causing edema to develop in supraglottic structures, the epiglottis, and the arytenoids.[3,5] Each of these mechanisms, or both in combination, can compromise spontaneous ventilation and hinder attempts to mask ventilate, place a supraglottic airway device, or intubate. The second mechanism also explains why cutting sutures to decompress the wound does not always relieve the symptoms.

Potential airway management scenarios and discussion

In the case described above, we have several choices to make.

The first choice is: Should we attempt to relieve the symptoms by cutting the sutures in the skin and pre-tracheal layer for decompression?

This approach should always be considered, but the decision depends solely on clinical judgment, and there is no guarantee that this maneuver will help. The respiratory distress may be caused by edema secondary to hematoma-induced impairment of venous return from the larynx rather than by the hematoma itself. In this case, the practitioners decided not to cut the sutures before securing the airway. An immediate decompression should be attempted, and can be lifesaving, if the hematoma is causing respiratory or cardiac arrest.[2]

The second choice is: Should this patient be anesthetized before securing the airway, or should the patient's airway be managed while the patient is awake and breathing spontaneously?

To answer this question, we must understand that tracheal intubation *after* induction of general anesthesia should be considered only when success with the chosen device(s) can be predicted![6] In the present case, we *cannot* predict that intubation will be successful after induction of anesthesia; thus, we should proceed with awake intubation. Awake intubation has many other advantages in this patient. (1) Mask ventilation and placement of a supraglottic airway device could easily prove to be impossible, and the obstruction is likely to be at the glottic level. Therefore, even after successful placement of a supraglottic airway, ventilation might still be impossible. (2) The patient can sit up, which was necessary for this patient in respiratory distress. (3) The patient can actually help the airway manager by opening her mouth, protruding her tongue, and taking a deep breath. (4) Intubation is often easier in the awake patient because in anesthetized patients the loss of muscle tone leads to tissue collapse. One should not hesitate to choose awake intubation when indicated, as it causes discomfort in only a minority of patients[7] and can be performed in a few minutes by an experienced airway manager.[8]

The third choice is: With which techniques should we secure the airway while the patient is awake? Awake tracheostomy should always be considered, but it is likely to be very difficult in this sitting patient who has anterior swelling of the neck and is in respiratory distress. Therefore, we chose tracheal intubation but had to decide which technique to use.

In principle, all techniques for intubation can be used for awake intubation, but some are more appropriate than others for the case described here. In this case, retrograde intubation is relatively contraindicated owing to the large hematoma obscuring the landmarks, and intubation via a supraglottic airway device may fail because the obstruction is likely to be at the level of the glottis. Video laryngoscopy is a well-described technique and has the advantage that it may cause less airway obstruction than a flexible scope in a severely narrowed airway. However, it is very difficult to perform video laryngoscopy in a sitting patient with respiratory distress. Furthermore, video laryngoscopy has the disadvantage that it will not allow us to ensure that the tip of the tube is located distal to the tracheal compression.

We chose to use a flexible optical scope for intubation. This technique allowed us to keep the patient sitting up, to choose between oral and nasal access, and to see exactly where the tip of the tube was in the trachea in relation to the tracheal compression. We chose oral access to avoid nasal bleeding and used a flexible scope with a large video screen attached, allowing simultaneous observation by the airway manager and the surgeon.

Even when performing awake intubation, it is possible to lose control of the airway, and the airway provider should always be prepared to change strategy to perform a best attempt at ventilation and intubation. Before initiating airway management, the airway manager should identify and mark the cricothyroid membrane. Additionally, equipment for emergency percutaneous airway access and a person trained in using it should be readily available. If the trachea and the cricothyroid membrane cannot be identified by palpation, they can be identified with ultrasonography if time permits.[9]

Algorithms/pathways to follow and alternate airway devices/resources

Timing and clinical judgment are crucial elements in the management of airway hematomas. As we saw in the case described above, the patient's arterial oxygen saturation on room air was normal. However, both hypoxia and hypercarbia are late signs of severe airway obstruction, and we should not wait for these signs to occur. We are thus faced with *clinical judgment* and must evaluate the degree of stridor and respiratory distress, the swelling, the choking sensation, the sensation of dyspnea expressed by the patient, dysphagia, voice changes, the respiratory rate, and the position of the patient. Patients with hematoma prefer the upright position with the head slightly extended.[2] Imaging procedures to diagnose the hematoma can significantly delay treatment and are generally not necessary or recommended.[2]

An airway hematoma is a *dynamic* condition that evolves over time, the duration of which can vary substantially. We must judge whether or not the condition is immediately life-threatening. *If* we judge that the hematoma can evolve into a health-threatening airway obstruction, it is extremely important to secure the airway *before* such an obstruction occurs.

If the condition is immediately life-threatening

In this situation, the patient may already be unconscious. We must immediately administer 100% oxygen via non-rebreather facemask and initiate bag-mask ventilation if necessary. A decompression of the hematoma should be attempted either before attempting to intubate the trachea[2] or immediately after a failed attempt at intubating the trachea. We should prepare equipment for emergency cricothyrotomy/tracheostomy while preparing for intubation. The attempt at tracheal intubation should be made by the most skilled person available, preferably with a Macintosh-shaped video laryngoscope and a 6-mm internal-diameter endotracheal tube that is already mounted with a stylet. The use of a Macintosh-shaped video laryngoscope is recommended because it combines the benefit of a wider viewing angle from the video part with the direct laryngoscope's ability to actually lift the tongue and thus create space.[10] It is important to cut the sutures in both the skin and the pre-tracheal layer. Reopening the wound in this way will not always help because massive internal edema caused by the compression may persist.

If the condition is *not* immediately life-threatening

In this situation we have different management options and have time to perform an airway evaluation. Administer 100% oxygen via non-rebreathing facemask or high-flow nasal cannula and thereafter perform a thorough airway examination. We may diminish or delay the symptoms by administering a mixture of oxygen and helium, administering nebulized epinephrine, and elevating the head of the patient. Glucocorticoid injection may help, but the onset is slow.

We must consider bedside decompression of the hematoma or removal of the hematoma under local anesthesia. In many cases, the initial evacuation of the hematoma can be performed with the patient under local anesthesia in the operating room with the head of the operating table elevated 45–60 degrees. The wound is reopened to below the level of the strap muscles. At this level, the trachea is accessible for emergent tracheostomy, should it become necessary, or intubation can be performed at this time if more extensive surgery is required.[2]

If it is decided not to open the wound before anesthesia, we must perform an *airway evaluation* and predict the likelihood of failure or success with the different airway techniques: mask ventilation, supraglottic airway device ventilation, and tracheal intubation. During the evaluation, we should judge the ease of performing a percutaneous emergency airway access[6] and determine the pre-anesthetic location of the trachea and cricothyroid membrane, if necessary with ultrasonography.[9] We must also judge if the level of the airway compression is above or below the level of the cricothyroid membrane. An emergency cricothyrotomy is unlikely to be effective if the airway compression is distal to the level of the cricothyroid membrane. If the level of compression is at the level of the trachea, even a tracheostomy may be ineffective until the hematoma has been evacuated.

Tracheal intubation after induction of general anesthesia should be considered only when success with the chosen device(s) can be predicted.[6] Thus, we should continue with awake intubation if we have doubt regarding our ability to intubate the patient, or if we cannot count on being able to perform a percutaneous emergency airway access.

For awake intubation, we should choose a flexible optical intubation if the patient needs to sit up and if there is a suspicion that the compression from the hematoma extends beyond the glottic opening. Otherwise we can choose a video laryngoscope or an alternative technique (for example retrograde intubation) for intubation.

If it is decided that general anesthesia will be induced before tracheal intubation, the initial attempt at intubation can be performed ideally with a Macintosh-shaped video laryngoscope, as it allows a lifting motion that might help to create space in the oral and pharyngeal cavity. At the same time, it improves vision of the glottis.

Post-management care and follow-up

It must be remembered that extubation, as opposed to the initial airway management, is an *elective procedure*. It should not be carried out with unnecessary risk to the patient. Even if the initial hematoma has been successfully removed, edema may remain that can compromise the airway postoperatively. Therefore, postoperative observation in the intensive care unit is mandatory until the edema has resolved. Before extubation, the airway provider must evaluate the likelihood that the patient will need reintubation and the likelihood of difficult reintubation, should the need arise. A thorough evaluation, including internal inspection of the airways, should be performed before extubation, and the cricothyroid membrane should be located so that the team is prepared for emergency airway access. An airway exchange catheter can be used if any doubt exists regarding the ease of a potential reintubation.

It is advisable to have a dedicated postoperative anesthesia care unit (PACU) in the vicinity of the operating suite, where this kind of surgical patient can be observed frequently by both the surgical and anesthesia teams. It is also advisable to have dedicated PACU nurses trained to watch for potential hematomas of the neck and the accompanying symptoms. Many of the complications arise within the first 6 hours after surgery[4] and therefore may be observed by the PACU nurses.

References

1. Teoh WH, Yeoh SB, Tan HK. Airway management of an expanding soft palate haematoma in a parturient. *Anaesthesia and Intensive Care*. 2013;**41**(5):680–1.

2. Dixon JL, Snyder SK, Lairmore TC, Jupiter D, Govednik C, Hendricks JC. A novel method for the management of post-thyroidectomy or parathyroidectomy hematoma: a single-institution experience after over 4,000 central neck operations. *World Journal of Surgery*. 2014;**38**(6):1262–7.

3. Palumbo MA, Aidlen JP, Daniels AH, Thakur NA, Caiati J. Airway compromise due to wound hematoma following anterior cervical spine surgery. *The Open Orthopaedics Journal*. 2012;**6**:108–13.

4. Burkey SH, van Heerden JA, Thompson GB, et al. Reexploration for symptomatic hematomas after cervical exploration. *Surgery*. 2001;**130**(6):914–20.

5. Rosenbaum MA, Haridas M, McHenry CR. Life-threatening neck hematoma complicating thyroid and parathyroid surgery. *American Journal of Surgery*. 2008;**195**(3):339–43; discussion 43.

6. Law JA, Broemling N, Cooper RM, et al. The difficult airway with recommendations for management – part 2 – the anticipated difficult airway. *Canadian Journal of Anaesthesia (Journal canadien d'anesthesie)*. 2013;**60**(11):1119–38.

7. Schnack DT, Kristensen MS, Rasmussen LS. Patients' experience of awake versus anaesthetised orotracheal intubation: a

controlled study. *European Journal of Anaesthesiology.* 2011;**28**(6):438–42.

8. Kristensen MS, Fredensborg BB. The disposable Ambu aScope vs. a conventional flexible videoscope for awake intubation – a randomised study. *Acta Anaesthesiologica Scandinavica.* 2013;**57**(7):888–95.

9. Kristensen MS, Teoh WH, Graumann O, Laursen CB. Ultrasonography for clinical decision-making and intervention in airway management: from the mouth to the lungs and pleurae. *Insights Imaging.* 2014;**5**(2):253–79.

10. Teoh WH, Saxena S, Shah MK, Sia AT. Comparison of three videolaryngoscopes: Pentax Airway Scope, C-MAC, GlideScope vs. the Macintosh laryngoscope for tracheal intubation. *Anaesthesia.* 2010;**65**(11):1126–32.

Extubation of the difficult airway

Richard M. Cooper

Case presentation

A 50-year old, obese, diabetic male is admitted to the emergency department with chest pain and hypotension. While being assessed, he goes into cardiac arrest and requires repeated defibrillation and chest compressions. Direct laryngoscopy is unsuccessful. On the third attempt with a video laryngoscope, the larynx is seen and intubation is achieved. Before being transported to the coronary care unit (CCU) he recovers consciousness and resumes spontaneous ventilation. When, where, and how should extubation be performed?

Introduction

In the case described above, intubation was emergent; however, extubation was, and always should be, elective. It should be performed when circumstances minimize the likelihood that reintubation will be required. Reintubation may be required when oxygenation or ventilation is inadequate, airway protection or patency is compromised, or pulmonary toilet cannot be achieved. Among adult surgical patients, the likelihood of reintubation is approximately 0.1–0.2%.[1] This figure is in stark contrast to that for intensive care unit (ICU) patients, who have minimal reserves and may require reintubation 10–35% of the time.[1] Reintubation is inherently more risky than elective intubation because patients are less stable, information may be incomplete, and medications that facilitate laryngoscopy and intubation may be unavailable, poorly tolerated, or considered too risky by the care provider. Morbidity increases significantly when multiple intubation attempts are required.[2,3] Knowledge that an elective intubation has been performed without difficulty provides a measure of reassurance but does not guarantee that an emergent reintubation will be equally easy. On the other hand, if an elective intubation required multiple attempts, operators, or techniques; provided limited laryngeal exposure; or was associated with other complications, then both extubation and reintubation can be expected to pose additional challenges and carry additional risks.

Based on these considerations, the concept of an extubation risk continuum has two components: (1) the risk of extubation failure necessitating reintubation and (2) the risk that the reintubation will be difficult. Unfortunately, the prediction of these risks is imprecise, but the clinician's tolerance for risk is made on the patient's behalf. This author assumes that the patient has limited risk tolerance when the consequences of difficulty or failure are very high.

Cases in Emergency Airway Management, ed. Lauren C. Berkow and John C. Sakles. Published by Cambridge University Press. © Cambridge University Press 2015.

The past two decades have witnessed a reduction in adverse outcomes related to tracheal intubation. Minor complications after extubation, such as breath holding, laryngospasm, coughing, transient hemodynamic instability, and oxygen desaturation, are probably more common than those accompanying intubation. Although important, they relate more to the quality of care than to a genuine threat to life. However, brain injury, death, an emergent surgical airway, and intensive care admission resulting from complications after extubation continue to occur at a high rate.[4,5] The purpose of this chapter is to identify the patients at increased risk of these more serious complications and propose a strategy to mitigate adverse outcomes.

Failure of extubation

An extubation failure occurs when the removal of a tracheal tube is followed by the need to reintubate. To define its occurrence, some arbitrary timeframe is necessary, such as failure within 24 hours. The likelihood of extubation failure is more properly defined along a risk continuum than a low/high dichotomy. For example, a patient who requires pressure support ventilation of 15 cm is more likely to fail than one who needs only 5 cm; likewise, a patient who requires a high concentration of supplemental oxygen or positive expiratory pressure is at a higher risk than a patient who does not require such support. Patients with reduced reserves are at a higher risk, but it is often difficult to know how high that risk is. Higher-risk patients are more likely to have impaired oxygenation, diminished alveolar ventilation (or rapid, shallow breathing), thick or increased secretions, or persistent pain. Pain may cause diaphragmatic splinting or necessitate opioid analgesics that can result in respiratory depression or airway obstruction. Our strategy in managing these patients is aimed at minimizing the specific risk factors and optimally timing their extubation.

Failure of reintubation

Attempts at reintubation might prove difficult or impossible, particularly if the initial or primary intubation was difficult. Prolonged intubation; multiple attempts; generalized edema; localized obstruction (e.g. macroglossia, hematoma, angioedema); or insufficient information, equipment, drugs, or assistance might also complicate reintubation. Additionally, a deteriorating, agitated patient may induce performance anxiety that results in judgment errors and imperfect execution.

Identification of the high-risk patient

The preceding paragraphs have addressed, in general terms, patients at a greater risk of failing extubation or reintubation. A detailed discussion is beyond the scope of this chapter but may be found elsewhere.[1,6,7] Once a high-risk patient is identified, we can focus our efforts at risk reduction by optimally timing extubation and maximizing the probability that reintubation or tracheal tube exchange will succeed. Optimal timing requires a consideration that all of the criteria mandating intubation have been reversed – can the patient maintain oxygenation, ventilation, clearance of secretions, and airway patency without an artificial airway? If not, can measures be implemented to make these capabilities more likely in the near future? If the decision is made to postpone extubation, an appropriate strategy should be created to address the risk criteria, such as continuous positive airway pressure (CPAP)/positive end-expiratory pressure (PEEP), recruitment, positioning, suctioning, diuresis, pain control, improvement in the level of consciousness, or recovery from neuro-muscular blockade. When extubation is deferred and the patient is transferred to the care of another team, it is essential to communicate the concerns identified and the difficulties encountered and anticipated. The same level of expertise should attend extubation that is expected of intubation.

Extubation strategies

The risk of necessary reintubation may be reduced but not eliminated by optimal timing. If reintubation is expected to be difficult, there should be in place a strategy that maximizes the probability of success. We should always be prepared to reintubate if necessary. Preparation includes the immediate availability of necessary drugs, supplies, personnel, and expertise. If an alternative technique was required, it would seem prudent to ensure that the device and required expertise is available to facilitate reintubation.

A "cuff-leak test" may be performed as follows: the oropharynx is suctioned and the cuff is slowly deflated. An audible leak around the endotracheal tube is reassuring; the larger the difference between the inspired and expired volumes as measured by a spirometer, the less swelling or obstruction between the soft tissues and the tracheal tube. The value of the cuff-leak test is open to question. However, a large leak is reassuring, and the absence of a leak is reason to question the appropriateness of extubation.

The use of steroids to combat swelling around the airway is also controversial. Suffice it to say, the role is probably marginal and it likely takes several hours to achieve a beneficial result. Head-up positioning may be helpful in promoting venous drainage and reducing swelling.

It is difficult to assess the airway with a tracheal tube *in situ*. Laryngoscopy may be stressful and produce misleading information. Flexible endoscopy from within the tracheal tube provides no useful information regarding the larynx or hypopharynx. Assessment of the periglottic structures requires withdrawal of the tracheal tube and endoscope to a supraglottic position. Unfortunately, a conscious patient is likely to swallow, cough, or attempt to dislodge the endoscope. However, the flexible endoscope may serve a useful function in two circumstances. First, it may prove useful in converting a nasal tube to an oral tube or vice versa. In such circumstances, it is probably best to introduce an endoscope, preloaded with the replacement tube, into the trachea alongside the existing tube. With the patient rendered unconscious and relaxed, the existing tube is carefully withdrawn, and the replacement is advanced over the endoscope. The second use, as described below, involves an airway assessment performed through a supraglottic airway (SGA).

Two other approaches should be considered, both of which have been designated as "advanced techniques."[7] Although neither is difficult, the airway manager should become familiar with them in nonthreatening settings. These include the substitution of an SGA for the existing tracheal tube (Bailey maneuver) and extubation over an airway exchange catheter. Variations of these techniques have been described and may be found elsewhere.[1,6–8]

Bailey maneuver

Substitution of an endotracheal tube for an SGA offers several advantages: it permits an assessment of spontaneous ventilation and airway patency and enables the provider to easily enrich the inspired oxygen, support ventilation, control the depth of sedation with volatile anesthetic agents, and sequester secretions away from the airway to permit an unhurried bronchoscopic evaluation of the upper and lower airway. It also provides a conduit for reintubation should it become necessary. This maneuver can be performed several ways, but it must be done with an adequate depth of anesthesia (and muscle relaxation) to minimize the risk of laryngospasm. The patient should be properly positioned and preoxygenated, and the oropharynx should be gently suctioned. A deflated SGA is introduced behind the endotracheal tube, its position is confirmed, and its cuff is inflated. The cuff of the endotracheal tube is deflated and the tube is removed, taking care not to dislodge the SGA. If a bite block is not an integral part of the SGA, one should be placed. After the provider ensures that the SGA is placed properly, the neuromuscular blockade can be reversed and the patient permitted to resume spontaneous breathing.*

This technique, as originally described, used the Laryngeal Mask Airway™ Classic, but it has been used with a variety of SGA devices. If the SGA is used as a conduit for reintubation, it is recommended that the technique be performed under bronchoscopic guidance using an Aintree Intubation Catheter® (Cook Medical, Bloomington, IN) when appropriate.

Airway exchange catheter

An airway exchange catheter is a device that is introduced into an endotracheal tube and remains in place after tracheal extubation is performed. If required, reintubation can be achieved by using the exchange catheter as a guide over which the replacement tracheal tube is railroaded. Early devices were solid and therefore could not be used for oxygenation or ventilation. Now, several commercial products of various lengths and external diameters are available. They are rigid, thermostable, and generally fabricated from polyurethane; some have removable Luer-lok jet adapters and/or 15-mm connectors. Most have distance markings, a radiopaque marker, and a distal-end hole as well as side holes. Examples of such devices are the Cook Airway Exchange Catheter, the Arndt Airway Exchange Catheter (Cook Medical), and the ETVC® (CardioMed Supplies, Lindsay, ON, Canada). Mort[9] has demonstrated that reintubation over a tube exchanger greatly increases first-pass success, thereby reducing the occurrence of hypoxemia, bradycardia, esophageal intubation, and the need for a rescue technique.[9]

A few simple measures will increase the safety of this simple device:

- Suction the oropharynx before introducing the exchange catheter.
- Ensure that the exchange catheter is not advanced beyond the endotracheal tube. This is easily achieved by aligning the distance markings on the exchange catheter with those of the endotracheal tube and making certain that the catheter is not advanced as the endotracheal tube is withdrawn (Figure 17.1).
- Fix the exchange catheter to the nares or in the center of the mouth to prevent dislodgement.
- Use sedation and neuromuscular blockade to facilitate reintubation.
- It is helpful to minimize the disparity between the outer diameter of the tube exchanger and the inner diameter of the replacement tracheal tube so as to minimize tube passage difficulties over the catheter. Thus, if a tube exchange is anticipated, it is preferable to use

---

* An alternative approach is to remove the endotracheal tube before inserting the SGA. This method makes the latter somewhat easier to achieve but leaves the patient with an insecure airway during the exchange. Either approach can lead to loss of the airway if difficulties are encountered while placing the SGA.

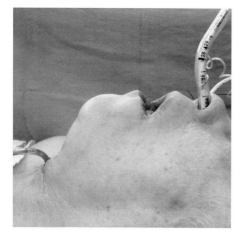

Figure 17.1 This photograph shows the alignment of the distance markings on a 14 F airway exchange catheter with those of a 6.5-mm nasotracheal tube. The patient had undergone a transoral composite resection and free radial forearm flap reconstruction. She also has a nasogastric tube in the contralateral nares

a larger-size tube exchanger. If reintubation is required in the presence of a smaller exchange catheter, a smaller-size tracheal tube can be selected.

- Use a tube exchanger in conjunction with an indirect laryngoscope (e.g. GlideScope, Airtraq®, or McGrath): conversion from "no view" to a full or near-full laryngeal view of the reintubation (48/51 cases) reduced the risk of impingement at the glottic chink and buckling of the device.[10] If an indirect laryngoscope is not available, a direct laryngoscope is still helpful in providing retraction of the tongue.

These devices are generally well tolerated and permit the patient to talk, cough, and ambulate. If the catheter is poorly tolerated, the depth should be rechecked before administering a local anesthetic or removing the device. They are frequently removed prematurely. Mort found that although all patients who required reintubation did so within 24 hours, only 41% of the exchange catheter reintubations occurred within 2 hours of extubation.[9] Most (30/51) extubation failures occurred between 2 and 10 hours after extubation. Because reintubations in patients with known difficult airways are much safer when performed with an airway exchange catheter, these should not be removed until it seems unlikely that reintubation will be required. An arbitrary time period is unlikely to be useful; this author assumes that if the patient is deemed suitable for discharge from a high-vigilance area such as a postoperative recovery room or ICU, it is reasonable to remove an airway exchange catheter. These devices should be used only in locations where it is understood that they are airway catheters, not feeding tubes.

The impetus for developing hollow exchange catheters was to permit oxygen insufflation, jet ventilation, and capnography.[11] However, there have been recent reports of patients suffering life-threatening or fatal barotrauma from these devices. Oxygen supplementation should not be undertaken lightly. It should be considered only when the patient's life is endangered by deteriorating oxygen levels and the airway manager is thoroughly familiar with the technique and its possible complications. The airway manager should also be certain about the location and depth of the catheter.[12] In general, the airway should be patent, the patient should be fully relaxed, the catheter should be proximal to the carina, and the lowest driving pressure that produces chest expansion should be used. Exhalation time should permit chest recoil to an appropriate end-expiratory volume and as few breaths as possible should be provided.

When it is unlikely that safe extubation and reintubation can be accomplished, extubation should be deferred or an elective, temporary tracheostomy should be performed. Extubation may be deferred for several days if resolution of the difficulties is anticipated. If, however, respiratory support, pulmonary toilet, airway access, patency, and protection are unlikely to recover, elective surgical management rather than an emergent intervention may be a safer alternative. This approach might be considered, for example, in a patient with an unstable cervical spine and significant upper airway or neck swelling that is unlikely to resolve within a few days. When extubation and reintubation (despite an exchange catheter) may not succeed, a multidisciplinary team should discuss the relative risks and benefits of elective tracheostomy.

If the decision is made to defer extubation, the reasons should be clearly documented, particularly if patient care must be transferred to another physician. The difficulties previously encountered or anticipated with extubation or reintubation should be clearly described in the patient's medical record and communicated directly to the receiving medical team.

Two strategies may be immediately helpful to avert the need for reintubation when moderate obstruction exists – the use of helium–oxygen and nebulized racemic epinephrine. Helium–oxygen (heliox) is less dense than air or oxygen and improves flow when turbulent conditions exist. A typical mixture is 30% oxygen–70% helium, though more oxygen can be blended if required. Nebulized racemic epinephrine (0.5 mL of 2.25% diluted in 3 mL normal saline) may also provide prompt relief, but the adverse effects, such as tachycardia, arrhythmias, ischemia, and rebound swelling may limit administration.

The Difficult Airway Society has recently published guidelines for the management of tracheal extubation that include three extubation algorithms relating to the planning, preparation, performance, and post-extubation care of "low-risk" and "at-risk" patients.[7] Planning consists of classifying the patient with respect to risk. In their formulation, at-risk patients should not be extubated while still unconscious. Preparation of the low-risk patient addresses the *patient factors* (cardiovascular, respiratory, metabolic, and neuromuscular) and *other factors* (location, skilled assistance, monitoring, and equipment). The performance includes preoxygenation, appropriate suctioning, insertion of a bite block, reversal and assessment of neuromuscular blockade, and assessment of consciousness, responsiveness, spontaneous ventilation, and airway patency.

In preparation for the extubation of the at-risk patient the airway provider must be satisfied that it is safe to proceed with extubation rather than to postpone or perform an elective surgical airway (Figure 17.2). If extubation is performed, the provider should consider the use of an "advanced technique" such as the Bailey maneuver, use of an exchange catheter, or extubation during a remifentanil infusion. A low dose of remifentanil (0.01–0.03 μg/kg per minute) may reduce agitation, coughing, and the hemodynamic stimulation associated with extubation but does not facilitate reintubation should this be required. This technique may be helpful in patients at cardiovascular or neurologic risk but must be used cautiously to avoid excessive sedation and hypoventilation.

Illustrative case (continued)

The 50-year-old obese, diabetic male who survived a witnessed cardiac arrest and was intubated by video laryngoscopy after two unsuccessful attempts has now recovered consciousness and resumed spontaneous ventilation. The airway provider should assess the adequacy of his oxygenation and spontaneous ventilation, his level of consciousness and

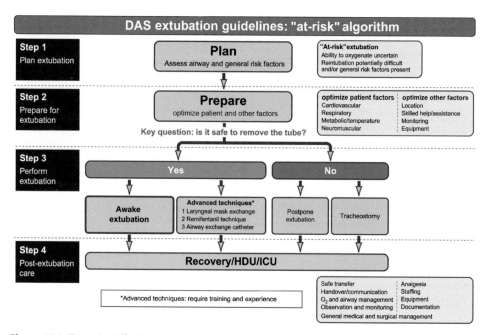

Figure 17.2 This is the Difficult Airway Society extubation algorithm for the "at-risk" patient. Reproduced with permission from Popat M. *et al.* Anaesthesia 2012;67(3);318–40.[7]

ability to protect his airway, his risk of aspiration, and his hemodynamic and metabolic stability. In this case, it is important to consider whether procedures are contemplated that might require sedation and/or neuromuscular blockade (such as diagnostic imaging).

The patient will be admitted to the CCU, a significant distance from the emergency department. Both the cardiology and neurology departments will assess the patient for cardiac catheterization and coronary intervention as well as possible brain imaging. Although he has woken up, he is still agitated and not purposeful. He likely has a full stomach and significant potential for further cardiovascular instability during coronary catheterization and agitation during neurologic scanning. A decision is made to defer extubation. A note is made in the hospital chart that describes the airway difficulties encountered and recommends that extubation be delayed until the patient is more stable, awake, and in the presence of a skilled airway provider. At such a time, the use of an airway exchange catheter would be a reasonable option.

References

1. Cooper RM, Khan SM. Extubation and reintubation of the difficult airway. In Hagberg C, editor. *Benumof and Hagberg's Airway Management*, 3rd edn. Philadelphia, PN: Elsevier-Saunders; 2012. pp. 1018–46.

2. Mort TC. Emergency tracheal intubation: complications associated with repeated laryngoscopic attempts. *Anesthesia & Analgesia*. 2004;**99**(2):607–13.

3. Sakles JC, Chiu S, Mosier J, Walker C, Stolz U, Reardon RF. The importance of first-pass success when performing orotracheal intubation in the emergency department. *Academic Emergency Medicine*. 2013;**20**(1):71–8.

4. Peterson GN, Domino KB, Caplan RA, Posner KL, Lee LA, Cheney FW. Management of the difficult airway: a closed claims analysis. *Anesthesiology*. 2005;**103**(1):33–9.

5. Cook TM, Woodall N, Frerk C. Major complications of airway management in the UK: results of the Fourth National Audit Project of the Royal College of Anaesthetists and the Difficult Airway Society. Part 1: anaesthesia. *British Journal of Anaesthesia.* 2011;**106**(5):617–31.

6. Cavallone LF, Vannucci A. Review article: extubation of the difficult airway and extubation failure. *Anesthesia & Analgesia.* 2013;**116**(2):368–83.

7. Popat M, Mitchell V, Dravid R, Patel A, Swampillai C, Higgs A. Difficult Airway Society guidelines for the management of tracheal extubation. *Anaesthesia.* 2012;**67**(3):318–40.

8. Ellard L, Cooper RM. Extubation of the difficult airway. In Glick DB, Cooper RM, Ovassapian A, editors. *The Difficult Airway: An Atlas of Tools and Techniques for Clinical Management.* New York, NY: Springer-Verlag; 2013.

9. Mort TC. Continuous airway access for the difficult extubation: the efficacy of the airway exchange catheter. *Anesthesia & Analgesia.* 2007;**105**(5):1357–62.

10. Mort TC. Tracheal tube exchange: feasibility of continuous glottic viewing with advanced laryngoscopy assistance. *Anesthesia & Analgesia.* 2009;**108**(4):1228–31.

11. Cooper RM. The use of an endotracheal ventilation catheter in the management of difficult extubations. *Canadian Journal of Anaesthesia.* 1996;**43**(1):90–3.

12. Duggan LV, Law JA, Murphy MF. Brief review: supplementing oxygen through an airway exchange catheter: efficacy, complications, and recommendations. *Canadian Journal of Anaesthesia.* 2011;**58**(6):560–8.

Management of blunt and penetrating neck trauma

Erik G. Laurin

Case presentation

A 25-year-old man is brought to the emergency department (ED) by ambulance after having been stabbed in the anterior neck 15 minutes earlier. He is otherwise healthy. He is intoxicated and agitated and difficult to fully assess. Paramedics visualized a 2-cm wound just left of midline at the level of the thyroid cartilage.

On arrival at the ED he has a firm hematoma and minimal active external bleeding. Blood intermittently bubbles from his wound with respirations, but he exhibits no audible stridor or active hemorrhage. The thyroid prominence is palpable, but tracheal anatomy is otherwise distorted from the hematoma. He has no other wounds. His vital signs show a heart rate of 130 beats per minute, blood pressure of 150/90 mmHg, respiratory rate of 26 breaths per minute, and oxygen saturation of 100% on a non-rebreather facemask at 15 L/min flow rate.

The decision is made to perform rapid sequence intubation (RSI) with a "double setup" preparation for cricothyrotomy because of the acuity of the situation and need for rapid airway control. While he is sitting upright, the patient is preoxygenated with a non-rebreather facemask at 15 L/min flow and then administered intravenous etomidate and rocuronium. Upon sedation and apnea, he is placed supine, and the anterior neck is prepped with chlorhexidine for a surgical airway, should it become necessary. The initial attempt at video laryngoscopy reveals a grade 3 Cormack–Lehane view with only the tip of the epiglottis visible and displaced to the right; a substantial amount of blood is in the airway. No better view is obtained with repositioning of the patient, and the pulse oximeter decreases to 88% saturation during an unsuccessful attempt at endotracheal tube (ETT) passage. An intubating laryngeal mask airway is attempted with a poor seal but some successful ventilations, and the pulse oximeter rises to 93%. After 10 breaths, the anterior neck develops significant subcutaneous emphysema. Blind intubation through the laryngeal mask airway is unsuccessful. The saturation is still 93%.

A more experienced intubator takes a second attempt at video laryngoscopy as the first practitioner prepares for cricothyrotomy. A Cormack–Lehane grade 3 view is again seen, with glottic deviation to the right. An intubating stylet (gum-elastic bougie) is gently advanced, and tracheal rings are palpated, with resistance to advancement at 35 cm. An ETT is advanced over the intubating stylet, cuff inflated, and stylet withdrawn. Capnography shows a normal waveform, and the oxygen saturation rises to 100% with no bubbling of air from the neck wound.

Cases in Emergency Airway Management, ed. Lauren C. Berkow and John C. Sakles. Published by Cambridge University Press. © Cambridge University Press 2015.

Discussion

Managing the airway in a patient with neck injuries is one of the most challenging scenarios for an airway practitioner. Vital structures are in close proximity, and external appearance is a notoriously poor predictor of significant internal injuries. Although common themes emerge in the evaluation and management of airways with blunt and penetrating neck injuries, there are also some important differences. In penetrating neck injury (PNI), the main focus is identification of aerodigestive and vascular injuries that may compromise the airway. In blunt neck injury (BNI), management is centered on evidence of direct airway trauma and the avoidance of secondary injuries from airway management techniques. Because of this difference, penetrating and blunt neck injuries will be discussed separately. However, a common algorithm can be utilized to approach these patients regardless of the mechanism of injury (see Figure 18.1). Although this algorithm will not capture every possible airway management technique (e.g. a neck laceration involving the trachea in which the ETT is placed directly through the wound into the trachea on first attempt), practitioners can appropriately follow the algorithm for the vast majority of injuries encountered.

After airway control, the overall management of neck trauma has shifted away from zones of injury dictating workup because many injuries cross zones and fail to predict the underlying pathology. "Hard signs" (active hemorrhage, expanding hematoma, bruit/thrill, massive hemoptysis or hematemesis, unstable airway) of significant aerodigestive or vascular injury require surgical exploration in the operating room. All others with symptoms receive computed tomography angiography imaging and intervention based on the findings. Patients with no symptoms may be observed.[1,2]

PNI

Penetrating injuries to the neck are most often from gunshot and stab wounds; only 1–5% involve the airway.[2] Signs and symptoms of airway involvement include dyspnea, hoarseness, cough, hemoptysis, drooling, subcutaneous emphysema, and tracheal deviation.[2] The decision to intubate patients with PNIs remains a clinical judgment in which the practitioner must balance the desire for early intubation with the likelihood that an injury will progress to the point of causing airway compromise. Most PNIs will not affect the airway at all. These circumstances will not be discussed here because airway management, if required, may proceed according to standard procedure.

There is no single accepted approach to airway management in PNI. Initially, the method of intubation varies based on immediate or delayed need for intubation, presence and location of aerodigestive tract involvement, amount of blood in the airway, and practitioner comfort level with advanced airway techniques. In patients who present with potentially difficult airways from PNIs, the single most important factor that affects the choice of method is the amount of time before the airway must be secured. Generally speaking, there are three broad categories of patients. First, the unresponsive patient, who has no airway reflexes and requires immediate intubation. Second, the emergent patient, who has airway reflexes, needs immediate airway management, and will require medications to facilitate intubation. Third, the urgent patient, who will need intubation, but for whom the practitioner has 10–20 minutes to fully prepare.

The first group of presenters are called, for simplicity, "unresponsive PNI" patients. Note the important distinction of the term "unresponsive": these patients are not just unconscious; they are perimortem, flaccid, and thought to be *physiologically unresponsive* to laryngoscopy

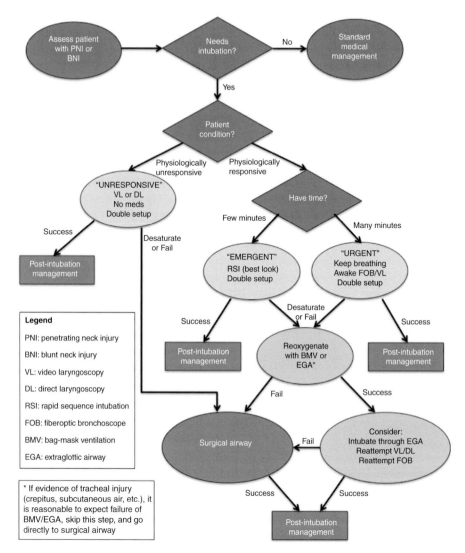

Figure 18.1 Algorithm for airway management in PNI and BNI

(i.e. would have no gag reflex or hemodynamic response). These patients should undergo immediate direct or video laryngoscopy and ETT placement without any medications. Because airway obstruction and hypoxemia may be the cause of arrest, rapid ETT placement to maintain the airway and prevent further obstruction is paramount. If available, video laryngoscopy should be used instead of direct laryngoscopy because it provides a better glottic view and the ability to facilitate intubation.[3–5] In addition, video laryngoscopy allows airway assistants to see the glottic view and help the intubator with positioning, suction, intubating stylet passage, and external laryngeal manipulation to successfully pass the ETT.

The second group of presenters are "emergent PNI" patients. They are critically ill and in need of rapid airway management. These patients have impending airway obstruction, airway hemorrhage, and altered mental status with either somnolence or combativeness. The best method of establishing a definitive airway is with a double setup.[6] RSI controls the patient quickly and allows the best possible glottic view by removing muscle tone. Every attempt should be made to administer 3 minutes of maximal preoxygenation to prolong apnea time, including high-flow oxygen (> 30 L/min by non-rebreather mask) and upright positioning to recruit alveoli.[7] If the patient is still hypoxemic despite these maneuvers, positive end-expiratory pressure (PEEP) with a bag-mask and PEEP valve can be used for preoxygenation. If there is concern for tracheal injury, such as subcutaneous emphysema or crepitus, the practitioner should monitor the patient closely to ensure that positive airway pressure does not cause massive neck subcutaneous emphysema, which may make intubation more difficult. Preoxygenation before paralysis is so important that the presence of subcutaneous emphysema in a hypoxic patient is not a strict contraindication to positive-pressure ventilation, but practitioners should attempt to limit the amount of additional subcutaneous emphysema during preoxygenation by putting direct pressure on the tracheal injury site (e.g. finger plugging the tracheal laceration). On the other hand, if tracheal injury is less of a concern than impending obstruction from hematomas, then positive-pressure ventilation may stent the airway open and provide improved oxygenation and ventilation. Prevention of desaturation during laryngoscopy should be addressed with a nasal cannula placed at 5–15 L/min flow for apneic oxygenation. An intubating stylet (bougie) is often helpful for finding the airway when glottic views are poor or obstructed. The small diameter of the intubating stylet increases "steerability" within the hypopharynx to maximize success in reaching the glottic opening, and tactile confirmation of tracheal placement – even without visual confirmation – ensures successful intubation.[8]

If initial attempts fail and the patient needs reoxygenation, bag-mask ventilation or an extraglottic airway (EGA) should be used with extreme caution. The cuff of the EGA may not seal if the glottic anatomy is distorted from hematomas, and subcutaneous emphysema of the neck may develop from even very small tracheal injuries. With the neck prepped and ready for cricothyrotomy, a surgical airway can proceed quickly if oxygenation fails or orotracheal intubation is deemed impossible. This technique is called a "double setup" because the airway is ready to be secured through the oropharynx or, if unsuccessful, through a cricothyrotomy.

The third group of presenters are called "urgent PNI" patients. These patients will require intubation but can be fully prepped for 10–20 minutes prior to ETT passage. They should undergo the preferred method, intubation with a fiberoptic bronchoscope (FOB). The FOB, when introduced orally or nasally, allows the practitioner to visualize the upper airway, determine the extent and location of injury, traverse deviated glottic openings, visualize the tracheal mucosa for signs of injury, and advance an ETT over the FOB to a confirmed depth in the trachea. FOBs are especially useful if the patient has a tracheal injury because the scope can be carefully advanced, under direct visualization, past the location of injury to secure a path for the ETT; the concern is that pushing an ETT into a lacerated trachea can convert a partial injury into a complete, circumferential injury, in which case the inferior portion of the trachea may retract, making intubation impossible.

Performing a FOB intubation takes time. Proper preparation involves anesthetizing three main areas: the mouth or nose (depending on which route is selected), the posterior pharynx, and the hypopharynx. Lidocaine is the preferred agent and is administered by atomizer, nebulizer, gel, and/or paste to the various portions of the airway. Systemic sedation or ketamine dissociation is also often required, but the airway practitioner must be very judicious to prevent respiratory depression or loss of airway muscle tone through oversedation. Therefore, backup plans must be discussed in case of failed FOB intubation. Typically, these include video laryngoscopy, direct laryngoscopy, EGAs, or surgical airway.

Several factors may make FOB intubation difficult, including excessive blood or secretions, poor patient cooperation, and inability to advance the FOB into the trachea. In some cases, the patient will have enough airway bleeding to prevent FOB use but not so much hemorrhage to require immediate airway control. In these situations, it may be possible to perform an awake intubation with a video laryngoscope or direct laryngoscope. Topical anesthesia, mild systemic sedation or ketamine dissociation (only if needed), plenty of suction, and an intubating stylet are vital. Laryngoscopes, especially video laryngoscopes, can provide glottic views in the presence of far more blood than a FOB can. Again, backup plans of EGA or surgical airway must be discussed and ready for use.

Because some time is available for urgent PNI patients, it is often best to transport them to the operating room for airway control. Multiple specialists with expertise in difficult FOB intubations and challenging surgical airways can be at the patient's bedside.

In the overall management of unresponsive, emergent, and urgent PNI patients, it is important to recognize that if a difficult airway is anticipated and does not need immediate control, the preferred method of intubation is awake, with either a FOB or a video laryngoscope. Spontaneous breathing maintains oxygen saturation and airway muscle tone, preventing obstruction. If excessive sedation or paralytics are used for airway management, the airway practitioner needs to be aware that "the bridge is burned" and, if intubation fails and reoxygenation is required, many pitfalls exist that may necessitate a surgical airway.

If a surgical airway is required, no particular technique has been shown to be more effective than others. Possible methods include the standard surgical ("no-drop") technique, rapid four-step technique, bougie-guided technique, and Melker percutaneous technique. A few scenarios should be considered:

- Tracheal landmarks easily palpated. Any method should be successful.
- Tracheal landmarks obscured. Perform a vertical midline skin incision and find tracheal landmarks with fingertips. Once identified, perform the cricothyrotomy with the technique of choice. Alternatively, if time permits, ultrasound may be used to find the tracheal landmarks, and the surgical airway can proceed with the desired method.
- Stab wound with visible airway penetration. In these rare cases, a tracheostomy tube or 6.0 mm ETT can be placed through the wound and into the trachea. To prevent false tract formation and confirm tracheal location, advance an intubating stylet into the wound first to confirm tracheal placement, and then place the ETT.
- Cricothyroid disruption. If the cricothyroid region is fractured or landmarks are impossible to determine, and tracheal intubation is unsuccessful from above, then a low surgical airway, or emergency tracheostomy, may be indicated. Ideally, this procedure should be performed in the operating room by experienced surgeons. If time does not permit patient transport, then it can be performed in the ED with an open surgical technique. Anticipate having to cut deep to get to the trachea, as the trachea is not a superficial structure in the lower neck. An intubating introducer may be advanced into the deep incision to confirm tracheal placement – with tactile clicks and stop sign (see 'Special considerations for PNI') – before a 6.0 mm ETT is threaded over it. Alternatively, a Melker (Seldinger method) percutaneous cricothyrotomy may be

favored, owing to the depth of the trachea near the sternal notch, and finding it with a midline needle may be more appealing than with deep scalpel incisions. Note that this is not a "needle tracheostomy," but instead involves the use of a Melker kit in which a proper tracheostomy tube is placed in the trachea.

With any surgical airway, the practitioner should anticipate poor or no visualization of airway structures. Blood typically fills the surgical field and forces the practitioner to do the procedure under tactile guidance alone. Universal precautions are vital, including complete eye and face protection, as any ventilation attempts during cricothyrotomy can aerosolize blood from the neck incision onto the practitioner. These procedures should be practiced under similar strenuous conditions with full universal precautions to simulate realistic clinical conditions.

Special considerations for PNI

Intubating stylet: The use of an intubating stylet is important in any patient with PNI who may have tracheal disruption. The intubator can advance the intubating stylet carefully and gently down the trachea, feeling tracheal rings ("tactile clicks"), until the stylet reaches a small bronchus and cannot be advanced further ("stop sign"). The intubating stylet secures a track for the larger ETT, which is advanced over the intubating stylet into the trachea. If the ETT makes contact with the tracheal walls and causes more tracheal disruption, at least the intubating stylet is far past the carina and may guide the ETT into the distal segment of the trachea to successfully establish an airway.

Blind nasotracheal intubation: Although now uncommon for emergency airway management, this technique may still be useful for practitioners experienced in this skill. A 2004 study found an overall success rate of 90% in PNI patients, with a mean number of attempts of 1.1 (range 1–4).[9] It is reasonable to consider this technique if no other option exists and the patient needs intubation. The risk is that manipulating hematomas may cause hemorrhage or further disruption of the airway.

Blind digital intubation: In cases of severe airway hemorrhage, direct and video laryngoscopy sometimes fail. It is possible to digitally intubate if the patient is paralyzed and unable to bite, and the practitioner has long enough fingers. This procedure is best performed with an intubating stylet because it is easier to manipulate in a small space than an ETT is. It also provides tactile feedback (tactile clicks and stop sign) of successful placement in the trachea before an ETT is advanced.

Cervical spine immobilization: Patients with neurologic deficits from PNIs should be placed in cervical immobilization, but patients without deficits do not require immobilization. The risk of unstable cervical spine injuries in PNIs is very low, and the deficits typically occur at the time of the injury. It is exceedingly unlikely for a neurologically intact patient to have an unstable spine injury or for the practitioner to cause further injury in the absence of a cervical collar. More likely, the collar will cause harm by obscuring an expanding hematoma or other significant findings of a PNI.[10]

BNI

Blunt trauma to the neck resulting in airway injury is rare, and if the airway is compromised, the injuries are usually fatal at the scene. The most common mechanism of injury is a motor vehicle collision, with external crushing of airway structures between the automobile (dashboard, steering wheel, seat belt, or airbag) and the cervical vertebrae. Other common methods of injury are hanging, chokeholds, direct blows, and clothesline injuries on vehicles or bicycles. Other than direct blunt force trauma to the airway, vascular injuries from blunt force trauma can cause hematomas that then compress the airway and cause obstruction.[2]

Signs and symptoms of airway involvement include dyspnea, hoarseness, cough, hemoptysis, drooling, subcutaneous emphysema, laryngeal crepitus or asymmetry, and tracheal deviation. In the absence of clinical instability requiring operative exploration, the overall management of BNI involves securing the airway and using computed tomography angiography to delineate the injuries.

The overall approach to the airway in patients with BNI is similar to that in patients with PNI. "Unresponsive BNI" patients (perimortem, flaccid, no airway reflexes) receive direct or video laryngoscopy without medications. "Emergent BNI" patients who require immediate intubation receive RSI with a double setup. In both cases, a surgical airway is anticipated and equipment is open and ready.

"Urgent BNI" patients are more stable but still require intubation in 10–20 minutes. FOB intubation is the preferred method for visualizing and securing the airway, as long as the patient can cooperate and blood is not excessive. Use of a FOB allows the airway practitioner to evaluate the level of injury, steer through damaged tissue to find the lumen of the trachea, and provide a path for an ETT to follow, thereby preventing the ETT from creating a false passage.

The location and severity of injury are the most important factors in assessing a difficult airway from BNI. Unlike for PNI, in which airway obstruction, deviation, hemorrhage, or laceration are the most worrisome findings, airway compromise in patients with BNI is often caused by crushing of the airway, laryngeal fractures, and massive subcutaneous air. Manual in-line stabilization of the cervical spine is required because an unstable cervical spine injury is possible, making laryngoscopy technically more difficult.

The intubator should closely assess the location of injury. If the injury is at the level of, or superior to, the larynx, then laryngoscopy may be difficult or impossible. If the injury is inferior to the larynx, then laryngoscopy may be possible, but ETT passage may be disrupted below the vocal cords – an area very difficult to assess with direct or video laryngoscopy.

Maximal preoxygenation is especially important in patients who have BNI and any signs of airway injury because tracheal perforation or rupture will make reoxygenation with positive-pressure ventilation extremely difficult owing to anatomical distortion from subcutaneous air. Therefore, practitioners should use high-flow oxygen and a "head-up" reverse Trendelenburg position with cervical spine precautions. This is the best method to recruit alveoli and provide a reservoir of oxygen in the lungs for the patient to draw upon during apnea. Additionally, apneic oxygenation with a nasal cannula at 5–15 L/min flow is highly recommended. These interventions will minimize the risk of desaturation and the need for attempts at reoxygenation.

If a surgical airway is necessary, then distortion of anatomical landmarks is the typical challenge. As in PNI, data are insufficient to clearly support one surgical technique over another. However, with the specific issues of laryngeal fracture and tracheal disruption, an intubating-stylet-guided technique may be the most theoretically advantageous because the intubating stylet may help practitioners to identify the lumen of the trachea through clicks and a stop sign; it also allows a 6.0 mm ETT to pass over it without creating a false passage. If the glottic area has major disruption, then using a Melker kit for a tracheostomy below the level of injury may be the method of choice.

Special considerations for BNI

Intubating stylets: These are useful in BNI as in PNI for similar reasons. Poor visualization may be overcome by passing the intubating stylet as anteriorly as possible and confirming tracheal placement tactilely. Likewise, the intubator can take advantage of the small diameter and tactile feedback to navigate an intubating stylet down the trachea gently – while paying close attention to tactile clicks and a stop sign at 30 to 40 cm depth to confirm tracheal placement – rather than unknowingly entering a tracheal laceration, creating a false passage from excessive force, and ending up with a paratracheal ETT placement.

Cervical spine movement and laryngoscopic device: The choice of device to intubate patients with BNI and potential cervical spine injury is often discussed. Further neurologic deterioration or secondary injury through excessive cervical spine movement has been studied well with many devices, and the incidence of further injury with intubation is exceedingly low.[11] The only method that may potentially minimize cervical spine movement during intubation is FOB intubation, but this technique requires time and a cooperative patient. Video laryngoscopy, regardless of device, along with lighted stylets or intubating EGAs, likely does not offer much clinically significant benefit over direct laryngoscopy for minimizing cervical spine movement.[11] This research is difficult to perform because of the infrequency of unstable injuries and variability of injury type. Additionally, it is difficult to establish a causal relationship between device and injury in the presence of other confounding factors, such as the quality of manual in-line stabilization. Furthermore, specific patient characteristics and situations may make one particular device more successful than another. Therefore, with all of these factors to consider, no one device can be recommended for the highest first-attempt success with the least cervical spine movement.

Summary

Airway practitioners who care for patients with penetrating and blunt neck injuries must thoroughly assess the nature and location of injury before deciding on the proper approach to secure the airway. Although no single device or technique has been shown to be clearly superior, different situations may favor one approach over another. Flexible bronchoscopic awake intubation is preferred in stable patients because it enables the intubator to find the airway and visualize injuries. For patients who require immediate intubation, video laryngoscopy has many advantages over direct laryngoscopy, including improved glottic views. Whichever method is used, maximizing preoxygenation to prevent desaturation, using intubating stylets for difficult or disrupted airways, and early preparation for a surgical airway are the mainstays of clinical care.

Successful management of these patients requires significant preparation by the individual practitioner, and a consistent, systems-level approach. A multidisciplinary protocol should be established that involves emergency medicine, anesthesiology, trauma surgery, and otolaryngology. If time permits, airway management is often best performed in the operating room with multiple highly trained airway specialists present. If the airway must be secured immediately, then airway management should occur in the ED. Each hospital needs its own unique strategies regarding which personnel will respond and which techniques will be utilized based on provider training and availability, expertise with advanced airway equipment, and familiarity with difficult airway management.

References

1. K. Inaba, B. Branco, J. Menaker, *et al.* Evaluation of multidetector computed tomography for penetrating neck injury: a prospective multicenter study. *J Trauma* 2012; **72**(3): 576–84.

2. N. Rathlev, R. Medzon, M. Bracken. Evaluation and management of neck trauma. *Emerg Med Clin North Am* 2007; **25**: 679–94.

3. M. Kaplan, C. Hagberg, D. Ward, *et al.* Comparison of direct and video-assisted views of the larynx during routine intubation. *J Clin Anesth* 2006; **18**(5): 357–62.

4. J. A. Law, N. Broemling, R. Cooper, *et al.* The difficult airway with recommendations for management – Part 2 – the anticipated difficult airway. *Can J Anaesth* 2013; **60**: 1119–38.

5. C. Brown, A. Bair, D. Pallin, *et al.* Improved glottic exposure with the video Macintosh laryngoscope in adult emergency department tracheal intubations. *Ann Emerg Med* 2010; **56**(2): 83–8.

6. D. Mandavia, S. Qualls, I. Rokos. Emergency airway management in penetrating neck trauma. *Ann Emerg Med* 2000; **35**(3): 221–5.

7. S. Weingart, R. Levitan. Preoxygenation and prevention of desaturation during emergency airway management. *Ann Emerg Med* 2012; **59**(3): 165–75.

8. Y. Daniel, S. de Regloix, E. Kaiser. Use of a gum elastic bougie in a penetrating neck trauma. *Prehosp Disaster Med* 2014; **29**(2): 212–13.

9. N. Weitzel, J. Kendall, P. Pons. Blind nasotracheal intubation for patients with penetrating neck trauma. *J Trauma* 2004; **56**(5): 1097–101.

10. J. Brywczynski, T. Barrett, J. Lyon, B. Cotton. Management of penetrating neck injury in the emergency department: a structured literature review. *Emerg Med J* 2008; **25**: 711–15.

11. A. Robitaille. Airway management in the patient with potential cervical spine instability: continuing professional development. *Can J Anaesth* 2011; **58**: 1125–39.

Airway management of patients with smoke inhalation

Jarrod M. Mosier

Case presentation

A 22-year-old male is brought into the emergency department (ED) by ambulance after being rescued from a house fire near the university campus. The patient was at a college party when the house fire started and was trapped inside the building for approximately 30 minutes before emergency medical services arrived. On presentation, the patient's respiratory rate is 32 breaths per minute, heart rate is 112 beats per minute, blood pressure is 111/68 mmHg, and oxygen saturation is 87% on a non-rebreather. On examination, the patient has no areas of burned skin. Head and neck examination show no soot in the nares or singed nasal hairs; however, oral examination reveals some soot in the oropharynx. Airway examination reveals no change in voice or stridor; however, wheezing can be heard throughout all lung fields.

Introduction

Patients with smoke inhalation present a diagnostic and therapeutic challenge to the physicians who care for them. Smoke inhalation has varying pathophysiology, and its effects are difficult to predict clinically. Most deaths at the scene of a fire (60–80%) result from smoke inhalation, likely owing to the inhalation of asphyxiants carried by the smoke.[1] Up to one-third of patients who present to the hospital with inhalational injury have acute airway obstruction.[2] Thus, the dilemma when diagnosing smoke inhalational injury is predicting which patients require emergent airway stabilization.

Smoke inhalation causes three distinct pathophysiologic processes: (1) thermal injury to the structures of the upper airway (mouth, oropharynx, larynx); (2) tracheo-bronchial and parenchymal injuries from toxicity induced directly or indirectly by chemicals carried in the smoke; and (3) metabolic asphyxiation induced by tissue hypoxia from asphyxiants, such as cyanide or carbon monoxide carried in the smoke.[3] The mucosal surface area of the upper airway (nasopharynx and oropharynx) allows for rapid dissipation of heat with each breath. However, smoke carries more thermal energy than dry air does. Consequently, it overwhelms the upper airway and damages the structures. As such, thermal injury to the upper airway is most immediately concerning in the first 12 to 24 hours after inhalation because patients are at risk of acute airway obstruction.[2,4]

Cases in Emergency Airway Management, ed. Lauren C. Berkow and John C. Sakles. Published by Cambridge University Press. © Cambridge University Press 2015.

Table 19.1 Symptoms and physical examination

Finding	Risk of intubation	Existing data*,¶
Facial burns	High	65% of patients with inhalation injury had burns to the face.[5] 37% (7/19) of patients with burns to the face required intubation.[6]
Soot in nose or mouth	High	Present in 44% of patients with inhalation injury.[5] Soot in the nose was not associated with intubation (22%, 6/27); however, soot in mouth was (55%, 6/11).[6]
Vocal fold edema	High	Laryngoscopic examinations performed on only 20 of 108 patients, yet laryngeal edema was present 60% of the time.[5] Edema of the true vocal cords was associated with intubation in 75% (6/8) of cases; edema of the false vocal cords was associated with intubation in 57% (4/7) of cases.[6]
Stridor	Moderate	Present in only 5% of patients;[5] however, required intubation 33% (1/3) of the time.[6]
Drooling	Moderate	Associated with intubation in 50% (1/2) of cases.[6]
Dysphagia	Moderate	Associated with intubation in 50% (1/2) of cases.[6]
Voice change	Low	Present in 19% of patients with suspected inhalation injury,[5] yet only required intubation in 25% (4/16) of patients.[6]

* Review of 108 patients with diagnoses of "burn," "smoke exposure," or "smoke inhalation" admitted to a burn center over a 10-year period.[5]

¶ Review of 41 patients over a 5-year period in which otolaryngology was consulted to perform indirect laryngoscopy on patients with suspected inhalation injury.[6]

Diagnosis

Diagnosis of thermal upper airway injury is difficult because the classic signs and symptoms can be unreliable. The classic symptoms of stridor, voice change, dysphagia, and drooling are present in only a minority (3–19%) of patients with inhalational injury.[5,6] Physical examination findings of facial burns, carbonaceous sputum or soot in the nose or mouth, and wheezing are present in many patients with inhalational injury.[5] However, only burns to the face and soot in the oropharynx have been shown to be associated with a need for intubation.[6] Unfortunately, data on this topic are lacking, and it is difficult to draw definitive conclusions regarding clinical practice from the data that are available (Table 19.1). As history and physical examination are unreliable, a fiberoptic examination of the airway is warranted. Edema of either the true or false vocal cords suggests an impending upper airway obstruction and is significantly associated with the need for intubation.[6] Carbon monoxide and carboxyhemoglobin levels should not be used to predict the need for intubation as they are metabolic asphyxiants rather than indicators of the degree of thermal upper airway injury.

Airway management

If smoke inhalation injury is a concern, intubation is indicated for several reasons. Patients who present with altered mental status may be intoxicated from substance use prior to the smoke exposure or, more seriously, may have encephalopathy from inhaled asphyxiants. Thus, these patients should have their airway secured if there is any concern for airway protection or further mental status deterioration. Intubation is indicated for patients who have respiratory failure secondary to lower airway and parenchymal injury caused by caustic smoke particulates and chemicals. Intubation allows for improved pulmonary hygiene, airway clearance, and frequent bronchoscopy, which is needed because of mucosal sloughing, coagulation, and thick mucus formation. Patients with large body-surface-area burns should be intubated regardless of smoke inhalation, as large-volume resuscitation often leads to respiratory failure from pulmonary edema. Deciding whether to intubate a patient for thermal injury to the upper airway, either prophylactically or therapeutically, is difficult. Figure 19.1 provides a clinical pathway for airway management in patients with smoke inhalation.

Because acute airway obstruction can occur within minutes of smoke inhalation, patients with facial burns, large body-surface-area burns, soot in the nose or mouth, and signs or symptoms of inhalation injury (i.e. stridor, hoarseness, wheezing, dysphagia) should be considered for prophylactic intubation. Waiting until the condition progresses can lead to an intubation that is procedurally more difficult. Medication choice for intubation of these patients is not without consequence. Patients with burns are generally volume depleted. Consequently, they may have a profound hypotensive response to intubation and transition to positive-pressure ventilation. Ketamine is an attractive induction agent for patients with smoke inhalation because it has sympathomimetic effects and can be administered during an awake airway examination. Neuromuscular blockers may improve overall intubating conditions and, if rapid sequence intubation is chosen, either rocuronium or succinylcholine can be used. Despite the concern for critical hyperkalemia in burn patients, succinylcholine is safe in the first 24 hours after a burn.

The device choices for intubation are many. In the absence of tongue or epiglottis swelling, direct laryngoscopy can be used. However, if tongue or epiglottis swelling is present, video laryngoscopy will likely provide a better view of the airway and allow for intubation in patients who would previously have required cricothyrotomy. Flexible fiber-optic bronchoscopes allow for either transoral or transnasal access to the airway. If a flexible bronchoscope is used, the patient should remain upright and breathing spontaneously. A neuromuscular blocker should not be used. During intubation, patients can be sedated with an opioid such as fentanyl and small doses of a sedative (ketamine, midazolam); a topical anesthetic should also be used. If possible, the transoral approach should be used because it permits the use of larger tracheal tube sizes, which are useful for airway clearance as tracheal tubes in inhalational injury patients are prone to obstruction due to secretions and mucosal sloughing. A laryngoscope (either direct or video) can be used to compress the tongue and displace the epiglottis while a second operator uses a fiberoptic bronchoscope as a stylet to intubate around the laryngoscope. This approach is an excellent option for several reasons: (1) it allows for increased sedation and neuromuscular blockade, (2) it allows for transoral intubation in patients who have upper airway edema and in whom operators find it difficult to visualize the airway with direct laryngoscopy or direct the tube to the airway with video laryngoscopy, and (3) it can be performed relatively easily by operators with little skill in flexible fiberoptic intubations. Cricothyrotomy is indicated if the patient has airway

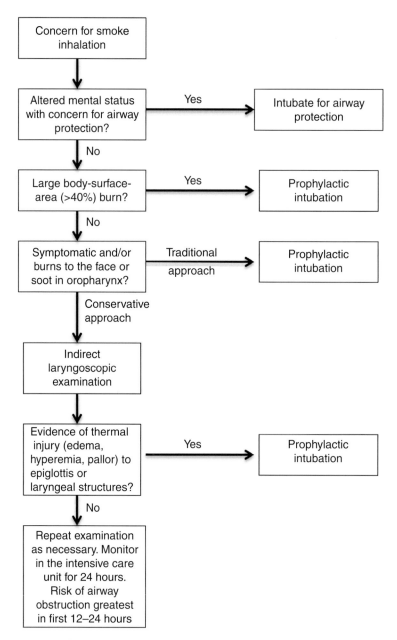

Figure 19.1 Algorithm for airway management in smoke inhalation

obstruction caused by laryngeal edema or the operator cannot visualize the airway or direct the tracheal tube through the glottic entrance.

For a more conservative approach, clinicians can also perform a laryngoscopic examination in asymptomatic patients without large surface-area burns, patients with isolated facial burns, symptomatic patients, or patients with soot in the oropharynx. The nasopharynx can be anesthetized with topical anesthesia (e.g. 4% lidocaine gel or atomized lidocaine in each nostril), and lubricated to allow easy access to the airway through the transnasal route. A fiberoptic endoscope is then inserted into the naris and advanced until a view of the airway is obtained. The clinician should evaluate for edema, hyperemia, or pallor of the epiglottis and laryngeal inlet. Patients who have edema of the epiglottis or vocal cords will likely have airway obstruction and should be intubated. Because the airway edema from thermal injuries peaks at 24 hours, repeated examinations may be necessary.

Post-intubation care of patients with smoke inhalation injury is critical. Properly securing the endotracheal tube is important, as loss of the airway can be catastrophic. Adhesive will likely not adhere to facial skin that has been burned; therefore, cotton ties should be used and must be checked frequently as facial and neck edema worsens. The airway should be cleared by frequent suctioning and/or bronchoscopy because the tracheal tube frequently becomes occluded by coagulated blood, sloughed mucosa, and thick mucus. Acetylcysteine and bronchoscopic lavage may be helpful for secretion management. Mechanical ventilation management should be aimed at limiting tidal volume (V_T) and plateau pressures to lung protective goals (V_T 6 mL/kg, plateau pressure < 30 cm H_2O). Bronchodilators may be helpful if the patient has wheezing caused by smooth muscle irritation and edema from smoke inhalation. Rescue modes of ventilation (i.e. airway pressure release ventilation) may be needed for refractory hypoxemia.

Case resolution

Although the patient has altered mental status, it is difficult to determine if he has ingested alcohol or drugs at the college party or if he has inhaled metabolic asphyxiants. His tachypnea and tachycardia suggest moderate critical illness systemically, and his persistent hypoxemia despite the non-rebreather mask indicates the presence of shunt physiology. Because of his wheezing, the shunt physiology is likely caused by ventilation–perfusion mismatch with bronchospasm and secretions induced by either chemical irritation from the smoke particles or chemical injury from toxicants in the smoke. He was administered bronchodilators, which improved the wheezing and oxygen saturation, and was placed on a high-flow nasal cannula at 30 L/min for preoxygenation. Given the wheezing and signs of lower airway injury, physicians were concerned that he may have upper airway involvement. Therefore, they anesthetized the nasopharynx with 4% lidocaine gel and performed indirect laryngoscopy with a fiberoptic bronchoscope. Bronchoscopy revealed soot in the oropharynx and vocal cords, as well as edema and hyperemia of the vocal cords and epiglottis, all signs of thermal injury. They decided to intubate using rapid sequence intubation and secured the airway. The patient developed significant tongue and epiglottis swelling, and then, 18 hours after admission, he developed acute respiratory distress syndrome owing to parenchymal injury and capillary leak. He remained intubated for 5 days in the intensive care unit.

References

1. Anseeuw K, Delvau N, Burillo-Putze G, et al. Cyanide poisoning by fire smoke inhalation: a European expert consensus. *Eur J Emerg Med.* 2013;**20**(1):2–9.

2. Cochran A. Inhalation injury and endotracheal intubation. *J Burn Care Res.* 2009;**30**(1):190–1.

3. Cancio LC. Airway management and smoke inhalation injury in the burn patient. *Clin Plast Surg.* 2009;**36**(4):555–67.

4. Antonio AC, Castro PS, Freire LO. Smoke inhalation injury during enclosed-space fires: an update. *J. Bras Pneumol.* 2013;**39**(3):373–81.

5. Clark WR, Bonaventura M, Myers W. Smoke inhalation and airway management at a regional burn unit: 1974–1983. Part I: diagnosis and consequences of smoke inhalation. *J Burn Care Rehabil.* 1989;**10**(1):52–62.

6. Madnani DD, Steele NP, de Vries E. Factors that predict the need for intubation in patients with smoke inhalation injury. *Ear Nose Throat J.* 2006;**85**(4):278–80.

Airway management in cervical spine injury

Jaime Daly and Keith J. Ruskin

Case presentation

A 27-year-old male cyclist is brought to the emergency department after a high-speed collision with a car. On admission, he is awake and alert with a heart rate of 115 beats per minute, blood pressure of 142/78 mmHg, respiratory rate of 20 breaths per minute, and oxygen saturation of 99% on a 4-L nasal cannula. A cervical collar, placed by the paramedics, is correctly positioned. He also has a left-sided open femur fracture. The patient is neurologically intact but complains of severe pain from his femur fracture. His medical history is unremarkable.

Introduction

Traumatic spinal cord injury occurs in the United States at a rate of 28 to 50 injuries per million people per year. Most of these injuries occur after motor vehicle collision, but they also occur in falls, diving injuries, and sports injuries. Approximately 55% of spinal injuries occur in the cervical region, and approximately 10% of patients with a cervical spine fracture have a second, noncontiguous vertebral column fracture.[1] The anatomy of the cervical spine is shown in Figure 20.1.

Several types of cervical spine injuries can occur. The first is atlanto-occipital dislocation. Patients with this injury suffer craniocervical disruption and rarely survive. This type of dislocation results from severe traumatic flexion and distraction of the cervical spine from the skull. The second is the atlas (C1) fracture. Fractures of the atlas represent around 5% of acute cervical spine fractures. Also, approximately 40% of C1 fractures are associated with fractures of the axis. The most common C1 fracture is a burst fracture. This type of injury is usually caused by an axial loading injury, meaning that either a heavy load lands on the head of the patient or (more commonly) the patient falls and lands on his head, such as in a diving accident. This injury is best seen on the axial views of a computed tomography (CT) scan. A burst fracture is considered unstable even though the spinal cord is rarely injured. Patients with this type of injury must wear a cervical collar. A unilateral ring or lateral mass fracture of C1 is not unstable but is treated as an unstable fracture until proven otherwise. The third type of cervical spine injury is C1 rotary subluxation. This injury is most often seen in children with torticollis. The head should not be forced to midline but instead immobilized in the rotated position.

Cases in Emergency Airway Management, ed. Lauren C. Berkow and John C. Sakles. Published by Cambridge University Press. © Cambridge University Press 2015.

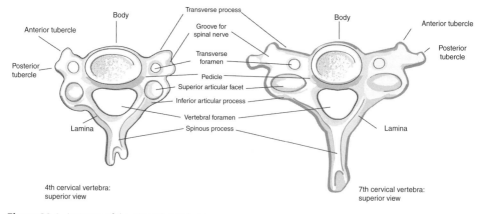

Figure 20.1 Anatomy of the cervical vertebrae

The fourth type of fracture is an axis (C2) fracture. The axis is the largest cervical vertebra and is the most unusual in shape. Acute fractures of C2 represent 18% of all cervical spine injuries. Odontoid fractures are often secondary to motor vehicle accidents or falls and make up 60% of C2 fractures. The odontoid process is a peg-shaped protuberance of the axis that is usually in contact with the anterior arch of C1. It is held in place mostly by the transverse ligament. This injury can be seen on axial CT scans. Type 1 odontoid fractures involve the tip of the odontoid and are rare. They are most often treated with a hard C collar for 6–8 weeks. Type II odontoid fractures occur through the base of the dens and are the most common type of odontoid fractures. These fractures can be managed either medically or surgically. A halo vest is often used for this type of injury and remains in place for 12–16 weeks. Type III odontoid fractures occur at the base of the dens and extend into the body of C2. These fractures require surgical management.[2]

The *hangman's fracture* (posterior element fracture of C2) represents 20% of all C2 fractures and usually is caused by an injury that results in overextension such as a high-speed motor vehicle collision during which the head impacts the windshield. This injury is considered to be an unstable fracture. The remainder of the C2 injuries are composed of fractures of the pedicle, lateral mass, laminae, and spinous processes.[2]

The fifth type of injury includes fractures and dislocations of C3–C7. C3 and C4 fractures are relatively uncommon, possibly because these vertebrae are less mobile than are C5–C7, which act like the fulcrum of the cervical spine. The greatest amount of flexion and extension occur at C5 and C6. In adults, cervical vertebral fractures occur most commonly at the level of C5. Subluxation occurs most commonly at C5 on C6. Rarely will a ligamentous injury occur in this part of the spine without an associated fracture. It is also noteworthy that in this part of the spine facet dislocation is associated with an increased incidence of neurologic injury.

Determining the presence and severity of a cervical spine injury

It is possible to rule out a cervical spine injury in a neurologically intact patient who is awake and alert with no other distracting injuries. The absence of pain or tenderness along the cervical spine virtually excludes the presence of a significant injury. It is also important to rule out a neurologic deficit such as weakness, numbness, and/or tingling of the extremities. Palpating the spine and having the patient demonstrate a full range of neck motion usually reveals whether or not an injury is present. Pain associated with a secondary injury may distract the patient, rendering the physical examination less accurate. Knowing the mechanism of injury and obtaining CT imaging is important in the evaluation of cervical spine injury. Immobilization is required until an injury can be determined by physical examination or by CT imaging if physical examination is inconclusive, the Glasgow Coma Scale (GCS) is reduced, or a distracting injury is present.[3]

Diagnostic tests to evaluate cervical spine injury

Cervical spine imaging is required for all trauma patients who have midline neck pain, tenderness on palpation, or neurologic deficits referable to the cervical spine. Patients who are intoxicated or have an altered level of consciousness (GCS 14 or less) should also undergo radiologic imaging to rule out injury.[3] CT scans of the cervical spine may be used to determine the presence of an unstable cervical spine injury. Significant instability is unlikely if CT images are normal. Magnetic resonance imaging (MRI) can detect ligamentous injury and is indicated if a neurologic deficit is present, but MRI is not usually available in the acute trauma setting. CT and MRI images must be of good quality and should be interpreted by a qualified radiologist.

Evaluation of the airway in patients with a suspected cervical spine injury

Respiratory complications are the most common cause of increased morbidity and mortality in patients with cervical spine injuries. Therefore, it is critical to evaluate the patient's airway and breathing. The first step is to determine whether or not a patient can speak. A patient who can communicate coherently and speak in a normal voice is unlikely to be in immediate danger. The initial assessment in an unconscious patient should include evaluation for impaired respiration. If airflow is absent, the airway should be opened by jaw thrust and not head tilt, as this can exacerbate an existing cervical spine injury. A recent study showed that there was almost twice as much angular motion in all planes of the cervical spine during a head tilt as during a jaw thrust.[4] Specifically, subluxation was greater at the site of spinal injury during a head tilt.

The oral pharynx should be cleared of any foreign bodies, secretions, or dislodged teeth. Breathing should be assessed by observing the patient for bilateral and coordinated chest wall movement. Placement of a pulse oximeter and end-tidal CO_2 monitor can also be helpful to assess oxygenation and ventilation. Patients who are not breathing adequately must be assisted with supplemental oxygen and bag-mask ventilation while they are prepared for definitive airway management.

Effect of injury location on respiratory status

Spinal injuries above the level of C3 cause diaphragmatic paralysis, severely compromising inspiratory and expiratory muscle function after injury. This patient population will become permanently ventilator dependent. Lower cervical spine injuries at the level of C4–C5 usually result in disruption of diaphragmatic and inspiratory muscle innervation and can also cause respiratory compromise. A recent study showed that delayed apnea developed hours after injury in patients with mid to lower cervical spine injuries. This may have been caused by edema of the ascending spinal cord, which subsequently involved higher cervical nerve roots.[1] Patients with complete cervical spine injury above C6 are likely to require tracheostomy.[2]

When and where should the airway be managed?

If the patient is stable, his or her airway should ideally be managed in the operating room or other controlled environment. If that patient is unstable or deteriorating, however, it may be necessary to manage the airway in the emergency department. Skilled personnel and a variety of airway tools (e.g. fiberoptic bronchoscope, video laryngoscope, cricothyrotomy set) should be immediately available. The surgical team should be available if attempts at intubation are unsuccessful and a surgical airway is urgently required. If time permits, all personnel on the team should be briefed on the airway management plan as well as all contingency plans.

Securing the patient's airway

Orotracheal intubation, when performed correctly, permits the airway to be controlled rapidly and safely.[5] Awake intubation with a fiberoptic bronchoscope results in the least manipulation of the neck but requires a cooperative and stable patient. Other video-assisted devices, such as a video laryngoscope, may improve the Cormack–Lehane grade and increase the success of intubation in a patient who is asleep.[6] An intubating stylet is also a good option because it requires less forceful laryngoscopy. Manual in-line stabilization (MILS) is recommended with each of the above approaches. The clinician responsible for securing the airway should use an approach with which he or she is experienced and comfortable.

Protecting the patient's neck during intubation

Trauma patients should be assumed to have a cervical spine injury until proven otherwise. MILS has been the standard approach to cervical spine stabilization during intubation of patients with suspected or known cervical spine injuries. The goal of MILS is to apply support to the head and neck sufficient to reduce movement that might occur during intubation. MILS requires having an assistant at the head or side of the bed. The patient is supine with his/her head and neck in a neutral position. The assistant at the head of the bed grasps the mastoid process with his fingertips and supports the occiput with the palms of his hands. Alternately, an assistant who is positioned on the side of the bed can cradle the mastoids and support the occiput. Once the patient's head has been stabilized with MILS, the anterior portion of the collar is removed in order to allow the mouth to be opened widely. During laryngoscopy, the assistant is ideally providing appropriate counterforce to keep the patient's cervical spine in a neutral position. Multiple studies have shown that although the cervical spine can move during MILS, the movement is less than that when intubation is attempted while a cervical collar is in place (Figure 20.2).[6]

Multiple studies have shown that MILS increases the rate of failed intubations.[6] Studies carried out in nontrauma patients have shown that the incidence of Cormack–Lehane grades 3 and 4 increases when MILS is used in patients who would otherwise have a grade 1 or 2 view without MILS.

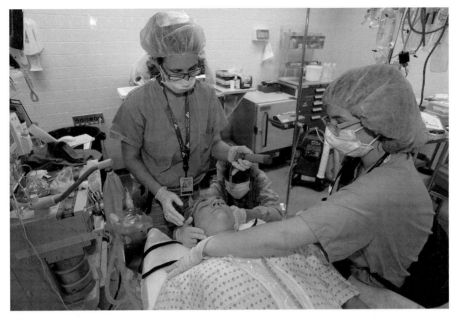

Figure 20.2 In-line stabilization. One assistant stabilizes the neck while the second assistant holds the shoulders

When to use rapid sequence intubation (RSI)

Most trauma patients are best managed with RSI because it is safest to assume that all trauma patients have full stomachs. It should be noted that swelling or bleeding in the airway can make intubation physically difficult. Suction should be immediately available. RSI is indicated in a patient who may deteriorate quickly and require urgent intubation but who will not tolerate intubation without general anesthesia. RSI is generally not required in a patient who is unconscious and apneic, for example. Absolute contraindications to RSI include total upper airway obstruction and the absence of facial or oropharyngeal landmarks (e.g. due to hematoma). Both of the above scenarios require a surgical airway.

Anesthetizing the airway for an awake intubation

The entire airway, including the nasopharynx, the posterior pharyngeal wall, the hypopharynx, and the trachea should be adequately anesthetized before attempting an awake intubation. Swabs soaked in viscous lidocaine or lidocaine ointment can be placed within the bilateral nasal passages. Slowly progress the swabs over 5 minutes until resistance is met. To treat the posterior pharyngeal wall, place more lidocaine-treated swabs at the base of the palatine arches by tracking along the side of the tongue. Do not push further if the patient starts to gag; let the lidocaine anesthetize the area for a few minutes. Finally, to treat the hypopharynx, drip a lidocaine solution down the back of the tongue or spray the back of the throat with benzocaine spray. Most importantly, work slowly and allow the local anesthetics to take effect. This approach will make placement of the breathing tube much easier because the patient will be cooperative and as comfortable as possible.

Risks of an awake fiberoptic intubation

Airway management in the awake patient requires more time and a cooperative patient and it is possible that the airway or mental status could deteriorate suddenly. If topical anesthesia of the airway is ineffective, patients can become agitated, combative, or uncooperative. In such cases, the practitioner may become over-dependent on intravenous sedation, which may lead to respiratory depression and desaturation. Uncommon complications from awake intubations are injury to the nerves and vessels during nerve blocks, toxicity from local anesthesia administration, and direct injury to the laryngeal or pharyngeal mucosa. Additionally, awake fiberoptic intubation may increase the risk of aspiration in patients with a full stomach for two reasons: (1) awake intubations take more time and (2) topical anesthesia of the pharynx and vocal cords can lessen the protective reflexes of the airway. These theoretical risks should not dissuade an experienced airway manager from proceeding with an awake intubation if RSI might not be successful.

Options for an asleep intubation

Options for an asleep intubation in a patient with a suspected cervical spine injury are the same as those for an uninjured patient. However, it is important to recognize how airway devices affect the alignment of the cervical spine. One cadaver study compared the effect of cervical spine movement with conventional laryngoscopy (Macintosh blade) to that with laryngeal mask airway (LMA) and other airway devices.[7] The authors found that conventional direct laryngoscopy caused greater extension of the C1 segment of the C spine in relation to the occipital condyles. To have an ideal view during conventional direct laryngoscopy, the atlanto-occipital and C1–C2 joints must be extended and the C2–C5 joints minimally displaced. The choice of laryngoscope blade (Miller vs. Macintosh) does not have a clinically significant effect on the degree of cervical spine movement during intubation.[8] Studies have also shown that even with MILS, movement of the cervical spine is unavoidable.[9]

An LMA should be used only if the patient cannot be mask ventilated and cannot be intubated immediately. The reason that an LMA should be avoided is that every time the airway is manipulated, it puts stress on the cervical spine. A cricothyrotomy is an option if respiratory failure is imminent, but the cervical spine should be stabilized by means such as MILS during the procedure. A general surgeon or otolaryngologist should also be available to assist with a surgical airway.

Medication options for asleep intubation

Sedative-hypnotics and short-acting neuromuscular blocking agents are commonly used to secure the airway of patients who present with cervical spine injury and during the anesthetic management of ensuing surgery. Etomidate is a reasonable choice in elderly patients or those with known cardiovascular disease. Ketamine is usually suitable in otherwise healthy patients because it causes catecholamine release, but may cause hypotension in a patient who is hypovolemic and catecholamine depleted. Any patient that suffers cervical spine injury may be at risk for developing "spinal shock," which is characterized acutely with hypertension and bradycardia but quickly can transition into hypotension due to loss of sympathetic tone. Therefore, it is important to be able to correct hypotension quickly, usually with an alpha agonist such as phenylephrine.

Table 20.1 Induction agents

Anesthetic agent	Advantages	Disadvantages
Propofol	User familiarity Can be combined with vasoconstrictor to negate hypotension	Hypotension
Etomidate	Minimal cardiovascular depression	Potential adrenal suppression
Ketamine	Maintains cardiovascular stability in patients who have not depleted catecholamine reserve	Increases intracranial pressure May increase secretions

Succinylcholine is usually the preferred neuromuscular blocking agent for RSI because it rapidly produces ideal intubating conditions and is quickly metabolized unless the patient has atypical pseudocholinesterase or pseudocholinesterase deficiency. The risk of hyperkalemia with the administration of succinylcholine becomes clinically significant within a week following a denervating injury and can last between 6 months and 2 years.[10] Therefore, succinylcholine is safe during the first few days of a cervical spine injury but should not be administered after the third or fourth day. Succinylcholine should also be avoided in patients with crush injuries; rocuronium should be used instead if the patient is not at risk for difficult mask ventilation or intubation.

Identifying and treating neurogenic and spinal shock

Neurogenic shock is distributive in nature and is attributed to disruption of the autonomic pathways within the spinal cord. Patients with neurogenic shock present with hypotension, which is caused by a reduction of sympathetic tone and decreased systemic vascular resistance, and bradycardia, which is caused by unopposed vagal activity. A patient in neurogenic shock may require a vasopressor, such as phenylephrine, to counteract unopposed parasympathetic activity and maintain blood pressure. There is no single, ideal induction agent for patients with spinal shock; Table 20.1 lists commonly used medications, and each one should be administered slowly and in incremental doses to minimize the risk of hypotension.

Conclusion

Patients with cervical spine injuries present multiple airway challenges. The airway manager must recognize a potentially difficult airway and manage it safely by minimizing secondary injury while securing a safe and stable airway. RSI followed by endotracheal intubation with MILS of the head and neck remains the gold standard in patients who require urgent airway control. Airway adjuncts such as an awake fiberoptic intubation or surgical airway may be required when the patient is not acutely decompensating. In the case presentation at the beginning of the chapter, if airway management is required (if the patient decompensates or requires surgical repair of the femur fracture), awake or asleep fiberoptic intubation should be considered because stabilizing devices such as cervical collars can be left in place and there is less stress on the atlanto-occipital joint. These decisions require that the airway manager understand the risks and benefits of each option for management. The airway manager should be able to recognize the following: situations where cervical spine injuries are likely, signs of spinal shock and the results on hemodynamics, and instances such as upper airway obstruction when orotracheal intubation is contraindicated and a surgical airway must be obtained.

References

1. Hassid VJ, Schinco MA, Tepas JJ, et al. Definitive establishment of airway control is critical for optimal outcome in lower cervical spinal cord injury. *J Trauma* 2008; **65**: 1328–32.

2. Malik SA, Murphy M, Connolly P, O'Byrne J. Evaluation of morbidity, mortality and outcome following cervical spine injuries in elderly patients. *Eur Spine J* 2008; **17**: 585–91.

3. Fujii T, Faul M, Sasser S. Risk factors for cervical spine injury among patients with traumatic brain injury. *J Emerg Trauma Shock* 2013; **6**: 252–8.

4. Prasarn ML, Horodyski M, Scott NE, et al. Motion generated in the unstable upper cervical spine during head tilt–chin lift and jaw thrust maneuvers. *Spine J* 2014; **14**: 609–14.

5. Shatney CH, Brunner RD, Nguyen TQ. The safety of orotracheal intubation in patients with unstable cervical spine fracture or high spinal cord injury. *Am J Surg* 1995; **170**: 676–9; discussion 679–80.

6. Thiboutot F, Nicole PC, Trépanier CA, Turgeon AF, Lessard MR. Effect of manual in-line stabilization of the cervical spine in adults on the rate of difficult orotracheal intubation by direct laryngoscopy: a randomized controlled trial. *Can J Anaesth* 2009; **56**: 412–18.

7. Wendling AL, Tighe PJ, Conrad BP, et al. A comparison of 4 airway devices on cervical spine alignment in cadaver models of global ligamentous instability at C1–2. *Anesth Analg* 2013; **117**: 126–32.

8. LeGrand SA, Hindman BJ, Dexter F, Weeks JB, Todd MM. Craniocervical motion during direct laryngoscopy and orotracheal intubation with the Macintosh and Miller blades: an in vivo cinefluoroscopic study. *Anesthesiology* 2007; **107**: 884–91.

9. Lennarson PJ, Smith D, Todd MM, et al. Segmental cervical spine motion during orotracheal intubation of the intact and injured spine with and without external stabilization. *J Neurosurg* 2000; **92**: 201–6.

10. Martyn JA, Richtsfeld M. Succinylcholine-induced hyperkalemia in acquired pathologic states: etiologic factors and molecular mechanisms. *Anesthesiology* 2006; **104**: 158–69.

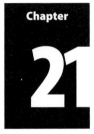

Airway management in facial trauma

Robert F. Reardon and Marc L. Martel

Case presentation

A 26-year-old man was an unrestrained driver in a high-speed motor vehicle collision and sustained significant head and facial injuries. En route to the hospital, the patient had gurgling respirations and copious bloody secretions. He was uncooperative and biting during attempts to suction his mouth. Paramedics applied oxygen via facemask, but he repeatedly removed the mask.

Upon arrival at the emergency department (ED) he is noted to have severe midface and mandibular injuries. He has a large amount of blood in his mouth and appears to be aspirating. He is immediately rolled onto his side but fights attempts to suction his mouth or reposition his mandible. His blood pressure is 120/60 mmHg, heart rate 140 per minute, and oxygen saturation 92%.

Evaluation of his airway reveals that he can open his mouth, but he will not cooperate with the examination. He has a short thyromental distance and his mandible appears to be fractured in multiple places. The anatomy of his anterior neck appears to be normal. He is moderately obese (5 feet, 10 inches (1.8 m) tall and 240 lbs (110 kg)), has a thick beard, and a cervical collar is in place.

Despite multiple indicators suggesting that this would be a difficult intubation, the decision is quickly made to proceed with rapid sequence intubation (RSI) due to his combativeness. Preoxygenation is initiated with facemask oxygen, and a nasal cannula is applied for apneic oxygenation.[1] Backup equipment, including suction, an endotracheal tube (ETT) introducer, supraglottic airway device, and a cricothyrotomy tray, is prepared. The anatomic landmarks of the anterior neck are identified by palpation and outlined with an indelible skin marker.

After approximately 3 minutes of preoxygenation and manual in-line stabilization (MILS), he is given etomidate and succinylcholine for induction and paralysis. Direct laryngoscopy is performed. Copious amounts of blood are suctioned from the posterior oropharynx, but the vocal cords cannot be visualized. However, the airway manager is able to visualize the epiglottis (Cormack–Lehane grade 3 view) by direct laryngoscopy (DL) and a bougie is placed. A size 7.5 mm ETT is placed over the bougie and rotated 90 degrees counterclockwise as the tip passes through the glottis.

On computed tomography (CT) scan, he was found to have a small epidural hemorrhage, an unstable teardrop fracture of the 5th cervical vertebra, and multiple severe facial

---

Cases in Emergency Airway Management, ed. Lauren C. Berkow and John C. Sakles. Published by Cambridge University Press. © Cambridge University Press 2015.

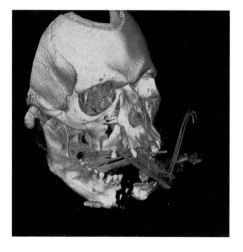

Figure 21.1 Smashed face. Comminuted fractures of the midface and mandible resulting in significant bleeding and potentially difficult bag-mask ventilation

fractures (Figure 21.1). He required multiple surgical procedures but made an excellent functional recovery.

Introduction

Facial trauma is a common presentation that precipitates some of the most difficult and intimidating airway management problems. Most of these problems can be managed by forethought, basic airway skills, and attention to detail. Airway managers should consider how different facial injuries are likely to complicate common airway techniques and develop a preconceived plan for dealing with specific injuries. Every airway manager has a different set of skills, experience, and availability of airway equipment, so management details will vary based on these factors. Common facial injuries include lacerations, fractures, and soft-tissue injuries that result in swelling or hematoma formation. It is useful to understand common facial injury patterns that affect airway management and then consider how each injury pattern will interfere with common emergency airway maneuvers.

Patterns of facial trauma and how they affect airway maneuvers

1. Smashed face – Significant deformity or loss of continuity of the midface, mandible, or facial soft tissue may make it difficult to get a good facemask seal, resulting in difficult or impossible facemask ventilation. Inability to perform effective bag-mask ventilation (BMV) is a significant problem that should not be overlooked. It is best to manage this situation by avoiding paralysis or planning to use a supraglottic airway device (SGA).
2. Floppy or swollen tongue – Injuries to the mandible may result in difficulty controlling the tongue (for both the patient and rescuers), leading to upper airway obstruction at rest and difficult BMV after the patient is sedated or paralyzed. Swelling of the tongue or the floor of the mouth may make it difficult for the patient to handle secretions and may make BMV and DL difficult. Counterintuitively, the most severe mandibular injuries (fractures with free floating segments) often make it easier to displace the tongue during laryngoscopy. An SGA should be considered in patients with difficult BMV or failed DL.
3. Severe bleeding – Severe bleeding is common in patients with midface injuries. These patients are at risk for significant aspiration, especially when they are unconscious, in a

supine position, or unable to clear secretions owing to a tongue or mandibular injury. These patients need optimal positioning and aggressive suctioning. An SGA should be considered when bleeding makes BMV or laryngoscopy difficult or impossible.

4. Trismus – Facial injuries often cause trismus, which significantly complicates airway assessment and management. Unfortunately, injuries that cause trismus may also cause a floppy or swollen tongue. This situation is often worsened by unconsciousness and the need for cervical spine immobilization. Trismus can usually be overcome by paralysis, but paralytic agents should be used with extreme caution and significant preplanning. Backup devices and surgical airway equipment should be immediately available. It may be reasonable to perform a primary surgical airway in these patients.

5. Laryngeal injury – The combination of facial trauma and laryngeal injury is one of the most daunting airway management scenarios because every common airway maneuver (BMV, DL, VL (video laryngoscopy), and SGA) may simultaneously fail. Providers should consider a primary surgical approach and be aware that a tracheostomy, rather than a cricothyrotomy, may be required.

General approach to airway management in facial trauma

Most patients with significant facial trauma have other potential injuries and are at high risk for cervical spine injury. Cervical spine immobilization makes intubation more difficult, especially if the patient has significant muscle tone or is actively fighting laryngoscopy. Many trauma patients also have a full stomach, so the risk of vomiting and aspiration with airway maneuvers must be carefully considered. To make matters worse, patients with facial trauma are frequently uncooperative and combative owing to head injury and/or intoxication. Thus, it may be impossible to get a good assessment of difficulty before managing the airway. In addition, many patients with severe facial injuries also have multisystem trauma, and airway compromise may be only one of many potential life-threatening conditions. Therefore, airway management must be completed expeditiously so that other injuries can be evaluated and managed in a timely manner. Because of these complicating factors, a difficult airway should be anticipated in most patients with significant facial trauma.

When managing these complex cases, one of the most important decisions is whether to use RSI or an awake approach. The decision is difficult and discussed in detail below but, regardless of which approach is used, the patient's safety and outcome are more likely to be related to whether the airway manager has good basic airway skills, a clear preconceived plan, and a good backup plan.

RSI usually allows the best chance for first-pass intubation success and is usually the best approach for immediate airway control in patients with facial trauma and potential multisystem injuries, even if they have difficult airway characteristics.[2–5] The widespread availability of modern airway devices, such as video laryngoscopes and SGAs, has helped to change the definition of difficult airway. Intubation with VL is often easy in cases where DL would be difficult or impossible, and SGAs have a high rate of success when BMV is difficult. Therefore, the "cannot intubate, cannot ventilate" scenario is extremely rare. Consequently, RSI has become the most common technique for emergency airway management and is the "go-to" airway management technique in trauma.[2–5]

Awake intubation is often considered a safer approach for managing patients with difficult airways, but this belief is unproven in the setting of significant facial or multisystem trauma. Before choosing an "awake" approach, the airway manager should have a clear understanding of the different ways to perform an awake intubation as well as the benefits and drawbacks of each. Variations of awake intubation include intubating the patient fully awake (with good topical anesthesia) or lightly sedated (still generally referred to as an awake intubation), or by using an "awake-look." These three "awake" approaches are very different and should not be confused. Fully awake intubation (usually with a fiberoptic bronchoscope) is rarely feasible in the acute setting in patients with significant facial trauma, especially if the patient is uncooperative, requires cervical spine immobilization, or has substantial bleeding. Intubation with only sedation is an option if a difficult airway is expected. This technique has the theoretical benefit of allowing the patient to breathe spontaneously and hopefully maintain oxygenation during intubation, but the risks and benefits of this technique have not been well established. Airway managers should be fully aware that sedation (without paralysis) of critically ill trauma patients may result in ineffective respirations, complete upper airway obstruction, and aspiration. It is clear that paralysis provides optimal intubating conditions and that sedation without paralysis provides poorer intubating conditions. In the acute setting the best option for an awake approach is probably an awake-look. This technique is essentially identical to an RSI procedure, but with an attempt at laryngoscopy just before administering the paralytic agent. The benefit of this technique is that it allows the intubator to get a better sense of the degree of difficulty of laryngoscopy before ablating spontaneous respirations. The downside, again, is that the patient may stop breathing, obstruct, or aspirate. When using this technique, the airway manager needs to have a clear plan for what to do next if the patient stops breathing or obstructs, or if the glottis cannot be visualized by laryngoscopy. The most important aspect of the awake-look procedure is that the details of preparation, preoxygenation, equipment readiness, and use of rescue devices are identical to those of the RSI procedure.

Regardless of whether the initial approach is RSI or an awake technique, the key to patient safety is careful attention to details, including a pre-procedural checklist, a clear plan (algorithm), techniques and equipment to help optimize the chance of first-pass intubation success, immediate availability and familiarity with backup techniques and equipment, and the willingness to quickly proceed to a surgical approach when necessary.

The following are critical details that increase the efficacy and safety of airway management in patients with significant facial trauma.

Call for help, who is "in charge," and where should care occur

Humility is the key to safe and successful management of the most difficult cases. Recognizing that an airway will likely be difficult and calling for proper help is critical. Very experienced and skilled airway providers may just need a few assistants, whereas less experienced providers should call the most experienced airway manager available. After the airway team has assembled, communication should be clear concerning the airway plan and the role of each team member. Depending on local practice patterns, the most experienced airway manager may be an emergency physician, an anesthesiologist, a certified registered nurse anesthetist, or a paramedic. Regardless of who is in charge of airway management, it should be clear who will make the decision to proceed and who will perform the procedure if a surgical airway is required. Also, it should be understood that optimal airway management depends on the availability of expertise and equipment, not the location of the care.

Facial Trauma Airway Algorithm

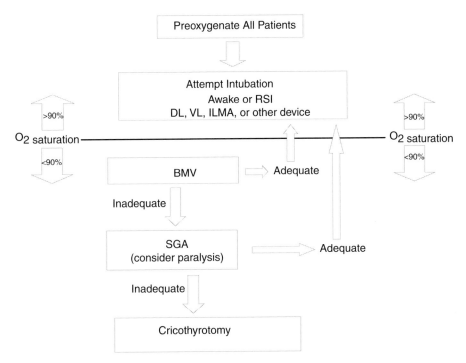

Figure 21.2 This algorithm stresses the importance of basic concepts such as ventilate/oxygenate (don't attempt intubation) if the O_2 saturation is below 90%. Also, if unable to ventilate/oxygenate there should be a rapid progression from BMV to SGA to a surgical approach. DL = direct laryngoscopy. VL = video laryngoscopy. ILMA = intubating laryngeal mask airway. BMV = bag-mask ventilation. SGA = supraglottic airway

Using an airway algorithm

By using a simple airway algorithm with well-proven techniques and carefully determining which techniques are likely to be difficult based on the patient's specific injuries, it is possible to estimate the degree of airway difficulty and determine the best course of action (Figure 21.2).

Using a pre-procedure checklist

Pre-procedural checklists improve the safety of intubation in trauma patients, especially when facial trauma is present and RSI is planned. Seemingly small details can make the difference between a straightforward intubation and a disaster. Details that may get missed without a checklist include ensuring that the intravenous line is running, ensuring that the suction is turned on, and ensuring that the laryngoscope light is functional. Using a checklist encourages a team approach to airway management and ensures that all members of the team are in accord. It also affirms the understanding that basic skills, techniques, and equipment are key to safe and effective airway management.

Preintubation checklist:

1. Oxygen mask and nasal cannula oxygen running
2. Suction working
3. BMV ready
4. Oral airway available
5. Laryngoscope functioning
6. ETT ready
7. SGA ready
8. Intravenous line functioning (and blood pressure cuff on opposite arm)
9. Assistant designated to provide MILS
10. Medications drawn up (including paralytic, even if not planning to use it)
11. Patient position optimized (if possible)
12. Airway plan verbalized with all personnel involved.

Awake-look

The concept of an awake-look is different from an awake intubation. An awake-look can be used before paralysis to assess how difficult laryngoscopy will be in patients who are potentially difficult or impossible to intubate. The preparation and technique are the same as for RSI, but the paralytic is held until the intubator attempts laryngoscopy while the patient is completely awake or after sedation alone. If the intubator is able to visualize the glottis then the paralytic (and/or the sedative) is administered. This technique is useful, especially when facial trauma is present, because paralysis provides the best intubating conditions, but predicting difficult intubation is challenging and prone to over- and under-estimation. An awake-look allows nearly the same approach as RSI without the risk of taking away spontaneous respirations. It is important to think of the awake-look procedure as essentially identical to RSI, with all of the same preparation, planning, and backups. Also, it is important to realize that if the patient's spontaneous respirations are inadequate, it is usually best to use paralysis to optimize the conditions for intubation, BMV, or placement of an SGA.

RSI

One of the most important decisions in trauma airway management, especially in the setting of facial trauma, is whether or not to paralyze the patient and use RSI. It is commonly taught that patients with difficult airways should not be paralyzed. The decision to use RSI in the setting of trauma is somewhat subjective because large studies show that most trauma patients are intubated via RSI, and nearly all trauma patients have some difficult airway characteristics.[2-5] The bottom line is that paralysis usually provides the best intubating conditions, and RSI usually allows the best chance for first-pass intubation success, even in patients with predictors of a difficult airway. Therefore, RSI has become the most common technique for emergency airway management.[2-5] The best approach to determine whether paralysis is safe is to realize that ventilation and oxygenation are critical and that intubation is a secondary consideration. Therefore, RSI should be strictly avoided in patients who will be difficult to intubate and difficult to ventilate.

Preoxygenation and apneic oxygenation

Preoxygenation is critical to success and safety of emergency intubation, especially when RSI is used. The best way to provide high fraction of inspired oxygen (FiO_2; 90%) for preoxygenation is by using a standard reservoir facemask with the oxygen flow rate set as high as possible (usually 60 L/min).[1] Preoxygenation with a bag-mask device is not recommended.[1] Ideally, patients should be preoxygenated for 3 minutes or 8 maximal capacity breaths if time is short. It is best to preoxygenate patients in a head-elevated position or in reverse Trendelenburg, especially if the patient is obese.

Apneic oxygenation is a relatively new concept that can help prevent oxygen desaturation during RSI. This is best accomplished by placing a nasal cannula (with an oxygen flow rate of 15 L/min) under the facemask during preoxygenation and leaving it in place during intubation.[1]

Positioning and opening the airway

Upper airway obstruction is common with facial trauma. Patients with copious bleeding, distorted anatomy, or difficulty controlling their tongue are at risk for complete airway obstruction if they are forced to wear a cervical collar or assume a supine position. In this situation, providers need to weigh the risks and benefits of strict cervical spine immobilization. It is usually better to allow awake patients to assume a comfortable position that allows them to open and protect their own airway. Cooperative patients may be allowed to perform self-suctioning with a suction device. Patients who are unconscious and supine should be expected to have some upper airway obstruction and will need help opening and clearing their airway. Those with low risk for cervical spine injury can be placed in the sniffing position and those at high risk in a neutral position. Oropharyngeal airways should be used liberally but nasopharyngeal airways should be avoided in patients with maxillary injuries. The jaw-thrust maneuver and aggressive suctioning are appropriate in all unconscious supine patients.

Suctioning equipment

When managing cases with significant oropharyngeal or nasopharyngeal bleeding and/or vomit, it is important to have the best available suction equipment. Most tonsil (Yankauer) and dental suction tips and standard ¼-inch suction tubing are easily clogged by blood clots or vomit, so suctioning equipment with a large-bore tip may be preferable. It is also reasonable to have two suction setups available in case one becomes clogged or malfunctions.

Bougie

The bougie is often recommended as an adjunct or backup in cases of failed intubation, but we recommend that it be used for every intubation attempt in trauma patients, especially those with facial trauma.[3] Evidence suggests that the bougie improves the chances of successful endotracheal intubation in patients with difficult airways.[2-5] The benefit of the bougie is that it can be used to successfully intubate the trachea even when the glottic structures are not well visualized and it provides immediate feedback that the tip is in the correct location even before the ETT is placed.

VL

DL has a high success rate, and the combination of RSI and DL is generally recommended as the primary approach in trauma airways.[2–5] However, recent studies comparing DL to VL have found that VL has a higher first-attempt success rate in patients with difficult airways, including those with cervical immobility, facial trauma, and blood in the airway.[6–8] In addition, the use of VL by emergency medicine residents significantly decreases their rate of esophageal intubation and associated complications.[6]

Optimal BMV

BMV may be difficult or impossible in patients with facial trauma. In this situation airway managers should do everything possible to optimize the mask ventilation technique. In apneic unconscious patients, a two-handed, two-person BMV technique is better than a one-handed technique. This method requires a second person to squeeze the ventilation bag, but it provides the patient with higher tidal volumes and decreases the chance of failed mask ventilation. The two-handed jaw-thrust technique allows the operator to create an optimal mask seal while simultaneously performing a jaw-thrust maneuver.

SGAs

Laryngeal mask airways (LMAs), and especially intubating LMAs, are critical backup devices for difficult trauma airways.[2,3,5,9] In particular, the intubating LMA Fastrach has proven to be an excellent primary backup device for failed RSIs, especially in patients with facial trauma. Several studies show that the LMA Fastrach has a high success rate in both known and unanticipated difficult airways.[5,9,10] In patients with difficult mask ventilation nearly all can be successfully ventilated with the LMA Fastrach.[5,10] Those with known difficult intubation or failed intubation can be intubated blindly through the device in more than 90% of cases.[5,9,10] The addition of flexible endoscopic guidance through the LMA Fastrach allows successful intubation in nearly all cases.[9] Other good SGA options include newer disposable intubating LMAs (air-Q, Ambu Aura-i, and igel).

King laryngeal tube

The King laryngeal tube (King LT™ and King LT(S)-D™) is a simple extraglottic device that has a high placement success rate, even in the hands of novices. It is used extensively in prehospital settings and is a reasonable temporizing device in patients with severe facial trauma.[11] It should be considered when an LMA fails due to high airway pressures or when the patient needs to be transferred with the device in place.

Cricothyrotomy

Cricothyrotomy is the first-line approach when oral or nasal intubation is thought to be too dangerous or impossible. Such cases are predictable, and airway providers should know which injury patterns are most likely to require a primary surgical approach.

Patients with significant facial trauma are at high risk for failed airways; therefore, surgical airway equipment should always be immediately available and opened before other airway techniques (especially RSI) are started. Palpation of the anterior neck anatomy and even marking of the cricothyroid membrane is also advisable before RSI is attempted. Detailed preplanning, including determining who will make the decision, who will perform the procedure, and exactly how the procedure will be performed is also critical to success.

Post-management care and follow-up

Ensuring proper ETT depth is crucial in patients with facial trauma because they often have progressive swelling that would make reintubation impossible if the tube is dislodged. The tube should be secured with twill tape, adhesive tape, or a commercially available device. Consider placing soft wrist restraints so that the patient cannot reach up to pull at the ETT. Sedate the patient as needed and consider paralysis during transport or diagnostic procedures. Notify the team providing ongoing care if the patient had a difficult airway, and have advanced airway equipment and a surgical airway tray at the patient's bedside in case of an unplanned extubation.

References

1. Weingart SD, Levitan RM. Preoxygenation and prevention of desaturation during emergency airway management. *Annals of Emergency Medicine*. 2012;**59**(3):165–75 e1.

2. Stephens CT, Kahntroff S, Dutton RP. The success of emergency endotracheal intubation in trauma patients: a 10-year experience at a major adult trauma referral center. *Anesthesia and Analgesia*. 2009;**109**(3):866–72.

3. Ollerton JE, Parr MJ, Harrison K, Hanrahan B, Sugrue M. Potential cervical spine injury and difficult airway management for emergency intubation of trauma adults in the emergency department – a systematic review. *Emergency Medicine Journal: EMJ*. 2006;**23**(1):3–11.

4. Mayglothling J, Duane TM, Gibbs M, *et al.* Emergency tracheal intubation immediately following traumatic injury: an Eastern Association for the Surgery of Trauma practice management guideline. *The Journal of Trauma and Acute Care Surgery*. 2012;**73** (5 Suppl. 4):S333–40.

5. Combes X, Jabre P, Margenet A, *et al.* Unanticipated difficult airway management in the prehospital emergency setting: prospective validation of an algorithm. *Anesthesiology*. 2011;**114**(1):105–10.

6. Sakles JC, Mosier J, Chiu S, Cosentino M, Kalin L. A comparison of the C-MAC video laryngoscope to the Macintosh direct laryngoscope for intubation in the emergency department. *Annals of Emergency Medicine*. 2012;**60**(6):739–48.

7. Mosier JM, Stolz U, Chiu S, Sakles JC. Difficult airway management in the emergency department: GlideScope videolaryngoscopy compared to direct laryngoscopy. *The Journal of Emergency Medicine*. 2012;**42**(6):629–34.

8. Aziz MF, Dillman D, Fu R, Brambrink AM. Comparative effectiveness of the C-MAC video laryngoscope versus direct laryngoscopy in the setting of the predicted difficult airway. *Anesthesiology*. 2012;**116**(3):629–36.

9. Ferson DZ, Rosenblatt WH, Johansen MJ, Osborn I, Ovassapian A. Use of the intubating LMA-Fastrach in 254 patients with difficult-to-manage airways. *Anesthesiology*. 2001;**95**(5):1175–81.

10. Combes X, Le Roux B, Suen P, *et al.* Unanticipated difficult airway in anesthetized patients: prospective validation of a management algorithm. *Anesthesiology*. 2004;**100**(5):1146–50.

11. Schalk R, Meininger D, Ruesseler M, *et al.* Emergency airway management in trauma patients using laryngeal tube suction. *Prehospital Emergency Care: Official Journal of the National Association of EMS Physicians and the National Association of State EMS Directors*. 2011;**15**(3):347–50.

Airway management in head injury

Christa San Luis and Athir H. Morad

Case presentation

A 38-year-old motorcyclist with past medical history of bipolar disorder presents to the emergency department via ambulance after being launched from his vehicle at high speed. The patient is initially combative, and his breath smells of alcohol. A rapid computed tomography (CT) scan reveals no evidence of any orthopedic or major organ injuries. However, an intracranial subdural hematoma is identified (Figure 22.1). The patient progressively becomes less responsive and requires intubation for airway protection.

Pertinent review of the medical problem/condition and relevant literature review

Isolated head injuries present several unique challenges to the approach of the airway. The most significant consideration is whether the patient has any signs of intracranial hypertension (Table 22.1).[1] The Monro-Kellie doctrine states that since the cranium is a rigid structure, the volumes of its contents (cerebrospinal fluid, blood, and brain tissue) are limited to an overall fixed capacity. Therefore, any increase in volume of one of the intracranial components must result in a decrease in volume of the other components. In the case of an expanding hematoma, once the size reaches a critical threshold, the brain begins to herniate through the foramen magnum and compress the brain stem. Brainstem compression may further result in irreversible global cerebral ischemia and cause physiologic havoc that is life-threatening.

When intracranial hypertension, classically defined as intracranial pressure (ICP) greater than 20 mmHg, is suspected clinically (Table 22.1) or on brain imaging (Figure 22.2), all attempts should be made to avoid cerebral herniation. Depending on the type of intracranial diagnosis, specific precautions during airway management should be considered (Table 22.2). While the immediate normalization of blood oxygen saturation is of upmost importance, hypercarbia must also be avoided because it increases the cerebral blood volume through vasodilation. Consequently, applying supplemental oxygen to a brain-injured patient without monitoring for ventilator insufficiency (respiratory rate decline, or CO_2 rise) can be harmful.

Indications for the intubation of brain-injured patients are generally the same as for non-brain-injured patients (Table 22.3).[2] Once the decision to intubate is made, the choice of patient positioning, proper intubating equipment, timing of the intubation sequence, pharmacologic induction agents, and ventilator settings becomes critical. When a patient's Glasgow Coma Scale (GCS) score falls below 9, guidelines from the Brain Trauma Foundation recommend that

Cases in Emergency Airway Management, ed. Lauren C. Berkow and John C. Sakles. Published by Cambridge University Press. © Cambridge University Press 2015.

Table 22.1 Signs and symptoms of high ICP

Early	Late
Headache	Pupillary changes, anisocoria or bilateral unreactive
Dizziness	dilated pupils
Loss of consciousness	Extensor or flexor posturing
Altered mental status	Absence of spontaneous venous pulsations on
Amnesia	fundoscopy
Memory loss	Cranial nerve IV and VI paralysis
Nausea	Contralateral or ipsilateral motor paralysis
Vomiting	Hypertension, bradycardia, and irregular respiration
Weakness or decreased sensation of	(Cushing's triad)
extremities	Apnea
Speech or swallowing difficulties	Coma

Derived from Marik P. *et al.* Management of increased intracranial pressure: a review for clinicians. *J Emerg Med* 1999; **17**:711–19.

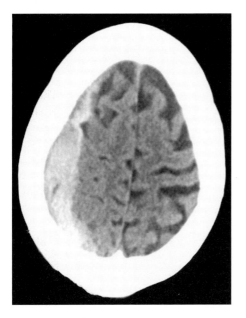

Figure 22.1 A right parietal hyperdense acute subdural collection

the airway be secured.[3] However, it is important to note that the GCS score is only part of the airway assessment and should be used in conjunction with other indications for intubation. Commonly, the cognitive impairment of these patients is so severe that they are unable to protect their airway and maintain adequate oxygenation and ventilation.

Potential airway management scenarios and discussion

Unlike scheduled surgical patients, patients with head trauma often present with full stomachs that pose a substantial risk of aspirating during intubation. In such patients, using a rapid sequence intubation technique would be an ideal way to prevent vomitus from

Table 22.2 Other precautions during airway management after a head injury

Scenario	Airway management precaution
Concomitant cervical spine injury	No neck movement is allowed, thus limiting ability to achieve view of vocal cords. For high cervical lesions, ventilation may be an emergent airway issue, even if the patient is awake, owing to spinal shock where there is absence of spinal reflexes below the level of the injury. This would include innervation to the diaphragm and intercostal muscles.
Seizures as the primary cause of head injury	In any acute head injury for which a CT scan shows another mass or blood of a different age (old blood or newly found tumor) a patient may be post-ictal as well. The urgency to intubate these patients may change depending on the speed of their recovery from both the seizure and head injury.
Traumatic intraparenchymal, subdural, and extradural hematomas	Patients with these types of injuries may deteriorate quickly in minutes owing to rapid expansion and mass effect caused by the blood. As the airway is being secured, care should be given in terms of simultaneously managing high intracranial pressure with mannitol or hypertonic saline and hyperventilating the patient as soon as possible.
Traumatic subarachnoid hemorrhage	Unlike aneurysmal subarachnoid hemorrhage, these patients do not typically develop vasospasm. Standard precautions for keeping normal cerebral perfusion pressure should be followed.
Concomitant facial fractures	In these patients, a possible surgical airway should be considered with the help of otolaryngology specialists or a specialized difficult airway team, as manipulating facial fractures for airway management may be more deleterious to the patient.

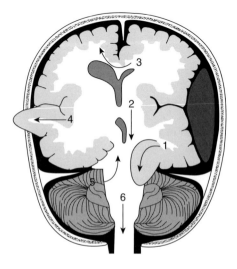

Figure 22.2 Types of brain herniation: (1) uncal; (2) central; (3) cingulate; (4) transcalvarial; (5) upward; and (6) tonsillar (http://commons.wikimedia.org/wiki/File:Brain_herniation_types.svg)

Table 22.3 Indications for early intubation after traumatic brain injury

Indications for early intubation	
Airway obstruction	Discretionary indications
Hypoventilation	Facial injury
Severe hypoxemia	Altered mental status
Severe cognitive impairment (GCS score ≤ 8)	Combativeness
Cardiac arrest	Respiratory distress
Severe hemorrhagic shock	Intoxication
	Preoperative management

Modified from Sise M. *et al.* Early intubation in the management of trauma patients: indications and outcomes in 1,000 consecutive patients. *J Trauma* 2009; **66**:32–40.

travelling into the trachea.[4,5] In traditional rapid sequence intubation, the inducing agent (propofol or etomidate in hemodynamically unstable patients) is administered in rapid succession with a muscle relaxant (depolarizer or non-depolarizer) in order to reduce the risk of any retching that could result in aspiration. Mask ventilation is avoided during induction to prevent insufflation of the stomach, while cricoid pressure is typically applied to prevent passive esophageal regurgitation. Typically, succinylcholine (a depolarizing agent) is used because it has rapid onset and short half-life. However, owing to concern over succinylcholine's theoretical ability to elevate ICP, practitioners often substitute non-depolarizing agents such as rocuronium. The decision to use a non-depolarizing agent is not without risk. The longer duration of apnea necessary to allow time for the non-depolarizing paralytic to take effect can cause an increase in ICP that may be riskier than the use of succinylcholine. Moreover, the relatively shorter half-life of succinylcholine allows for quicker recovery of the neurological examination compared to non-depolarizing paralytic agents.

Algorithms/pathways to follow if indicated, alternate airway devices/resources recommended

Two possible intubation plans that are reasonable when approaching the airway of patients with acute traumatic brain injury and full stomachs are:

1. traditional rapid sequence intubation with succinylcholine (described above); and
2. "modified" rapid sequence intubation with a non-depolarizing muscle relaxant (described below).

When using the modified rapid sequence technique, the patient is gently mask ventilated after induction until the neuromuscular blocking agent takes effect (30–120 seconds, depending on the agent). The application of cricoid pressure to prevent passive esophageal regurgitation or gastric insufflation may also be considered during this time. Mask ventilation serves to assure the clinician that the patient is salvageable should the intubation attempt fail. In addition, successful mask ventilation prevents hypercarbia from developing as a result of a longer induction time.

In addition to the choice of appropriate induction technique, all patients with elevated ICP should receive standard ICP management, which begins with positioning the head of the bed at 30 degrees. Such positioning results in proper drainage of venous blood and cerebrospinal fluid. However, elevating the head of the bed may pose a challenge for viewing angles when performing traditional intubation techniques with direct laryngoscopy. Therefore, video laryngoscopy may prove to be more useful in this unique patient population. An additional benefit of video laryngoscopy is to reduce angling of the neck in the case of unrecognized cervical injuries, particularly when the head is deliberately kept in a neutral position.[6] In addition to proper head positioning, care must be taken to avoid hypertension, which can cause elevations in ICP. Hypotension during intubation can be equally harmful, as the brain is most vulnerable to reduced perfusion pressures when ICP is elevated. Because perfusion pressure is derived from the difference between mean arterial pressure (MAP) and ICP, even small changes in blood pressure can have devastating effects on brain tissue viability. Finally, the patient should be prevented from coughing during intubation or "bucking" during mechanical ventilation because increased intrathoracic pressures can lead to spikes in ICP.

A simple algorithm to follow when approaching a trauma patient with brain injury is presented in Figure 22.3. First, determine whether the patient has any signs of elevated ICP

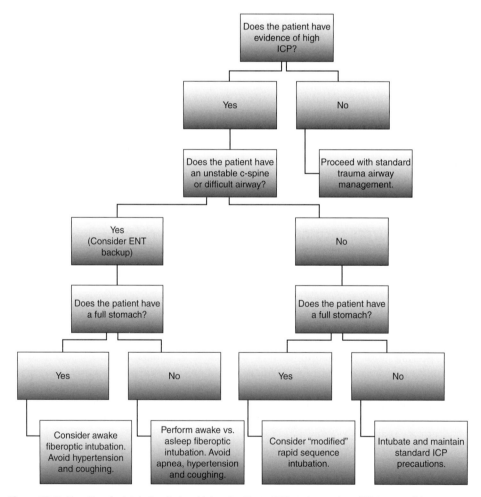

Figure 22.3 Algorithm for intubation in head-injured patients. ENT, otolaryngology; ICP, intracranial pressure

(Table 22.1). Next, determine whether the patient is at risk for having a difficult airway or cervical spine instability. If either of those scenarios is present, then consider obtaining backup from an otolaryngologist while performing an awake (full stomach) or asleep (empty stomach) fiberoptic intubation. Consider moving the patient to an operating room for the intubation because it will provide access to an adjustable operating room table, suction, electrocautery, and ample lighting, which may become necessary if emergent cricothyroidotomy/tracheostomy is needed. More important, the operating room has an abundance of staff that can lend support. Once a cervical spine injury is ruled out, the third question to address is whether the patient has a full stomach. In the most common scenario, it is unknown whether the patient has sustained a cervical injury or has a full stomach. In these circumstances, consider performing a modified rapid sequence intubation with the neck held in neutral positon but with the head of the bed at 30 degrees, exercising the standard ICP precautions described above.

Post-management care and follow-up if applicable

Once a patient is intubated, proper endotracheal tube placement must be confirmed immediately by auscultating both lung fields and over the epigastrium. End-tidal CO_2 must be detected, and a chest X-ray provides visual confirmation. In addition, the patient's vital signs must be surveyed to ensure that adequate blood oxygen saturation levels have been achieved and that the patient's hemodynamic parameters are stable and can provide adequate cerebral perfusion. The transition from hand ventilation to mechanical ventilation must also be monitored closely to avoid hypercarbia or elevated peak airway pressures, which would exacerbate intracranial hypertension. Ideally, the patients will proceed to a specialized neurointensive care unit for further management.

Conclusion

Patients with head injuries pose a unique set of challenges to the management of the airway. In addition to requiring a narrower window of opportunity for the successful establishment of an airway, these patients are less tolerant to supine positioning during preparation, and are at risk of hemodynamic instability during induction, prolonged apnea during the intubation attempt, and increased peak airway pressures once successfully intubated. Whenever possible, the intubation of such patients should be attempted by the most experienced airway provider available.

References

1. P. Marik, K. Chen, J. Varon, R. Fromm, Jr., G.L. Sternbach. Management of increased intracranial pressure: a review for clinicians. *J Emerg Med* 1999; **17**: 711–19.

2. M.J. Sise, S.R. Shackford, C.B. Sise, *et al.* Early intubation in the management of trauma patients: indications and outcomes in 1,000 consecutive patients. *J Trauma* 2009; **66**: 32–40.

3. Brain Trauma Foundation. Guidelines for the management of severe traumatic brain injury. *J Neurotrauma* 2007; **24**, Supplement 1.

4. R.M. Walls. Rapid-sequence intubation in head trauma. *Ann Emerg Med* 1993; **22**: 1008–13.

5. J.M. Ehrenfeld, E.A. Cassedy, V.E. Forbes, N.D. Mercaldo, W.S. Sandberg. Modified rapid sequence induction and intubation: a survey of the United States current practice. *Anesth Analg* 2012; **115**: 95–101.

6. M. Aziz. Use of video-assisted intubation devices in the management of patients with trauma. *Anesthesiol Clin* 2013; **31**: 157–66.

Airway management of pediatric congenital anomalies

Paul Baker and Natasha Woodman

Case presentation

A 33-year-old woman presented in her third pregnancy with an antenatal ultrasound scan showing a fetus with polyhydramnios, ear abnormalities, and severe micrognathia. Concern about potential airway obstruction in the fetus after birth led to the decision to deliver that child by an ex utero intrapartum treatment (EXIT) procedure at 37 weeks' gestation.[1]

The airway management plan during the EXIT consisted of a cascade of techniques, including direct laryngoscopy, rigid bronchoscopy, flexible bronchoscopy, retrograde intubation, and finally a tracheostomy. During the maternal general anesthetic and cesarean section, the EXIT procedure was performed with the fetus attached to the placenta. The head and shoulders were delivered for airway management, but the first attempt at tracheal intubation by direct laryngoscopy with a size 1 Seward blade failed. This attempt revealed severe microstomia, cleft palate, and a grossly hypoplastic mandible that caused the posterior third of the tongue to occupy the cleft palate, obstructing the oropharynx and obscuring a direct view of the larynx. Rigid bronchoscopy with a 2.5 mm 0 degree bronchoscope also failed to expose any anatomy beyond the tongue. The anesthesiologist then inserted a Classic laryngeal mask airway (cLMA™), providing a conduit for flexible bronchoscopy with an ultrathin flexible bronchoscope. Two 3.0-mm internal diameter endotracheal tubes (ETTs) were wedged end-to-end and mounted on the bronchoscope. Then, the anesthesiologist advanced the ETTs off the bronchoscope into the trachea and, using the proximal ETT as a holder, withdrew the cLMA over its length while keeping the distal ETT in position. The proximal ETT was then detached and the distal ETT secured. Correct placement of the ETT was confirmed by capnography and bilateral gas entry to the lungs. The trachea was intubated 20 minutes after beginning the EXIT procedure and, 4 hours after delivery, a tracheostomy was performed to establish a secure airway. The neonate had severe micrognathia, with jaw opening of 4 mm. This condition was diagnosed as isolated dysgnathia complex, which is a severe congenital airway anomaly associated with a very high perinatal mortality owing to airway obstruction (Figures 23.1 and 23.2).

The successful outcome of this case can be attributed to meticulous planning in the antenatal phase. A fetal medicine panel determined the likely outcome of the EXIT procedure and communicated with the parents. Radiology provided vital information about the

Cases in Emergency Airway Management, ed. Lauren C. Berkow and John C. Sakles. Published by Cambridge University Press. © Cambridge University Press 2015.

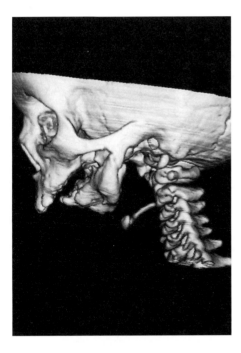

Figure 23.1 This three-dimensional reformatted computed tomography (CT) scan shows abnormal temporomandibular joints with rudimentary mandibular condyles articulating with the skull base. (Permission from publisher J. Wiley and Sons.)

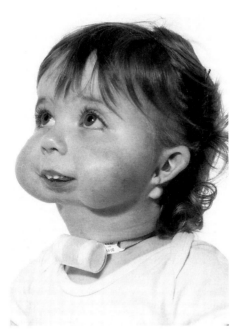

Figure 23.2 Clinical photograph of the child at 13 months of age showing the ear abnormality. Features included malformation of the external auricles with noncontiguous lobules dorsal to the rest of the auricles. (Photograph by permission from the parents and publisher J. Wiley and Sons.)

severity of airway obstruction, and multiple specialty teams worked together at the delivery to effect successive action plans for an anticipated difficult airway.

The EXIT procedure is indicated for fetal conditions that pose a significant risk of airway obstruction immediately after birth. These conditions include giant fetal neck masses, lung or mediastinal tumors, congenital high airway obstruction syndromes, EXIT to extracorporeal membrane oxygenation for certain congenital cardiac conditions, congenital cystic adenomatoid malformation, and severe micrognathia.

Introduction

Congenital anomalies, by definition, are conditions that are present from birth. This chapter will focus on congenital anomalies of the airway, particularly those that can cause respiratory compromise for the patient and management dilemmas for the airway practitioner.

The prevalence of congenital anomalies of the airway ranges between 1 in 10,000 and 1 in 50,000 live births.[2] The etiology of these anomalies is varied and includes genetic, infectious, neoplastic, and environmental causes. Neural tube defects, cardiac anomalies, and Down syndrome are the most common congenital anomalies and, like many other congenital anomalies, are associated with airway complications that can present with variable severity at any time after birth.

Congenital anomalies can affect any part of the airway and may compromise respiratory function at multiple levels. They are frequently associated with anomalies from other organ systems, including cardiovascular, gastrointestinal, and central nervous systems. This broad range of pathology creates a challenge for the airway practitioner.

In the assessment of congenital airway anomalies, it is essential to incorporate knowledge of syndromes and comorbidities for safe patient care. This is particularly true for infants and neonates in whom the incidence of difficult intubation is higher.[3] Whenever possible, management of the airway should be conducted by experienced practitioners in a safe operating environment, with the focus being on maintaining oxygenation and avoiding trauma. Careful planning is required at each stage, from presentation to postoperative care, and should always incorporate backup plans. Certain congenital airway anomalies, including mucopolysaccharidoses, mediastinal masses, Klippel Feil syndrome, CHARGE syndrome, and micrognathia associated with glossoptosis and cleft palate, are associated with high morbidity and mortality during airway management and anesthesia. Patients with these conditions should be assessed on admission and, provided they are stable, transferred to a specialist referral center. If the patient is unstable on admission, basic resuscitation should be provided and expert help should be requested. Multiple attempts at intubation should be avoided because of high morbidity. Transporting the unstable patient before establishing a definitive airway carries a high risk of airway obstruction in transit.

Anatomical approach to congenital airway anomalies

The following anatomical approach (Tables 23.1–23.7) considers congenital anomalies of the airway from the nose to the diaphragm.[4–6]

Several syndromes are associated with nasal anomalies (Crouzon, Apert, Piriform aperture stenosis, Pfeiffer syndromes, nasal dermoid cysts, gliomas, and encephaloceles). These patients present in childhood but can also require airway management as adults.

Mandibular hypoplasia and glossoptosis (posterior and superior displacement of the tongue) prevent palatal shelf fusion and result in a cleft palate. This condition gives rise to the diagnostic triad of micrognathia, glossoptosis, and cleft palate.

Tracheobronchomalacia (TBM) is the most common cause of airway collapse and obstruction in children.

Table 23.1 Nasal malformations

Condition	Syndromes	Implications	Suggestions
Isolated choanal atresia		Airways generally not difficult to manage	
Choanal atresia and stenosis		Severe airway obstruction and cyanosis when mouth closed or during breast feeding	During anesthesia, try positioning, oropharyngeal airway, SGA, or orotracheal intubation
Choanal atresia with other anomalies	CHARGE (Coloboma, Heart defects, Atresia of choanae, Retarded growth development, Genitourinary abnormalities, Ear defects) Treacher Collins	Airway difficulty, particularly with micrognathia and subglottic stenosis	Early tracheostomy to prevent hypoxic episodes Associated airway management might include awake insertion of SGA, tracheal intubation through SGA, use of small ETT for subglottic stenosis

SGA, supraglottic airway; ETT, endatracheal tube.

Table 23.2 Neck and head

Condition	Causes	Implications	Suggestions
Head anomalies	Hydrocephalus encephalocele	Difficulty positioning for BMV and gaining access for direct laryngoscopy	Try inverting an adult size five facemask for frontal encephalocele
Congenital cervical spine instability	Mucopolysaccharidoses (seven hereditary conditions including Hunter's, Hurler's, and Morquio's syndromes) Lysosomal enzyme deficiency leads to lysosomal deposits in tissues Down syndrome	Patients with OSA have a particularly high risk of airway obstruction during airway management[7] Airway complications with mucopolysaccharidoses become more frequent with age. Life expectancy has improved with hematopoietic stem-cell transplantation in the first 2 years of life and enzyme replacement therapy late in the	Ideally these patients should be managed in specialist referral centers. Airway management options include: • awake intubation with flexible bronchoscopy • sedation with ketamine and placement of an SGA for ventilation and intubation

Table 23.2 (cont.)

Condition	Causes	Implications	Suggestions
		clinical course. Death in the first two decades from cardiorespiratory failure is not uncommon, and patients rarely survive beyond 30 years. Older patients are prone to severe OSA owing to laryngeal or tracheal narrowing. Anesthesia for orthopedic, neurosurgery, and palliative care becomes more common Anesthetic morbidity of 20–30%	• gas induction of anesthesia and intubation by direct laryngoscopy, video laryngoscopy, or rigid or flexible bronchoscopy Avoid neuromuscular blockers Careful tracheal intubation is required because of potential for cervical cord compression
Congenital fusion of cervical vertebrae	Klippel Feil syndrome (congenital fusion of two or more cervical vertebrae) can be associated with facial asymmetry, cleft lip, malformed laryngeal cartilages, micrognathia, and congenital heart disease	Progressive syndrome with disc degeneration and cervical stenosis Airway may not be difficult until late childhood; can present in adults	Past history of easy intubation is an unreliable predictor of future safety Minimize cervical spine movement Patients have been successfully intubated with the Bullard laryngoscope, light wand, flexible bronchoscope, and, less so, with the GlideScope video laryngoscope and Macintosh direct laryngoscopy
Congenital tumors	Cystic hygroma, dermoid cysts, teratoid cysts, true teratomas	May present as maternal polyhydramnios owing to in utero airway obstruction Risk of severe respiratory obstruction at birth	Ideally diagnosed antenatally; use EXIT procedure in extreme cases
Congenital microstomia	Freeman–Sheldon (whistling face), Hallerman–Streiff, otopalatodigital syndromes	Laryngoscope insertion and tracheal intubation may be difficult	Flexible bronchoscopy and an SGA can be used as alternative airway strategies

Table 23.2 (cont.)

Condition	Causes	Implications	Suggestions
Macroglossia	Congenital tumors, hemangioma, lymphangioma Metabolic, glycogen storage disease, lipid storage disease, neurofibromatosis, Beckwith–Wiedemann syndrome Down syndrome	Down syndrome is also associated with OSA, predisposing patients to airway obstruction Patients may also have cervical instability and a tendency for bradycardia (with or without congenital heart disease) Can present in adults	Careful airway planning, particularly immediately after induction of anesthesia and in the recovery phase Consider a "double setup" in which macroglossia, macrocephaly, and mandibular anomalies coexist Treat bradycardia with an anticholinergic

BMV, bag-mask ventilation; EXIT, ex utero intrapartum treatment; OSA, obstructive sleep apnea; SGA, supraglottic airway.

Table 23.3 Mandibular hypoplasia

Condition	Implications	Causes	Suggestions
Triad of micrognathia, glossoptosis, cleft palate	Poor laryngoscopic views and difficult tracheal intubation Glossoptosis causes tongue base obstruction, OSA, and respiratory distress	Pierre Robin, Treacher Collins, Goldenhar, and Nager's syndromes[8]	Maintenance of oxygenation and ventilation can often be established with an SGA Use an SGA as a conduit for flexible bronchoscopy and tracheal intubation after local anesthetic spray to the airway

OSA, obstructive sleep apnea; SGA, supraglottic airway.

Airway management techniques

Overview of airway management

Managing a child with a congenital airway anomaly requires careful planning, skill, and experience. Important decisions need to be made concerning when, by whom, how, and where to manage the airway. If the patient is stable and time allows, an experienced team should manage the airway under ideal conditions. This strategy allows for unexpected difficulty, which may necessitate a range of airway techniques performed by experienced pediatric practitioners in the operating room. After initial airway management, the patient may require controlled ventilation or continuous positive airway pressure (CPAP) and

Table 23.4 Laryngeal anomalies

Condition	Implications	Causes	Suggestions
Laryngomalacia (60%)	Most common cause of stridor in newborns Mainly self-limiting		15% require supraglottoplasty, 3% require tracheostomy[2] With an experienced team, laryngomalacia, in isolation, does not pose serious difficulty during airway management
Vocal cord paralysis (15–20%)	Stridor, breathy cry, feeding difficulty, aspiration	Central nervous system Trauma Idiopathic	Most recover spontaneously without surgical intervention
Subglottic stenosis (10–15%) Subglottic diameter < 4 mm in term neonate, < 3 mm in premature neonate	Biphasic stridor Recurrent or prolonged croup	Subglottic hemangiomas (rare congenital vascular lesions, grow rapidly in the first month of life, stabilize at 12 to 18 months, and involute by 5 years of age)	Use careful endoscopic assessment Avoid the trauma of an oversized ETT Patients with severe hemangiomas may require tracheostomy to prevent airway obstruction
Laryngeal cysts	Airway obstruction risk BMV and tracheal intubation may be difficult	Saccular cysts Vallecular cysts Thyroglossal cysts Ductal cysts Laryngoceles	A planned surgical airway may be required
Laryngeal webs and atresia	Dysphonia		With complete atresia, the patient needs an emergency tracheostomy or planned EXIT procedure
Recurrent respiratory papillomatosis (most common benign neoplasm of larynx in children)	Hoarseness Complete airway obstruction can occur on induction of anesthesia Can present in adults	Infectious disease contracted during birth from mothers infected with human papilloma virus (HPV 6 and 11)	CO_2 laser microlaryngoscopy Gas induction, with topical anesthesia of the larynx and spontaneous ventilation, is a common airway management technique

BMV, bag-mask ventilation; EXIT, ex utero intrapartum treatment.

Table 23.5 Congenital tracheal anomalies

Causes	Presentation	Suggestions
Primary isolated TBM Secondary TBM associated with other abnormalities; esophageal atresia and tracheoesophageal fistula Extrinsic compression neoplasms, cysts, vascular or cardiac conditions	Cough, expiratory stridor, rarely cyanosis, apnea, cardiopulmonary arrest during feeding	Moderate to severe TBM can be treated with CPAP by creating a "pneumatic stent" Rarely, premature and term infants require a tracheostomy for severe TBM[6]

CPAP, continuous positive airway pressure; TBM, tracheobronchomalacia.

Table 23.6 Congenital esophageal atresia/tracheoesophageal fistula (TEF)

Presentation	Risk factors for airway complications	Suggestions
Choking during feeding, excessive salivation, practitioner unable to pass a suction catheter 9–10 cm down the esophagus Prenatal diagnosis and ultrasound yield is poor	1. Fistula within 1 cm of carina 2. Fistula below carina 3. Fistula larger than 3 mm 4. More than one fistula 5. Concomitant airway anomalies TEF is associated with coexisting congenital anomalies in up to 50% of presentations	Isolated esophageal atresia, without a fistula to the trachea, poses few airway problems Tracheal intubation above a small (< 1 mm) proximal fistula is generally safe, with low risk of gastric distension Endobronchial intubation past a distal fistula risks misplacement of the tube into the fistula. Use preoperative rigid bronchoscopy to delineate the airway anatomy and determine safe tube placement and ventilation[9]

careful weaning with extubation in intensive care. After extubation, pulse oximetry and apnea monitoring should continue if intubation was prolonged and traumatic, or if airway obstruction and respiratory arrest are possibilities. Many of these children are at risk of obstructive sleep apnea or rare complications such as post-obstructive pulmonary edema.

If the patient arrives in the emergency department in respiratory distress, call for help and commence immediate resuscitation. Oxygenation is the priority with optimum bag-mask or supraglottic airway (SGA) ventilation. Avoid repeated intubation attempts because of the high risk of complications.

Bag-mask ventilation (BMV)

Airway narrowing is the main cause of difficult ventilation, and children with a collapsible upper airway, such as that seen in laryngomalacia, will benefit from CPAP, which stents the airway and increases functional residual capacity. Creating an adequate mask seal can be

Table 23.7 Congenital thoracic anomalies

Causes	Implications	Suggestions
Congenital tumors *Anterior compartment* Congenital thymomas Teratomas *Middle compartment* Congenital pericardial teratomas *Posterior compartment* Descending aorta, esophagus, autonomic ganglia, and thoracic lymph nodes (site for most congenital mediastinal masses, including neurogenic and germ cell tumors)	Direct compression of the bronchi, trachea, heart, and great vessels Anterior mediastinal masses are associated with airway obstruction and hemodynamic instability	Risk of airway management depends on the site, type, and size of the lesion The patient may be difficult to ventilate, and anesthesia should be avoided, if possible Patient posture is important: sitting, reverse Trendelenburg, or even prone position may relieve airway obstruction Gas induction with sevoflurane and oxygen–helium mixture (20:80%) may be prolonged and is conducted in the best breathing position for the patient Maintain spontaneous ventilation, avoid muscle relaxants, consider rigid bronchoscopy, and plan for femoral–femoral bypass[9]
Congenital lobar emphysema Congenital high airway obstruction (CHAOS) Congenital diaphragmatic hernia Congenital cystic adenomatoid malformation (CCAM) Bronchopulmonary sequestration Bronchial atresia Congenital bronchogenic cysts	Can cause severe or complete airway obstruction May be associated with hypoplastic lungs	Antenatal diagnosis by ultrasound or MRI could indicate that an EXIT procedure, or EXIT to ECMO, should be used to avoid severe airway obstruction immediately after birth

ECMO, extracorporeal membrane oxygenation; EXIT, ex utero intrapartum treatment; MRI, magnetic resonance imaging.

challenging during BMV for children with dysmorphic features and distorted anatomy. Thomas and Ciarallo achieved a mask seal in a term infant with a frontonasal encephalocele by the novel approach of using an inverted adult size five facemask over the infant's face.[10] Maintaining a patent airway during inhalation induction of anesthesia can be difficult in infants with micrognathia. Optimum BMV techniques include jaw thrust, head tilt, and chin lift. Of these, jaw thrust is the most effective for opening the obstructed airway in an anesthetized child.[11] Airway obstruction in neonates during induction of anesthesia can be avoided by inserting an SGA after topicalization of the upper airway.[12]

Tracheal intubation

Although the incidence of difficult laryngoscopy is lower in children than in adults (1.37% vs. 9%), the incidence in infants is significantly higher than that in older children (4.7% vs. 0.7%).[3] The incidence of difficult laryngoscopy is doubled in children undergoing cardiac anesthesia owing to the relatively high incidence of concomitant congenital syndromes such as CHARGE and DiGeorge.[13] Difficulty to intubate can change as the child matures. Children with Treacher Collins syndrome, for example, become more difficult to intubate with age, whereas those with Pierre Robin syndrome become easier to intubate.[8]

Direct laryngoscopy and tracheal intubation, aided by a bougie and optimum external laryngeal manipulation, can be successful in the hands of experienced practitioners. For example, a straight blade paraglossal approach with a bougie was successful for infants with Pierre Robin syndrome.[14] Alternative options such as flexible bronchoscopy, rigid bronchoscopy, optical stylet, video laryngoscopy, or surgical airway need to be available in the event of failure.

Direct laryngoscopy attempts may be prolonged for infants with congenital airway anomalies, increasing the likelihood of patient awareness, trauma, and hypoxia. The use of nasal or buccal oxygen during intubation helps to avoid hypoxia, but intubation should be limited to three attempts to minimize the risk of trauma and other adverse events. Small tracheal tubes should be available for unexpected subglottic tracheal stenosis. Video laryngoscopes are useful adjuncts for rigid bronchoscope intubation in children.

Supraglottic airways

SGAs have multiple applications in the management of patients with congenital airway anomalies. They can be used as a primary airway; a conduit for tracheal intubation; a rescue ventilation device during resuscitation; and rescue during a failed airway. These devices can be used for extended periods of time for various surgical and medical indications.[15] Absolute contraindications to SGA use include increased risk of pulmonary aspiration, airway obstruction beyond the glottis, and high airway pressure. Relative contraindications include a partially collapsible lower airway, restricted access to the airway, and inexperience using an SGA.[16]

Awake intubation

An awake intubation technique in children is usually impractical because of poor patient cooperation; however, variants of this technique can be used in neonates and infants. Using an SGA for awake intubation of neonates with a predicted difficult airway is safe for early establishment of an airway. This technique avoids hypoxia during induction of anesthesia and has been used successfully in patients with Pierre Robin syndrome and Treacher Collins syndrome.[17] First, local anesthetic is applied, and the SGA is inserted. Then, the neonate receives gas induction followed by tracheal intubation with an ultrathin, flexible bronchoscope and an appropriate-size ETT.[12]

Muscle relaxants

Muscle relaxants can be beneficial for patients who have functional airway obstruction, such as laryngospasm. In patients who are mask ventilated and endotracheally intubated, conditions may improve with muscle relaxants. Conversely, patients with distal airway obstruction, including tracheomalacia, mucopolysaccharidosis, and mediastinal masses, should not be paralyzed. Paralysis in these patients exacerbates extrinsic airway compression, eliminates diaphragmatic movement, increases large airway compression, and decreases expiratory flow rates.

Conclusion

Patients with congenital airway anomalies are often challenging. Airway management requires a systematic approach and a thorough knowledge of syndromes and their comorbidities. Because some airways deteriorate with age, the airway practitioner should not rely on the security of a good past history. Given the frequency of airway-related problems associated with congenital anomalies, it is wise to plan for a difficult airway in these patients. Safe airway management is ideally conducted by an experienced team using preplanned strategies to maintain oxygenation and avoid trauma.

References

1. Baker, P. A., S. Aftimos, and B. J. Anderson, Airway management during an EXIT procedure for a fetus with dysgnathia complex. *Paediatric Anaesthesia*, 2004. 14(9):781–6.

2. Monnier, P., Congenital anomalies of the larynx and trachea. In P. Monnier, editor, *Pediatric Airway Surgery*, 2011, Springer, pp. 99–157.

3. Heinrich, S., T. Birkholz, H. Ihmsen, *et al.*, Incidence and predictors of difficult laryngoscopy in 11,219 pediatric anesthesia procedures. *Paediatric Anaesthesia*, 2012. 22(8):729–36.

4. Jain, R. R. and M. Rabb, The difficult pediatric airway. In C.A. Hagberg, editor, *Airway Management*, 2013, Elsevier, pp. 723–760.

5. Baum, V. C. and J. E. O'Flaherty, *Anesthesia for Genetic, Metabolic and Dysmorphic Syndromes of Childhood*, 2nd edn., 2007, Lipponcott Williams and Wilkins.

6. Isaacson, G., *Congenital Anomalies of the Head and Neck: Otolaryngologic Clinics of North America, Volume 40*, 2007, Saunders.

7. Walker, R., K. G. Belani, E. A. Braunlin, *et al.*, Anaesthesia and airway management in mucopolysaccharidosis. *Journal of Inherited Metabolic Disease*, 2013. 36(2):211–19.

8. Hosking, J., D. Zoanetti, A. Carlyle, *et al.*, Anesthesia for Treacher Collins syndrome: a review of airway management in 240 pediatric cases. *Paediatric Anaesthesia*, 2012. 22(8):752–8.

9. Duwe, B. V., D. H. Sterman, and A. I. Musani, Tumors of the mediastinum. *Chest*, 2005. 128(4):2893–909.

10. Thomas, J. J. and C. Ciarallo, Facemask ventilation with a frontonasal encephalocele. *Anesthesiology*, 2015. 122(3):698.

11. von Ungern-Sternberg, B. S., T.O. Erb, A. Reber, *et al.*, Opening the upper airway – airway maneuvers in pediatric

anesthesia. *Paediatric Anaesthesia*, 2005. 15(3):181–9.

12. Jagannathan, N. and C. T. Truong, A simple method to deliver pharyngeal anesthesia in syndromic infants prior to awake insertion of the intubating laryngeal airway. *Canadian Journal of Anaesthesia*, 2010. 57(12): 1138–9.

13. Heinrich, S., *et al.*, Incidence and predictors of poor laryngoscopic view in children undergoing pediatric cardiac surgery. *Journal of Cardiothoracic & Vascular Anesthesia*, 2013. 27(3):516–21.

14. Semjen, F., M. Bordes, and A. M. Cros, Intubation of infants with Pierre Robin syndrome: the use of the paraglossal approach combined with a gum-elastic bougie in six consecutive cases. *Anaesthesia*, 2008. 63(2):147–50.

15. Jagannathan, N., L. Sequera-Ramos, L. Sohn, *et al.*, Elective use of supraglottic airway devices for primary airway management in children with difficult airways. *British Journal of Anaesthesia*, 2014. 112(4):742–8.

16. Asai, T., Is it safe to use supraglottic airway in children with difficult airways? *British Journal of Anaesthesia*, 2014. 112(4):620–2.

17. Asai, T., A. Nagata, and K. Shingu, Awake tracheal intubation through the laryngeal mask in neonates with upper airway obstruction. *Paediatric Anaesthesia*, 2008. 18(1):77–80.

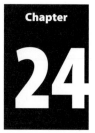

Management of post-tonsillectomy hemorrhage

Nicholas M. Dalesio

Case representation

A 12-year-old male presents on postoperative day 10, after tonsillectomy, which was performed for treatment of recurrent tonsillitis. He has been vomiting copious amounts of blood. On physical examination, he is pale and tachycardic, but he is conversant, alert, and oriented. Currently, he is not vomiting and has old blood present in his mouth.

Introduction

More than 530,000 children undergo tonsillectomies in the United States annually.[1] Adenotonsillectomy (AT) is most commonly performed to treat sleep-disordered breathing and obstructive sleep apnea (OSA) in children; however, AT is also performed to treat recurrent tonsillitis and chronic sinus infections. The most common, and potentially life-threatening, complication after tonsillectomy is postoperative hemorrhage. The frequency is estimated to be less that 3% in children,[2,3] but higher frequencies are seen with increased use of coblation techniques (11.1%)[4] and in older adults, especially those over 70 years of age. In children less than 3 years of age, post-AT hemorrhage can lead to severe dehydration, decreased oral intake, and worsening of breathing problems. In addition to losing fluids from active bleeding, young patients may be extremely intravascularly depleted from lack of oral intake before the bleeding. Therefore, fluid resuscitation must be aggressive.

Postoperative hemorrhage is classified as primary (occurring less than 24 hours after surgery) or secondary (occurring more than 24 hours postoperatively). Primary bleeding occurs in < 1% of patients but is considered more dangerous owing to a higher likelihood of brisk bleeding from an arterial source.[5,6] Secondary hemorrhage is more common, and brisk bleeding can occur well beyond 24 hours after surgery. In fact, secondary hemorrhage can occur up to 2 weeks after surgery, with the peak of bleeding events occurring 5–8 days after tonsillectomy (Figure 24.1). The proposed mechanism of such secondary bleeding is retraction and sloughing of the eschar covering the healing tonsillar bed. The most common locations of postoperative bleeding are the tonsillar fossa (67%) and the nasopharynx (27%), with bleeding at both locations occurring only 7% of the time. Factors that appear to increase the risk for post-tonsillectomy bleeding include older age, male sex, and surgical indication of recurrent/chronic tonsillitis.

Cases in Emergency Airway Management, ed. Lauren C. Berkow and John C. Sakles. Published by Cambridge University Press. © Cambridge University Press 2015.

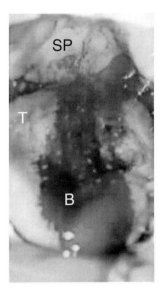

Figure 24.1 Image of the oropharynx with bleeding (B) originating from the tonsillar beds tracking along the anterior portion of the tongue (T). SP = soft palate

Airway management

Post-tonsillectomy bleeding is considered a surgical emergency, as concerns for both acute blood loss/hypovolemia and airway obstruction occur simultaneously, often in young children who may already be relatively dehydrated or have pharyngeal swelling from post-surgical issues. In the emergency department, nonsurgical treatments may help to slow the bleeding, such as clot removal from the tonsillar fossa followed by compression using epinephrine or cocaine-soaked sponges, cauterization, or ligation of bleeding vessels; however, pediatric patients often cannot tolerate these interventions.[7]

Securing the airway of these patients for airway management during surgical procedures to control bleeding can be quite difficult. Airway managers should review the previous anesthetic records of these postoperative patients to identify comorbidities that may make airway management more difficult and establish the methods used hours or days earlier during a successful induction of anesthesia. Even if the patient has a history of easy induction and intubation, copious amounts of blood and clot within the oropharynx, and/or pharyngeal swelling from postoperative changes, can turn a previously easy airway into a difficult one. The same comorbid conditions that predict respiratory compromise after AT in children should be red flags for difficulty maintaining airway patency, including diagnosis of Down syndrome, cerebral palsy and other neuromuscular diseases, sickle cell disease, obesity, severe OSA, young age (specifically age < 3 years), craniofacial abnormalities, and metabolic or genetic diseases.

Airway management of these patients is difficult even in the elective setting. An estimation of the quantity of blood vomited and duration of bleeding, in combination with a physical examination and acquisition of vital signs, can help clinicians determine the patient's blood volume status. Clinical signs that suggest hypovolemia include orthostatic hypotension, dizziness, and mental status changes, necessitating vigorous fluid resuscitation with crystalloid or colloid solutions. Clinical symptoms of hypovolemia may not present until 10–20% of a child's total blood volume is lost, and typically presents with narrowed pulse pressures due to elevations in diastolic pressure from compensating increases in systemic vascular resistance. Tachycardia may not be evident due to high heart rates at baseline in smaller children.

Before anesthesia is induced, the patient should receive fluid resuscitation to avoid hypotension and should have a type and cross-match of blood. Transfusion is rarely required, but blood needs to be available for the most extreme cases. Early intervention for children with bleeding after tonsillectomy can preclude the need for blood products and avoid the possible airway and physiologic consequences of blood loss.

Patients with oropharyngeal bleeding should be treated as non-fasted patients who likely have a stomach full of food/liquid/blood. Additionally, copious amounts of blood and/or clots in the posterior oropharynx can obstruct a view of the glottis and increase aspiration risk. Primary and secondary plans for airway exposure, intubation, and ventilation should be made prior to induction of anesthesia. Pharyngeal bleeding is often temporized by pharyngeal packing until the airway can be secured. Bleeding vessels may be controlled with ipsilateral compression to the carotid artery and careful suctioning, and aspiration risk can be reduced by maintaining the patient in a head-down position. Surgical exploration and ligation/cauterization is the definitive treatment; therefore, efforts to bring the patient to the operating room should be expedited. If the patient is in respiratory distress, unable to protect his/her airway, and additional assistance is not available, the airway should be secured by the airway practitioner immediately caring for the patient. Precautions should be taken in anticipation for a difficult airway (having immediately available multiple intubation devices, oral/nasal airways, and supraglottic airways) and surgical consultation and their presence should be requested if a "cannot intubate, cannot oxygenate" situation occurs. If time permits, and a difficult airway is known or suspected, an otolaryngology or pediatric surgeon should be present at the bedside prior to airway intervention.

Airway managers should place cardiopulmonary monitors and allow for adequate denitrogenation time before administering anesthesia agents. Intravenous access also should be established before induction of anesthesia, both for volume replacement and for administration of intravenous agents. Rapid sequence intubation should be performed if a review of comorbid conditions shows no contraindication and the anesthesia record does not suggest any previous difficulties with laryngeal exposure/intubation. The operating room should be stocked with multiple laryngoscope blades and handles, and several operational suction lines and canisters should be available to clear the oropharynx of blood. A styletted endotracheal tube (ETT), preferably one with a cuff to decrease aspiration risk, should be used during the intubation attempt. Medications that can be used include propofol 1–2 mg/kg, etomidate 0.1–0.3 mg/kg, or ketamine 1.5–2 mg/kg for induction, in combination with succinylcholine 1.5–2 mg/kg or rocuronium 1.2 mg/kg for prompt neuromuscular blockade, to rapidly expose the airway and allow intubation. If the patient is hemodynamically unstable, ketamine is the best choice, as etomidate or propofol can cause a decrease in blood pressure.

Difficult airway risk

In patients who have comorbidities that suggest a possible difficult intubation, the airway manager may want to attempt intubation while the patient is awake or asleep and spontaneously ventilating. If intubation is unsuccessful, the American Society of Anesthesiologists' (ASA) difficult airway algorithm should be used as a guide for airway management options.[8,9]

In a retrospective study, Fields *et al.* found that 2.7% of patients with post-tonsillectomy hemorrhage had difficult airways.[3] Most commonly, the difficult airway was related to the clinician's inability to see the glottis as a result of blood or clot in the oropharynx. None of these patients had airway difficulties at initial surgery.[3] All patients, however, were successfully intubated in subsequent intubation attempts. A supraglottic airway, such as a laryngeal mask airway (LMA) or an AirQ laryngeal airway, has been used successfully in management of oropharyngeal bleeding and should be considered early if ventilation and/or intubation are difficult.[10] The supraglottic airway device may tamponade areas of tonsil bleeding and partition the bleeding area away from the airway. Additionally, it provides a protective conduit to the glottis through which suctioning can be used to eliminate blood and clot obstructing the view of the vocal cords. Subsequently, the patient can be intubated with a fiberoptic laryngoscope through the supraglottic airway. Be sure to select a supraglottic airway through which the pilot balloon from a cuffed ETT can pass, especially when using small supraglottic airways for younger patients. Placement of a supraglottic airway is relatively contraindicated in patients with a surgically altered airway (e.g. laryngotracheal separation, tracheostomy, congenital or acquired laryngeal obstruction), full stomach, and where high airway pressures are necessary. However, in situations where tonsillar hemorrhage is uncontrollable and difficulty visualizing the glottis is likely, the supraglottic airway should be considered.

Bleeding risk

Repeated bleeding after surgery, specifically if no causative vessel is identified, suggests that the patient may have a previously undiagnosed coagulopathy or, in rare cases, a vascular injury. It has been suggested that prothrombotic factors are upregulated in patients with OSA and that patients with OSA may have some protection against post-tonsillectomy bleeding compared with patients who undergo AT for chronic tonsillitis.[11] Anesthesiologists or emergency department physicians should order measurements of prothrombin, partial prothrombin time, international normalized ratio, fibrinogen, and bleeding time to determine if a bleeding abnormality is present. More specialized testing can be directed by hematology consultants. Patients with severe or repeated bleeding should be held for observation and may be discharged with oral antifibrinolytics (aminocaproic acid), especially after two or three occurrences of re-bleeding. Embolization performed in interventional radiology may be considered as an adjunct or alternative to surgical control if bleeding continues after multiple surgical evaluations or the hemorrhage cannot be controlled through a transoral approach.[12]

Extubation

Extubation should be planned carefully in a patient who has been completely reversed from anesthesia and is ventilating spontaneously. Fields *et al.* reported that, based on their institutional experience, the majority of hypoxemic events occurred during airway management for extubation.[3] Patients may need to remain intubated if they do not meet extubation criteria (aspiration of blood leading to ventilation/perfusion defects, tachypnea, inability to return to baseline mental status, etc.) and if bleeding could not be controlled surgically. Patients unable to be extubated should be transported to the pediatric intensive care unit (PICU) for hemodynamic monitoring. If the child meets extubation criteria, they should be monitored in the hospital overnight if continued bleeding is expected; otherwise, the patient can be discharged from the hospital if surgical exploration and identification of a bleeding source was successfully controlled. Other complications associated with tonsillectomy, including upper airway obstruction, remain a postoperative concern.

Airway management summary

1. Previously determined easy airway and minimal bleeding.

   (a) Denitrogenate patient, place standard ASA monitors, and ensure otolaryngology or pediatric surgeon has been consulted and is present if possible before induction.
   (b) Perform rapid sequence intubation using a cuffed ETT.
   (c) After securing the ETT, suction the stomach.
   (d) Have supraglottic airway available as backup device.

2. Previously determined difficult airway, severe bleeding, and/or copious blood in the mouth.

   (a) Denitrogenate patient, place standard ASA monitors, and ensure otolaryngology surgeon is present before induction if the patient is hemodynamically stable and not in respiratory distress. If a surgeon is not available, preparation for an emergent surgical/needle cricothyrotomy is necessary.
   (b) Consider elective intubation through supraglottic airway while maintaining spontaneous ventilation.
   (c) After securing the ETT, suction the stomach.
   (d) Have a backup plan established, which may include a video laryngoscope.

References

1. Baugh RF, Archer SM, Mitchell RB, et al. Number of tonsillectomy surgeries in the US. *Otolaryngology – Head and Neck Surgery*. 2011 Jan;**144**(1):S1–30.

2. Windfuhr JP, Chen Y-S. Incidence of post-tonsillectomy hemorrhage in children and adults: a study of 4,848 patients. *Ear Nose Throat Journal*. 2002 Sep;**81**(9):626–8–630–632passim.

3. Fields RG, Gencorelli FJ, Litman RS. Anesthetic management of the pediatric bleeding tonsil. *Paediatric Anaesthesia*. 2010 Nov;**20**(11):982–6.

4. Windfuhr JP, Chen YS, Remmert S. Hemorrhage following tonsillectomy and adenoidectomy in 15,218 patients. *Otolaryngology – Head and Neck Surgery*. 2005 Feb;**132**(2):281–6.

5. Handler SD, Miller L, Richmond KH, Baranak CC. Post-tonsillectomy hemorrhage: incidence, prevention and management. *The Laryngoscope*. 1986 Nov;**96**(11):1243–7.

6. Windfuhr JP, Verspohl BC, Chen Y-S, Dahm JD, Werner JA. Post-tonsillectomy haemorrhage – some facts will never change. *European Archives of Otorhinolaryngology*. 2015 May;**272**(5):1211–18.

7. Steketee KG, Reisdorff EJ. Emergency care for post-tonsillectomy and post-adenoidectomy hemorrhage. *American Journal of Emergency Medicine*. 1995 Sep;**13**(5):518–23.

8. American Society of Anesthesiologists Task Force on Management of the Difficult Airway. Practice Guidelines for Management of the Difficult Airway. An updated report by the American Society of Anesthesiologists Task Force on Management of the Difficult Airway. *Anesthesiology*. 2003 May;**98**(5):1269–77.

9. Engelhardt T, Weiss M. A child with a difficult airway: what do I do next? *Current Opinions in Anaesthesiology*. 2012 Jun;**25**(3):326–32.

10. Go WH, Kim K-T, Kim JY, Choe WJ, Kim JW. The use of laryngeal mask airway in pediatric patient with massive post-tonsillectomy hemorrhage. *Korean Journal of Anesthesiology*. 2012 Aug;**63**(2):177–8.

11. Perkins JN, Liang C, Gao D, Shultz L, Friedman NR. Risk of post-tonsillectomy hemorrhage by clinical diagnosis. *The Laryngoscope*. 2012 Oct;**122**(10):2311–15.

12. Opatowsky MJ, Browne JD, McGuirt WF Jr., Morris PP. Endovascular treatment of hemorrhage after tonsillectomy in children. *AJNR American Journal of Neuroradiology*. 2001 Apr;**22**(4):713–16.

Fiberoptic intubation

William Rosenblatt and P. Allan Klock, Jr.

Case presentation

A 59-year-old female presents to the emergency department in respiratory distress. She has a 75-pack-year smoking history. Her oxygen saturation on 3 L nasal cannula oxygen is stable at 82%, and her respiratory efforts appear to be tiring. She has ankylosing spondylitis and her cervical spine is rigid. Her oral aperture is limited and her Mallampati class is 3. Close examination reveals a healed tracheostomy scar. After intravenous injection of a desiccant, 500 mg of lidocaine is applied to the airway. A tracheostomy set is brought to the bedside, and an on-call trauma surgeon is present. The airway manager intubates the patient's trachea using a flexible intubation scope. After proper tube position is confirmed with end-tidal CO_2 detection and auscultation, sedation is administered.

Introduction

The flexible intubation scope (FIS) is an important tool for airway management that may be used in elective and urgent situations. The FIS is a delicate device that demands substantial hand–eye coordination. Its use is often impaired by saliva, sputum, blood, and traumatic debris. Despite these shortcomings, the FIS is considered a gold standard in many difficult airway situations.

In the case described above, the patient, though failing, is maintaining a stable, albeit low, oxygen saturation. The presence of a tracheostomy scar and her fixed cervical spine suggest that the patient's trachea likely will be difficult to intubate by routine means. The airway management team made the wise decision to keep her spontaneously breathing and awake. An FIS was a good choice of instrumentation because her arthritic disease would likely prevent neck extension, hampering direct and video laryngoscopy. Despite their success, it was prudent to prepare for surgical airway access.

Mechanics

The classic FIS is referred to as a fiberoptic bronchoscope (FOB), reflecting its reliance on flexible glass fibers for image transmission and its use for inspecting the bronchi. The main structures of the FOB include the insertion cord, which contains a coherent image bundle, one or two noncoherent light-carrying bundles, a working channel, and control wires.

Distal chip, or "digital," intubation scopes employ a camera chip embedded at the objective end of the scope. Illumination is provided by one or more light-emitting diodes (LEDs).

Cases in Emergency Airway Management, ed. Lauren C. Berkow and John C. Sakles. Published by Cambridge University Press. © Cambridge University Press 2015.

In addition to traditional reusable FISs, single-patient distal chip intubation scopes are now available. These scopes may be used on one patient multiple times, but they cannot be cleaned or used on another patient. These scopes require considerably less capital investment than do traditional scopes, and they alleviate concerns related to FIS-facilitated cross-contamination of respiratory pathogens.[1]

The working channel, a continuous lumen that extends from the handle to the objective end, can be used to suction the airway, deliver drugs, pass wires or tools such as graspers, or insufflate oxygen. The size of the working channel is limited by the size of the insertion cord. The smallest FISs cannot accommodate a working channel.

Two control wires originate in the handle, where they attach to a finger-operated lever mechanism. Moving the lever, typically with the thumb of the left hand, results in movement of the distal end of the scope in the sagittal plane. The scope should be cleaned and inspected as dictated by the manufacturer before each use, and it should be stored vertically (i.e. hanging) between uses.

Advantages of video monitors

Whether FOB or electronic, systems that employ video monitors have several advantages, especially during management of a difficult airway. In particular, they have improved ergonomics and allow other practitioners to view the airway (Figure 25.1). When an FIS-dedicated video system is not available, most laparoscopic cameras or operating room video systems will interface with classic eyepiece-FOBs.

Difficult airway cart – what you need

The FIS is a complex device that requires careful handling and special equipment to protect it and facilitate its use. Typical FIS systems use a cart or workstation to store the adjunct equipment, light source, image processor, and video monitor and carry the FIS in a manner that prevents damage or cross-contamination (Figure 25.1). The American Society of Anesthesiologists (ASA) Task Force on Management of the Difficult Airway suggests that such a mobile workstation be outfitted with a variety of airway management devices (Box 25.1).[2]

Handling the FIS

The FIS is intended to be used so that the handle is held in the nondominant hand, with the directional lever facing the operator and the working channel control on the opposite side of the scope (Figure 25.2). The tip of the thumb is positioned on the directional lever. The tip of the first finger is positioned on the working channel control, if present. Upward motion of the lever results in posterior bending of the distal end of the FIS, and downward lever pressure results in anterior bending. An oxygen or suction source may be connected to the working channel control valve, if present (Table 25.1). The first finger will operate this valve to provide oxygen flow or apply suction.

The operator's dominant hand is positioned close to the objective end of the insertion cord. Most operators will find a comfortable hand position. The author prefers a pencil-like grip. This hand will manage fine insertion and retreat control, and delicate adjustments in yaw rotation. The operator's two hands work in concert to provide gross rotation along the entire insertion cord.

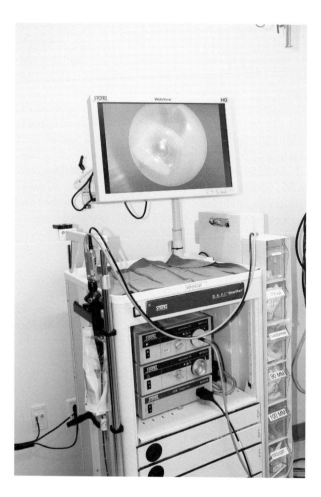

Figure 25.1 A difficult intubation cart equipped with a digital FIS. The FIS is stored in a single-use plastic shield (ProShield, Seitz Tech, Oxford, PA). A Karl Storz adult FOB with a digital image correlation camera light source coupler is also shown

Choosing the FIS outer diameter

FISs are manufactured in outer diameter (o.d.) sizes that range from 2 mm to 6 mm. Choosing the correct size is essential to airway management success. As a general rule, the clinician should first decide what size ETT is to be placed into the airway and then choose the FIS diameter that best matches that ETT's internal diameter (i.d.). Under ideal circumstances, the o.d. of the scope should be 1 to 1.5 mm smaller than the i.d. of the tube. For example, if a 7.0-mm i.d. ETT is chosen, a FIS no smaller than 5.5 mm o.d. should be used. The FIS should pass smoothly through the ETT, with or without a medical grade lubricant, depending on the recommendation of the manufacturer. The most commonly used FISs are in the 3.7 to 4.2 mm o.d. range.

Choosing an ETT size

During urgent or emergency care of a patient with a compromised or difficult airway, the clinician should consider using the smallest i.d. ETT that can oxygenate and ventilate the patient for the short term. After the airway has been secured and the patient's other

BOX 25.1 Equipment for a FIS and difficult airway workstation

ASA-suggested difficult airway workstation

- Rigid laryngoscope blades of alternate design and size from those routinely used; this may include a rigid fiberoptic laryngoscope
- Video laryngoscope
- Endotracheal tubes (ETTs) of assorted sizes
- ETT guides; examples include (but are not limited to) semi-rigid stylets, ventilating tube-changer, light wands, and forceps designed to manipulate the distal portion of the ETT
- Supraglottic airways (e.g. laryngeal mask airway (LMA) or intubating laryngeal mask airway (ILMA) of assorted sizes for noninvasive airway ventilation/ intubation)
- Flexible fiberoptic intubation equipment
- Equipment suitable for emergency invasive airway access
- An exhaled carbon dioxide detector

Suggested dedicated devices to facilitate FIS use

- Dedicated clean and "dirty," or disposable, transport receptacle
- Light source, image processor, video monitor mounting as needed
- Cable storage (e.g. universal cord)
- Electricity supply
- Water-soluble, medical-grade lubricant and/or medical silicone lubricant (for lubrication of insertion cord and/or ETT cuff)
- Defogging agent and/or alcohol: used on objective lens prior to use. Often available in laparoscopic suites
- Intubating oral airways: dedicated oral airways that provide a channel for FIS and ETT passage
- Nasal airways (variety of infant to adult sizes): often used to prepare the nasal channels or as a conduit for passage of the FIS

Equipment to facilitate awake intubation

- Variety of local anesthetics* – solution, viscous, ointment, gel
- Nasal vasoconstrictor agents (e.g. oxymetazoline)
- Gauze pads, cotton applicators
- McGill or Krause forceps
- Medication nebulizer
- Epidural catheters
- ETTs (variety of sizes and types)

* The authors prefer lidocaine as sole local anesthetic. This drug is available in a number of preparations and concentrations, making dose calculations simple.

Table 25.1 Comparison of oxygen versus suction application to the working channel

Oxygen		Suction	
Benefits	**Cautions**	**Benefits**	**Cautions**
Clear fogging	Damage to FIS if occluded	Removal of secretions	Requires adequately sized channel
Blows aside secretions	Reports of stomach rupture[3]	Clear fogging	Reduced inspired oxygen possible
Enriched inspired oxygen environment			

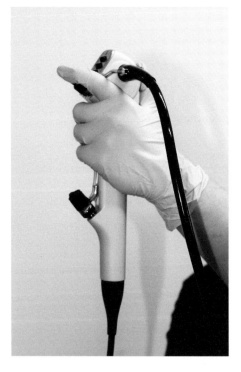

Figure 25.2 This picture demonstrates proper position of the hand and fingers while holding the fiberoptic scope

conditions stabilized, the clinical provider can make a controlled switch to another ETT, perform a surgical airway, or use expectant management.

Preparation of the fiberscope

Appropriate valves may need to be attached to the FIS handle (e.g. suction/oxygen valve, working channel diaphragm, stop-cock, or cap). Suction or an oxygen source may be attached to the valve, if available. The illumination source should be attached and tested. Image quality should be tested. Whether using eyepiece or video monitoring, a crisp, well-illuminated image should be produced. Image pixilation can occur as an artifact of the FIS

Table 25.2 Pitfalls during FIS-aided intubation

Pitfall	Resolution
Fogging	Suction/oxygen/prewarming or chemical solution
Secretions	Antisialagogue/suction/oxygen
White out (tissue contact)	Slow retreat
Epiglottis covering airway	Aggressive chin lift or jaw thrust
Unrecognized anatomy	Slow retreat
Unrecognized pathway	Aim toward obvious lumens and structures
Obstructing masses	Steer around masses
Multiple pathways without clear anatomic distinction	Investigation with FIS; observe air movement (e.g. bubbles)

mechanics. Slight "defocusing" will often improve the image. Often, a defogging agent will be applied to the objective lens or eyepiece, or the objective lens can be placed in warm water before use (Table 25.2).

An ETT is loaded onto the FIS (see Choosing an ETT size, above) with or without lubrication as discussed above. The ETT is loaded to the handle and may be secured with tape or a friction fitting.

Approach to the patient

In an emergency situation, especially when the patient's oxygenation and ventilation are inadequate, FIS-aided intubation may not be the best choice for airway management, as discussed above. Blood, traumatic debris, and uncontrolled secretions (sputum, saliva) will hinder visualization. Despite this, experienced operators who are using an FIS with an adequate working channel and access to suction or oxygen are often able to secure the airway with the FIS within a few seconds.

Level of consciousness

The clinical provider must decide whether to pursue airway management before or after induction of general anesthesia. When the patient is kept awake and is adequately prepared (discussed below), FIS-aided tracheal intubation can usually be pursued at a cautious pace and in a controlled manner while keeping the patient cooperative and self-oxygenating/ventilating. The patient should be kept at a depth of sedation that meets criteria for minimal or moderate sedation, especially if there are concerns regarding the aspiration of gastric contents or soiling of the trachea with blood or other material. FIS-aided intubation efforts can be safely aborted if proven impossible, and another method of airway management chosen. The advantages and disadvantages of awake management are listed in Table 25.3.

FIS-aided intubation can also be carried out in the unconscious patient regardless of whether the unconsciousness is drug-induced or pathologic. The advantages and disadvantages of managing airways in unconscious patients are also listed in Table 25.3.

Table 25.3 Comparison of awake versus asleep FIS-aided intubation

Awake FIS-aided intubation		Asleep FIS-aided intubation	
Advantages	**Disadvantages**	**Advantages**	**Disadvantages**
Oxygenation/ventilation patient self-maintained	Airway analgesia required	Does not require analgesic blocks	Intra-airway collapse
Intra-airway space maintained	Time and resource expenditure	Obtunded reflexes	Oxygenation/ventilation dependent on operator
Self-protection from aspiration			Aspiration risk

In patients who are partially obtunded, FIS-aided management may be particularly difficult and require expert help to open the airway with jaw-thrust or other maneuvers. An FIS-aided technique can require subtle and skilled manipulation of the airway and the device. An uncooperative or frankly combative patient is often difficult to manage. Forceful application of the device and lack of cooperation may result in airway trauma, failure to secure the airway, and/or damage to the FIS.

Route of airway access

The upper airway may be accessed through either the nose or mouth. Nasal access to the larynx is generally easier than oral access owing to the course of the airway (less-acute angles). Nasal access in the face-traumatized patient is safe in most circumstances because the course is being visually guided. A vasoconstrictor should be applied to the nasal cavities, if not contraindicated. Visual guidance through the nasal cavity ensures that the FIS and ETT follow the correct course. Nasal manipulation is often accompanied by bleeding, which may hinder not only FIS-aided intubation, but also other optical and image techniques.

Oral access requires an adequate aperture, not only for the FIS and ETT, but also for adjuncts such as intubating oral airways. Intubating oral airways have a dual purpose – they create a space for passage of the ETT through the potential space of the mouth (occupied by the tongue in the unconscious patient) and prevent damage to the FIS by the teeth. A variety of types and sizes of intubating oral airways are available.

FIS-aided tracheal intubation

The operator should assess the patient's airway, paying close attention to anatomic distortion and soiling. A highly soiled airway is unlikely to be amenable to FIS-aided management. If the patient has trismus or a high degree of oral trauma, including multiple broken teeth, nasal intubation may be favored over oral intubation. Facial trauma may favor oral intubation, though nasal intubation is not necessarily contraindicated.

The mouth and pharynx should be suctioned to remove blood and/or secretions. If time permits, an antisialogogue such as glycopyrrolate may be administered intravenously or intramuscularly. This drug will require 15 minutes to reach peak effect and should not be used if contraindicated by a history of tachyarrhythmias or glaucoma.

If oral intubation is chosen, an intubating airway may be placed. If nasal intubation is chosen, the operator may choose to use a soft, lubricated nasal airway coated with local anesthetic and a vasoconstrictor such as phenylephrine or oxymetazoline to improve the intranasal space. Blind placement is contraindicated in the face of trauma.

The operator either holds the FIS above the patient while standing behind him/her or holds the FIS in front of the patient while standing in front. The nondominant hand is positioned on the FIS handle, and the dominant hand is at the objective end. Throughout the intubation, the hands are kept maximally separated with slight tension applied to the insertion cord. This approach keeps the insertion cord straight and improves rotational control.

As the FIS is passed into the nose or mouth, the operator maintains an image of the anatomy. Slow and decisive scope movements are used. The operator should keep the anatomic target in the center of the image as the scope is inserted. Loss of image may be due to fogging, secretions, or contact with tissue. The application of suction/oxygen will remove the two former offenders. Contact with tissues should be treated with slow withdrawal until anatomy can once again be recognized. Progress toward the larynx is made slowly. A variety of pitfalls may be encountered and must be overcome (Table 25.2).

When the glottis is identified, the FIS is advanced into the larynx. Often the FIS must initially be steered toward the anterior commissure of the laryngeal inlet. When the tip of the scope is within a few millimeters of the commissure, the tip is directed posterior to the control lever and the scope is passed between the vocal cords. As the FIS enters the larynx, the operator should identify the cricoid cartilage, tracheal rings, and carina. The longitudinal striations of the posterior membranous part of the trachea should be appreciated opposite the arch of the tracheal rings. Failure to identify any of these structures may indicate esophageal position.

Once the carina is identified, the ETT is advanced along the insertion cord and into the larynx. Importantly, if the patient is awake, anesthesia should not be induced – tracheal intubation may still fail. At approximately 12 cm into the airway, the ETT bevel will encounter the larynx. Operators commonly encounter tissue impingement (also called hang-up), with entrapment of the right vocal cord and other structures in a gap between the FIS and ETT. If hang-up occurs, a 1-cm withdrawal of the ETT, followed by 90 degree counterclockwise rotation and reinsertion will most often be successful.

After the ETT has been passed through the laryngeal inlet, it should be possible to visualize the tube bevel above the carina. It is a good practice to image the carina and ETT simultaneously. The operator should then withdraw the FIS, inflate the endotracheal tube cuff, and begin ventilation. An end-tidal carbon dioxide detector and auscultation or ultrasonography should always be used to confirm tracheal position of the tube. If the patient is awake, unconsciousness may be induced, if necessary, only after confirmation of proper tube position. The ETT should be secured firmly in place.

Awake intubation (AI)

As discussed elsewhere in this text, tracheal intubation while the patient is still awake and cooperative is pursued in a number of circumstances where ablation of spontaneous respiration or airway reflexes may increase the risk of morbidity. The patient should understand the plan of AI. A patient who understands the process will better cooperate with it.

If not contraindicated, an antisialagogue is administered as early in the course as possible. Glycopyrrolate 0.2 mg or atropine 0.5 mg can be used. Dexmedetomidine and

Table 25.4 Common blocks

Location	Method	Dose*
Nose	Swabs or dripped LA	50 mg per side
Pharynx	LA swabs against palatoglossal arch, bilateral	50 mg per side
Hypopharynx/ larynx	Dripped LA	100 mg
	Superior laryngeal nerve block	2 mL, 4% lidocaine injected into the superior, posterior thyrohyoid membrane †
Larynx/trachea	LA injected via FIS	100 mg
	Trans-CTM block	100 mg injected via the CTM‡
Nebulized block all structures	LA solution is placed in a respiratory atomizer	400 mg or less

CTM, cricothyroid membrane; LA, local anesthetic.
* Doses are for lidocaine.
† In the superior laryngeal nerve block, the hyoid bone is palpated and manually deviated to the side to be blocked. The most lateral border of the hyoid is identified. LA is injected 1 cm medial to this position at the underside of the bone. The operator aspirates for air and blood, and anesthetic is injected in and around the membrane. The block is repeated on the contralateral side.
‡ The CTM block is really a topical anesthetic block performed invasively. A fine needle is passed through the CTM. When air can be easily aspirated from the larynx, the LA is injected. The patient should be warned of the ensuing stimulation (and likely cough), and the operator should secure the needle during injection.

scopolamine are also effective antisialagogues but may require more time and effort to achieve significant desiccation. Desiccation is used to improve both visualization in the airway and contact of topical anesthetics with the mucosa. If not contraindicated, a nasal mucosa vasoconstrictor is applied.

After desiccation, topical airway blocks are applied to the mouth, pharynx, hypopharynx, larynx, and trachea. Invasive blocks need not be held until drying occurs. Table 25.4 lists common blocks and their techniques. For swab techniques, local anesthetic (solution, viscous, or ointment) is loaded onto a swab or gauze and held against the appropriate anatomy. For drip techniques, an appropriate local anesthetic (e.g. 4% lidocaine) is delivered via syringe and spread over the anatomy. Whenever local anesthetic is applied to the structures of the mouth and pharynx or hypopharynx, it is helpful to control the patient's tongue by grasping it with a dry cotton gauze to reduce guarding of the structure and prevent swallowing. Local anesthetic can be applied below the cords by administration through the cricothyroid membrane (Table 25.4). A syringe and fine needle should be used for injections. The authors prefer to use lidocaine preparations. Lidocaine is marketed in a number of concentrations and preparations, and total dose can be recorded. For adult topical analgesia, 600–800 mg of lidocaine may be used, though it is rare that more than 500 mg will be necessary. If atomized lidocaine is used, the total dose from all applications should be limited to 400 mg.

Sedation must be used judiciously. Too often, excessive sedation is used in lieu of no, improper, or poor local anesthetic blocks. Deep sedation invites the risk of negating the careful decision-making and safety concerns that led to the choice of AI. Small doses of benzodiazepines (1–2 mg of midazolam) and rapidly acting opioids (25–50 mcg of fentanyl) are usually sufficient in the adult. Remifentanil (0.1–0.5 mcg/kg per minute) or dexmedetomidine (0.4–0.7 mcg/kg per hour) infusions have been used with great success.

Regardless of the rationale, the decision to pursue AI is based on patient safety, and few other factors, apart from rapid deterioration of the patient, should interfere with AI attempts. Though AI is very often performed with an FIS, virtually any tool used to secure the airway in an asleep patient may be used in the awake patient.[4]

The process of AI is multifaceted and should be pursued in a deliberate, methodical, and controlled way. In some urgent situations, AI may not be appropriate owing to rapid deterioration of other systems. When AI must be abandoned, the care team may need to secure the airway quickly using percutaneous or surgical techniques if airway management by other techniques fail.

Conclusion

The FIS is a versatile tool that should be familiar to all airway managers. Hospitals and appropriate departments need to invest in the proper maintenance, cleaning, storage, and distribution of these devices if they are to be used safely and effectively. Ongoing practice and training, including simulation, are vital to maintaining skills.

Likewise, AI is a key skill. Most airway managers agree that securing the airway while the patient is breathing spontaneously and maintaining his or her airway architecture is perhaps the safest way to care for a patient with a difficult-to-manage airway.

References

1. C.A. Diaz Granados, M.Y. Jones, T. Kongphet-Tran, *et al.* Outbreak of *Pseudomonas aeruginosa* infection associated with contamination of a flexible bronchoscope. *Infect Control Hosp Epidemiol* 2009; **30**: 550–5.

2. J.L. Apfelbaum, C.A. Hagberg, R. A. Caplan, *et al.* Practice guidelines for management of the difficult airway: an updated report by the American Society of Anesthesiologists Task Force on Management of the Difficult Airway. *Anesthesiology* 2013; **118**: 251–70.

3. N. Chapman. Gastric rupture and pneumoperitoneum caused by oxygen insufflation via a fiberoptic bronchoscope. *Anesth Analg* 2008; **106**: 1592.

4. C.V. Rosenstock, B. Thogersen, A. Afshari, *et al.* Awake fiberoptic or awake video laryngoscopic tracheal intubation in patients with anticipated difficult airway management: a randomized clinical trial. *Anesthesiology* 2012; **116**: 1210–16.

Video laryngoscopy
for emergency intubation

Kenneth P. Rothfield and John C. Sakles

Introduction

Direct laryngoscopy (DL) has long been the primary method to secure the airway under emergency circumstances. The problem with this technique is that it requires the operator to compress and displace the tissues of the upper airway so that a straight line of sight can been obtained between the operator's visual axis and the laryngeal inlet. Due to anatomical variations this is simply not possible in a substantial portion of the population. To overcome this limitation, video laryngoscopy (VL) was developed. Video laryngoscopes incorporate a micro-videocamera on the distal portion of the laryngoscope blade and thus bring a view of the glottis out of the patient's body to an external video monitor. This obviates the need to create a straight line of sight to the airway as the operator can now effectively "see around the corner." Instead of trying to displace the tongue the operator simply can look around it.

The first video laryngoscope introduced to the market was the GlideScope®, which became clinically available in 2001. The GlideScope® employs a miniature digital imaging chip and a cold light-emitting diode (LED) light source, incorporated into a steeply curved (60-degree angle) composite blade connected to a liquid crystal device (LCD) screen. These elements combined to create a video laryngoscope that is lightweight, simple to operate, and viewable by multiple providers simultaneously. Visualization of the glottis was predictable, even in patients with predictors of difficult laryngoscopy. Since that time several manufacturers have developed video laryngoscopes. These vary considerably in design. Some use highly angulated blades while others use conventional curved blades similar to the Macintosh blade. Some have built-in channels that guide the tube while others allow for free hand direction of the tube. Some have large external monitors to display the video image, while others have small displays that attach to the laryngoscope handle. This chapter will review the different types of video laryngoscopes and discuss their role in emergency intubation.

Advantages of video laryngoscopes

Video laryngoscopes have numerous advantages over direct laryngoscopes:

- They obviate the need to create a direct line of sight to the airway and thus require less force for intubation.
- They allow for better visualization of the airway during intubation thus improving the ability to recognize laryngeal pathology.

Cases in Emergency Airway Management, ed. Lauren C. Berkow and John C. Sakles. Published by Cambridge University Press. © Cambridge University Press 2015.

- They allow others helping with the procedure to see what the operator is seeing and thus improve the ability for them to help.
- They allow more experienced operators to supervise and assist less experienced operators.
- They allow for recording of both photos and videos, which can be placed in the medical record to augment documentation of the procedure.
- They allow for excellent teaching, both in real time during the intubation, and after the intubation by using video recordings.

Overview of video laryngoscopes

At first glance, there appears to be an overwhelming number of options in the video laryngoscope market (see Table 26.1). Many of the currently available devices possess more similarities than differences. The next section will review some of the key design elements that provide product differentiation.

Blade geometry

Both conventional and proprietary blade designs are available. A Macintosh-style video laryngoscope requires no alteration in technique, and can be used as a conventional direct laryngoscope or as a video laryngoscope. Some examples include the GlideScope® Titanium T3 and T4 (Verathon Medical Inc, Bothell, WA, USA), the Storz® C-MAC (Karl Storz, Tuttlingen, Germany), and the McGrath® MAC (Covidien, Mansfield, MA, USA). Proprietary blade designs, such as the GlideScope®, Storz® D-Blade, and McGrath X-blade incorporate a hyperangulated blade angle, and require a modification of technique. These blades require a midline insertion approach, without sweeping the tongue to the left. Because a more acute angle follows the anatomy of the posterior pharynx, less vertical lifting force may be required to view the vocal cords because the airway is not being straightened.[1] Evidence demonstrating the definitive superiority of one style of blade, however, is lacking.

Table 26.1 Features of video laryngoscopes currently available

Manufacturer/ distributor	Device	Blades available	Disposable blade option
Verathon	GlideScope® Titanium	Hyperangulated Titanium (T3, T4) Macintosh Titanium (Mac T3, T4)	Yes
Karl Storz	Storz® C-MAC	Hyperangulated (D-blade) Macintosh (Mac 2,3,4) Miller (0,1)	Yes
Aircraft Medical/ Covidien	McGrath® MAC	Hyperangulated (X-blade) Macintosh (Mac 2,3,4)	Yes
Pentax/Ambu	Pentax Airway Scope®	Hyperangulated Channeled	Yes
King Systems	King Vision®	Hyperangulated Channeled Hyperangulated Unchanneled	Yes
SonoSite	VividTrac®	Hyperangulated Channeled	Yes

Guiding channel

Several video laryngoscopes have abandoned stylets altogether and incorporate a guiding channel within the blade of the instrument. Guiding channels are featured in the Pentax Airway Scope® (Ambu A/S, Ballerup, Denmark), King Vision® (King Systems, Glen Burnie, MD, USA), and VividTrac® (SonoSite, Inc., Bothell, WA, USA) video laryngoscopes. In theory, this feature should simplify placement of the endotracheal tube (ETT), by eliminating the need for right-hand dexterity in steering the ETT through the glottis. However, precise alignment of the channel and the glottis remains a prerequisite to successful intubation. Although a guiding channel points the ETT in the right general direction, laryngeal structures such as the epiglottis or right arytenoid cartilage can catch the ETT and thwart intubation. The use of an angled bougie as a guide has been reported anecdotally to increase success with such devices. At the present time, however, there is no clear evidence of the superiority of channeled blades.

Integrated or detached display

Self-contained video laryngoscopes incorporate a miniature LCD or organic LED screen attached directly to the laryngoscope. For example, highly portable video laryngoscopes such as the McGrath® MAC, King Vision®, and C-MAC® Pocket Monitor are attractive for their portability compared with stand-mounted units and a separate monitor. Small screens, however, require the use of the operator's near-field vision, which declines – sometimes substantially – after age 40 years. Use of near-field vision requires that the operator maintains a fixed orientation to the screen, with associated head movements to maintain focus. Furthermore, miniaturized images may impair dexterity – fine manipulation of the ETT during attempted intubation may be hard to discern on a tiny screen. Finally, small screens impede group viewing of the image, making VL a single-operator technique.

In contrast, larger screens rely on the operator's far-field vision, require much less deliberate focusing, and permit operators to shift their gaze to other areas and back to the screen with ease. Because large screens present a magnified image of structures, dexterity may be improved because small motions and structures are seen clearly. Additionally, other team members can view the intubation on the large screen and thus assist the operator.

Single-use vs. reusable

Like many other medical devices, video laryngoscopes may pose a risk for cross-contamination and infection. For most of the emergency medical services (EMS) market, the need for sterilization is a deal breaker, as paramedic vehicles lack this capacity. Single-use blades or disposable sheaths are an attractive option in this setting. Single-use blades, however, may drive up cost. The decision to employ reusable video laryngoscopes that require sterilization between uses may impact the manner in which they are used, and impact the airway management culture. For example, to avoid unavailability in critical situations, organizations with a limited number of reusable video laryngoscopes may employ them only for rescue after failed DL.

Some manufacturers offer both single-use and reusable systems. The recently introduced GlideScope® Titanium can be used with a lightweight, reusable metal blade or a single-use composite blade. The fact that the camera chip and LED light source can be used in an inexpensive disposable product is evidence of how intense price competition in the consumer electronics market has driven down the cost of this technology.

Pole-mounted or portable

Cart or pole-mounted video laryngoscopes have the advantage of placing the display in a convenient, readily viewable location. Pocket-size devices, however, have instant appeal, particularly for providers who must travel to remote locations in a hospital. This convenience must be weighed against the risk of loss or damage.

Conventional or proprietary stylet

The steeply curved blades of several video devices follow a more natural path to the posterior pharynx, as opposed to flatter blades that compress and straighten the airway. However, hyperangulated blades may solve one problem but create a new one, requiring a change in the curve of the ETT stylet so that the tube tip is guided correctly to the glottis. For example, the manufacturer of the GlideScope recommends the use of their proprietary GlideRite® stylet – a rigid, steeply curved stylet. In the controlled setting of the operating room the standard malleable stylet was shown to work just as well as the GlideRite® rigid stylet, but in the emergency department it was demonstrated that operators using the GlideRite® stylet had a much higher first-pass success and lower incidence of complications as compared to those using a standard stylet.[2,3]

Capital vs. operational budget pricing

Although equipment priced above the capital threshold (varies by organization, typical range $5,000 to $10,000) may present an initial financial barrier, the ultimate cost per intubation may be quite low, depending on the frequency of use and usable lifespan of the product. This is especially true of devices that do not use a consumable, such as a disposable blade or cover. The cost of processing reusable blades, however, must be considered when calculating total financial impact.

A recent surge in availability of low-cost video laryngoscopes has increased access for providers. Many of these devices can be acquired with operational budget funding, and use a low-cost, consumable blade. In the case of the VividTrac single-use video laryngoscope, the entire product is disposed of after use. Because this channel-guided video laryngoscope connects via a USB port to a variety of displays, acquisition cost is extremely low. The cost per intubation, however, is relatively high. This strategy makes sense for organizations that perform relatively few intubations, but need devices available in multiple locations.

VL in context: outcomes

Without question, the video laryngoscope is the single biggest improvement in airway management since the introduction of direct laryngoscopy in the early twentieth century. Over 10 years worth of clinical data confirm the efficacy of these devices in routine and difficult airways.[4-8] Virtually all studies have demonstrated that video laryngoscopes provide a significantly improved view of the airway as compared to direct laryngoscopes.[9-11] Although the literature is conflicting on the efficacy of video laryngoscopes, all studies show that VL has a success rate higher than, or at least equal to, DL.[4,12-16] No study has shown that VL is inferior to DL in terms of first-pass success.

Review of the current literature on video laryngoscopes reveals studies that demonstrate the following:

- VL is superior to DL in the management of patients with difficult airways[4,17]
- VL is superior to DL in trauma patients with cervical immobilization[18]
- VL is superior to DL in inexperienced operators[19]
- VL is superior to DL for rescuing a failed airway[4,20]
- VL has a shorter learning curve than DL[21]
- VL decreases the rate of erroneous esophageal intubation compared to DL[6,22]
- VL improves the learning of DL.[23,24]

Using a video laryngoscope

Video laryngoscopes are used very differently than conventional direct laryngoscopes. The recommended approach is as follows:

1. Turn on the videolaryngoscope for a minute or two prior to use to allow it to warm up and minimize the risk of lens fogging. Wrapping the blade in a warm towel can also be effective.
2. Prepare an appropriate stylet by bending it into the approximate shape of the video laryngoscope blade. For hyperangulated blades, a 60- or 90-degree shape is recommended. If a proprietary stylet such as the GlideRite® rigid stylet is available it should be used.
3. Suction out the mouth completely prior to inserting the video laryngoscope.
4. Starting in the *midline*, insert the tip of the video laryngoscope blade into the mouth.
5. Hugging the tongue, navigate down the *midline* towards the epiglottis, taking care not to contaminate the micro-videocamera lens in the posterior oropharynx.
6. Advance the tip of the video laryngoscope in the vallecular to elevate the epiglottis. If this is not successful, directly lift the epiglottis with the tip of the video laryngoscope blade. Avoid inserting the blade too far or lifting too much, as this may enhance your view but make tube delivery more difficult as the larynx will be lifted further up.
7. Once an adequate view of the larynx is achieved on the video monitor, turn your attention back to the mouth and insert the styletted ETT under direct vision. Advance the ETT along the curvature of the video laryngoscope blade while looking directly in the mouth until the tip can just be seen on the video monitor.
8. Once the tip of the ETT can be seen on the video screen use the monitor to further advance the ETT through the laryngeal inlet.
9. Once the tip of the ETT passes between the vocal cords it sometimes engages the anterior tracheal wall and cannot be advanced any further. If resistance is felt at this point carefully withdraw the stylet 5–10 cm while advancing the ETT down the trachea.

Note: When using a channeled video laryngoscope the technique is similar to that described above, with the exception that a lubricated ETT without a stylet is preloaded into the channel before laryngoscopy. Once the laryngeal inlet is centered on the screen, the ETT can gently be advanced through the channel into the glottic inlet. Occasionally, the tip of the ETT will engage the right arytenoid, which can impede entry into the airway. If this occurs, the entire device can be moved slightly to the left and the ETT rotated counterclockwise as it is advanced through the channel.

Summary

Successful intubation on the first attempt is critical during emergency airway management. Several investigators have confirmed that the road to catastrophe is paved with multiple failed intubation attempts.[25,26] VL is typically associated with improved first-pass success compared to DL in a variety of settings, including the operating room, intensive care unit, emergency department, and prehospital setting.[4–6,15,19,27] Given this body of evidence, some investigators have envisioned a future in which DL is relegated to a legacy technique.[28]

References

1. Lee C, Russell T, Firat M, Cooper RM. Forces generated by Macintosh and GlideScope® laryngoscopes in four airway-training manikins. *Anaesthesia.* 2013;**68**(5):492–6.

2. Jones PM, Loh FL, Youssef HN, Turkstra TP. A randomized comparison of the GlideRite(R) rigid stylet to a malleable stylet for orotracheal intubation by novices using the GlideScope(R). *Canadian Journal of Anaesthesia (Journal canadien d'anesthesie).* 2011;**58**(3):256–61.

3. Sakles JC, Kalin L. The effect of stylet choice on the success rate of intubation using the GlideScope video laryngoscope in the emergency department. *Academic Emergency Medicine: Official Journal of the Society for Academic Emergency Medicine.* 2012;**19**(2):235–8.

4. Aziz MF, Dillman D, Fu R, Brambrink AM. Comparative effectiveness of the C-MAC video laryngoscope versus direct laryngoscopy in the setting of the predicted difficult airway. *Anesthesiology.* 2012;**116**(3):629–36.

5. Aziz MF, Healy D, Kheterpal S, *et al.* Routine clinical practice effectiveness of the GlideScope in difficult airway management: an analysis of 2,004 GlideScope intubations, complications, and failures from two institutions. *Anesthesiology.* 2011;**114**(1):34–41.

6. Mosier JM, Whitmore SP, Bloom JW, *et al.* Video laryngoscopy improves intubation success and reduces esophageal intubations compared to direct laryngoscopy in the medical intensive care unit. *Critical Care.* 2013;**17**(5):R237.

7. Niforopoulou P, Pantazopoulos I, Demestiha T, Koudouna E, Xanthos T. Video-laryngoscopes in the adult airway management: a topical review of the literature. *Acta Anaesthesiologica Scandinavica.* 2010;**54**(9):1050–61.

8. Paolini JB, Donati F, Drolet P. Review article: video-laryngoscopy: another tool for difficult intubation or a new paradigm in airway management? *Canadian Journal of Anaesthesia (Journal canadien d'anesthesie).* 2013;**60**(2):184–91.

9. Griesdale DE, Liu D, McKinney J, Choi PT. GlideScope® video-laryngoscopy versus direct laryngoscopy for endotracheal intubation: a systematic review and meta-analysis. *Canadian Journal of Anaesthesia (Journal canadien d'anesthesie).* 2012;**59**(1):41–52.

10. Healy DW, Maties O, Hovord D, Kheterpal S. A systematic review of the role of videolaryngoscopy in successful orotracheal intubation. *BMC Anesthesiology.* 2012;**12**:32.

11. Brown CA, 3rd, Bair AE, Pallin DJ, Laurin EG, Walls RM. Improved glottic exposure with the Video Macintosh laryngoscope in adult emergency department tracheal intubations. *Annals of Emergency Medicine.* 2010;**56**(2):83–8.

12. Sakles JC, Mosier J, Chiu S, Cosentino M, Kalin L. A comparison of the C-MAC video laryngoscope to the Macintosh direct laryngoscope for intubation in the emergency department. *Annals of Emergency Medicine.* 2012;**60**(6):739–48.

13. Platts-Mills TF, Campagne D, Chinnock B, *et al.* A comparison of GlideScope video laryngoscopy versus direct laryngoscopy intubation in the emergency department. *Academic Emergency Medicine: Official Journal of the Society for Academic Emergency Medicine.* 2009;**16**(9):866–71.

14. Yeatts DJ, Dutton RP, Hu PF, *et al.* Effect of video laryngoscopy on trauma patient survival: a randomized controlled trial. *The Journal of Trauma and Acute Care Surgery.* 2013;**75**(2):212–19.

15. Wayne MA, McDonnell M. Comparison of traditional versus video laryngoscopy in out-of-hospital tracheal intubation. *Prehospital Emergency Care: Official Journal of the National Association of EMS Physicians and the National Association of State EMS Directors.* 2010;**14**(2):278–82.

16. Kory P, Guevarra K, Mathew JP, Hegde A, Mayo PH. The impact of video laryngoscopy use during urgent endotracheal intubation in the critically ill. *Anesthesia & Analgesia.* 2013;**117**(1):144–9.

17. Sakles JC, Patanwala AE, Mosier JM, Dicken JM. Comparison of video laryngoscopy to direct laryngoscopy for intubation of patients with difficult airway characteristics in the emergency department. *Internal and Emergency Medicine.* 2014;**9**(1):93–8.

18. Michailidou M, O'Keeffe T, Mosier JM, *et al.* A comparison of video laryngoscopy to direct laryngoscopy for the emergency intubation of trauma patients. *World Journal of Surgery.* 2015;**39**(3):782–8.

19. Silverberg MJ, Li N, Acquah SO, Kory PD. Comparison of video laryngoscopy versus direct laryngoscopy during urgent endotracheal intubation: a randomized controlled trial. *Critical Care Medicine.* 2015;**43**(3):636–41.

20. Sakles JC, Mosier J, Patanwala AE, *et al.* The C-MAC video laryngoscope is superior to the direct laryngoscope for the rescue of failed first attempt intubations in the emergency department. *Journal of Emergency Medicine.* 2015 Mar;**48**(3):280–6.

21. Sakles JC, Mosier J, Patanwala AE, Dicken J. Learning curves for direct laryngoscopy and GlideScope® video laryngoscopy in an emergency medicine residency. *The Western Journal of Emergency Medicine.* 2014;**15**(7):930–7.

22. Sakles JC, Javedani PP, Chase E, *et al.* The use of a video laryngoscope by emergency medicine residents is associated with a reduction in esophageal intubations in the emergency department. *Academic Emergency Medicine.* 2015;**22**(6):700–7.

23. Howard-Quijano KJ, Huang YM, Matevosian R, Kaplan MB, Steadman RH. Video-assisted instruction improves the success rate for tracheal intubation by novices. *British Journal of Anaesthesia.* 2008;**101**(4):568–72.

24. Low D, Healy D, Rasburn N. The use of the BERCI DCI video laryngoscope for teaching novices direct laryngoscopy and tracheal intubation. *Anaesthesia.* 2008;**63**(2):195–201.

25. Mort TC. Emergency tracheal intubation: complications associated with repeated laryngoscopic attempts. *Anesthesia & Analgesia.* 2004;**99**(2):607–13, table of contents.

26. Sakles JC, Chiu S, Mosier J, Walker C, Stolz U. The importance of first pass success when performing orotracheal intubation in the emergency department. *Academic Emergency Medicine.* 2013;**20**(1):71–8.

27. Sakles JC, Mosier JM, Chiu S, Keim SM. Tracheal intubation in the emergency department: a comparison of GlideScope® video laryngoscopy to direct laryngoscopy in 822 intubations. *The Journal of Emergency Medicine.* 2012;**42**(4):400–5.

28. Rothfield KP, Russo SG. Videolaryngoscopy: should it replace direct laryngoscopy? A pro–con debate. *Journal of Clinical Anesthesia.* 2012;**24**(7):593–7.

Surgical airway management

Aaron E. Bair

Case representation

A 35-year-old man was assaulted with unknown objects to his face, neck, chest, and extremities in the early hours of the morning. He has undergone an initial evaluation in the emergency department (ED). The results of his various imaging studies reveal multiple injuries, including orbital wall, zygomatic arch, and mandibular fractures.

At the time of shift change, a consulting otolaryngology resident in the ED is repairing the various facial wounds using local anesthesia. The patient is supine and under a sterile field when he becomes agitated, sits up, and begins grasping at his neck in an effort to remove his cervical collar. The consultant immediately summons help. When the team arrives, they note the patient to be stridorous. He gasps and collapses as his heart rate plummets from approximately 120 beats per minute to the mid 40s. His pulse oximetry reading is no longer detectable.

Immediate efforts to provide oxygenation and ventilation with a bag-mask ventilation (BMV) device are unsuccessful. The patient's mouth is clenched. The team finds it impossible to insert a nasopharyngeal or oropharyngeal airway. He very quickly loses pulses, and chest compressions ensue. His intravenous access has been lost during the struggle. Initial attempts at laryngoscopy are quickly abandoned and, from the head of the bed, the airway manager is able to identify the relevant laryngeal anatomy – albeit significantly deviated laterally from midline. With tools immediately available in his pocket, the physician performs a rapid four-step technique (RFST) cricothyrotomy to place an endotracheal tube (ETT). From the time of initial palpation to incision and delivery of the first insufflation of oxygen, the procedure takes less than 30 seconds. With subsequent ventilations through the ETT, the patient regains pulses and his vital signs stabilize. Ultimately, he is admitted for surgical repair and close observation in the surgical intensive care unit.

The patient's airway obstruction was caused by progressive swelling of a perilaryngeal hematoma. His sudden obstruction was likely precipitated by aspiration of clotted blood. He was eventually discharged home from the hospital on day 10. Although his course was complicated by ethanol withdrawal, he went on to recover from his injuries uneventfully.

Cases in Emergency Airway Management, ed. Lauren C. Berkow and John C. Sakles. Published by Cambridge University Press. © Cambridge University Press 2015.

Airway management in context

Defining the failed airway

A failed airway can be defined in several ways. In general, a clinical scenario in which the patient is *unable to be intubated* (orally or nasally) and likewise, *cannot be oxygenated* (or ventilated) is sufficient to meet the definition.[1]

Additionally, a second form of failed airway exists when three attempts to intubate (by an experienced operator) have not resulted in successful ETT placement. It is important to highlight that three failed attempts meet the criteria for a failed intubation *even if ongoing efforts at BVM ventilation are successful*.[1] Likewise, it is worth noting that three attempts are *not required* if the attempts are obviously futile, as was the case in the scenario described above.

Various adjuncts and technological advances, such as video laryngoscopy, and wide adoption of extraglottic devices, have made cricothyrotomy an infrequently used rescue technique.[2] However, it remains the cornerstone of failed airway management. A quickly deployable approach to the failed airway is essential if hypoxic brain injury or death is to be avoided. In circumstances of anticipated difficult airway (e.g. glottic or supraglottic tumor or obstruction) cricothyrotomy might even be the initial approach to managing the airway.

If the airway has failed, the algorithm shown in Figure 27.1 may provide guidance regarding management.[1]

Approach to the failed airway

Cricothyrotomy is frequently regarded as the airway rescue technique of last resort. As such, it is often only attempted after multiple attempts or techniques have failed. Unfortunately, by the time the decision has been made, it can be too late to salvage the patient from hypoxic injury. Overcoming the inevitable cognitive inertia to end attempts at nonsurgical airway management is often the biggest challenge. The surgical procedure itself is fairly straightforward but can be associated with various complications (e.g. bleeding, cartilaginous injury, perforation of posterior trachea, creation of a false tract).[3,4] Often, the primary hurdle to performing a timely surgical airway is simply recognizing when it is necessary. Cricothyrotomy is indicated when an emergency airway is required and attempts to intubate orally or nasally have been unsuccessful. What follows are descriptions of various surgical techniques for airway access.

Surgical options

Surgical airway management is generally defined as the creation of an opening to the trachea by "invasive" or surgical means in order to provide oxygenation and ventilation. For purposes of this discussion, the techniques highlighted here are limited to several of those most commonly used. In particular, needle cricothyrotomy (with percutaneous transtracheal ventilation) is rarely done in adults and will not be covered here.

Open techniques

Rapid four-step technique

The RFST can be performed quickly and requires only a number 20 scalpel, hook, and cuffed tracheostomy tube.[5-7] For this technique, the operator stands at the head of

The failed airway algorithm ©

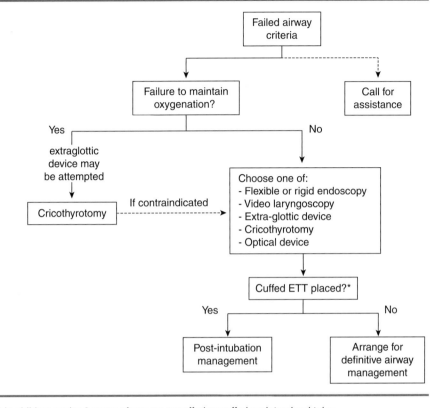

* In children under 8 years of age an uncuffed or cuffed endotracheal tube may be placed. In neonates, uncuffed endotracheal tubes should be placed.

Graphic 73112 Version 15.0

Figure 27.1 The failed airway algorithm. Reproduced with permission from: *Manual of Emergency Airway Management*, 4th edition, editors Walls, R. M. and Murphy, M. F., *Lippincott Williams & Wilkins*, 2012.

the patient in the same position as that used when attempting endotracheal intubation. Next, perform the following four steps in sequence.

Step 1: Identify the cricothyroid membrane by palpation. See Figure 27.2.

Step 2: Make a horizontal stab incision through both skin and cricothyroid membrane with the scalpel. See Figure 27.3a. The size of the skin incision is approximately 1 to 2 cm.

Step 3: Before removing the scalpel, place the hook along the handle of the scalpel and direct the hook inferiorly. See Figure 27.3b. Apply caudal traction to the cricoid cartilage to stabilize the larynx and widen the opening of the incision.

Step 4: Insert the tracheostomy tube into the trachea. See Figure 27.3c. The RFST can be modified by using a tracheal tube introducer (often referred to as a "bougie").[8] In this

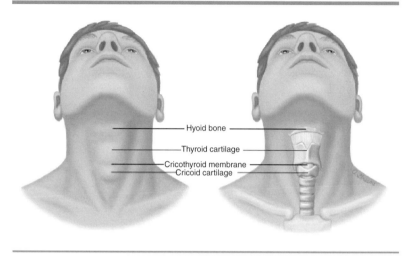

Anatomic landmarks for emergency cricothyrotomy

Hyoid bone

Thyroid cartilage

Cricothyroid membrane

Cricoid cartilage

Figure 27.2 Superficial anatomy of the anterior neck. (From UpToDate Chapter.)

technique, the introducer is inserted through the incision into the trachea after step 3 above. Then, an ETT is slid over the introducer.

Standard technique

Among the multiple techniques that have been described, the "standard" technique may be the most familiar. It is the basis on which the RFST was developed, although, with the RFST, certain time-consuming elements were eliminated (see Figure 27.4).

Step 1: Immobilize the larynx and palpate the cricothyroid membrane. Stand at the patient's right side if you are right-handed, or at the patient's left side if you are left-handed. Immobilize the larynx with the nondominant hand and perform the procedure with the dominant hand. The procedure is largely tactile, so proper finger position is essential. Place the thumb and long finger of the nondominant hand on either side of the thyroid cartilage to immobilize the larynx. Identify the cricothyroid membrane by palpating the laryngeal prominence at the midline of the cephalad rim of the thyroid cartilage with the index finger and then move caudally 1 to 2 cm until a small depression inferior to the thyroid cartilage is encountered. This is the cricothyroid membrane. Maintain manual control and immobilization of the larynx throughout the procedure to preserve the anatomic relationships (don't let go!). Proper stabilization and continuous palpation of the immobilized larynx serves as the foundation for the procedure, from which all other anatomic relationships are established. While immobilizing the larynx, palpate the cricothyroid membrane and complete the entire procedure by palpation. Do not waste time attempting to visualize the cricothyroid membrane.

Step 2: Incise the skin vertically. After palpating the cricothyroid membrane, make a midline, *vertical* incision 3 to 5 cm long through the skin overlying the membrane. The midline skin incision is intended to avoid vascular structures that might be inadvertently

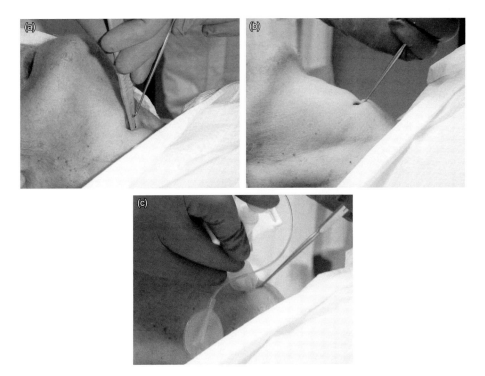

Figure 27.3 Key steps for the rapid four-step technique. (Previously published in R. J. Vissers and A. E. Bair, Surgical airway management, in *Manual of Emergency Airway Management,* 4th edition, editors R. M. Walls and Murphy, M. F., Lippincott, Williams & Wilkins, 2012, pp. 193–219.)

lacerated. The vertical orientation allows the incision to be extended superiorly or inferiorly should the initial location be too high or too low to provide adequate access to the membrane.

Step 3: Incise the cricothyroid membrane horizontally. Make a 1-cm *horizontal* incision in the cricothyroid membrane. Make the incision with care; excessive depth of placement can lead to injury of the posterior wall of the trachea. Aim the scalpel in a caudad direction to avoid the vocal cords. Once you have made the incision in the cricothyroid membrane, keep the tip of the index finger of the nondominant hand in the entry to the incision so as not to lose the opening. Continue to immobilize the larynx firmly, maintaining a triangle formed by the thumb and middle finger on opposite sides of the larynx and the index finger in the incision in the cricothyroid membrane. It is crucial not to let go at this point because there is often substantial bleeding that obscures the view of the membrane. If you are unable to stabilize the larynx because of obesity, edema, trauma, aberrant anatomy, or other reasons, you may wish to leave the scalpel in the incision until you place the tracheal hook so as not to lose the opening. In this case, be careful not to injure the back wall of the trachea with the scalpel.

Step 4: Insert the tracheal hook. Place the tracheal hook under the thyroid cartilage and ask an assistant to provide upward (i.e. cephalad) traction.

Step 5: Insert the Trousseau dilator and open it to enlarge the incision vertically. Squeeze the handles of the Trousseau dilator to open its jaws. The membrane is naturally wider in the horizontal direction, which makes the vertical direction the hardest to dilate.

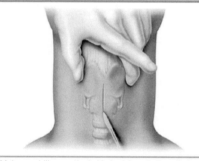

Make a midline vertical skin incision, 3–5 cm in length.

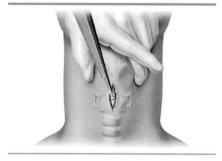

Incise the cricothyroid membrane transversely.

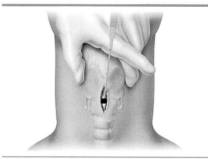

Insert the tracheal hook and ask an assistant to provide upward traction.

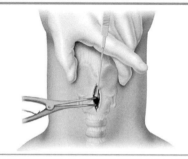

Insert the Trousseau dilator and open to expand the incision vertically.

Figure 27.4 Key steps for the standard technique. (Source Custalow, C. B., *Color Atlas of Emergency Department Procedures*, Elsevier Saunders 2005.)

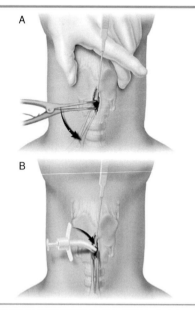

A) Rotate the dilator 90 degrees. B) Insert the tracheostomy tube, and advance the tube into the trachea.

Overcome the resistance from the thyroid cartilage as it retracts downward and the cricoid cartilage as it retracts upward against the dilator. Leave the Trousseau dilator in until the tube is placed; the thyroid and cricoid cartilages will spring back into place if the dilator is removed.

Step 6: Insert the tracheostomy tube. After dilating the opening, rotate the Trousseau dilator 90 degrees so that the handles are pointing toward the patient's feet. Then insert the tube between the jaws of the Trousseau dilator. If the Trousseau dilator remains in its original horizontal position, its inferior blade will prevent the tube from passing into the trachea. Once the tube is past the blades, advance it into the trachea. Remove the tracheal hook and Trousseau dilator. Pay particular attention not to puncture the balloon of the tube when withdrawing the sharp point of the tracheal hook.

Percutaneous techniques

Seldinger technique

Cricothyrotomy using a Seldinger technique has been described and shown to be faster than standard surgical technique.[9] However, it may also be prone to a higher failure rate.[10] Commercial cricothyrotomy kits are available that contain all essential equipment to perform the Seldinger technique. As an example, the Cook® Melker kit (Cook Medical Inc., Bloomington, IN) includes the following: a 6-mL syringe, an 18-gauge needle with overlying catheter (angiocatheter), a guide wire, a tissue dilator, a modified airway catheter, and tracheostomy tape. The procedure described here is based upon the Melker kit. Perform the procedure as follows (see Figure 27.5).

Step 1: Be certain that all equipment is present and functioning. Insert the dilator into the airway catheter. Palpate the cricothyroid membrane with the index finger of the nondominant hand while immobilizing the larynx with the thumb and middle finger.

Step 2: Attach the introducer needle to the syringe and, if time permits, fill it with a small amount of saline or water. Apply a small amount of negative pressure on the syringe and insert the needle carefully into the cricothyroid membrane at a 45-degree angle with the needle oriented caudad. Be careful not to insert it too far, as it may damage the posterior wall of the trachea. Watch for the appearance of bubbles in the water, or feel for the free flow of air into the syringe, which indicates that the needle is in the airway.

Step 3: When bubbles appear, remove the syringe and then remove the needle; leave the catheter in place with its distal tip in the trachea. Thread the guidewire through the catheter into the trachea. Remove the catheter by sliding it over the guidewire. Alternatively, using the needle without the catheter is acceptable. This may be faster as the wire can be placed directly through the needle without taking time to isolate the catheter.

Step 4: Make a 1- to 2-cm incision in the skin at the entrance point of the guidewire with a number 15 scalpel blade. Consider incising the cricothyroid membrane at this point, as it will allow for easier advancement of dilator and tube.

Step 5: Thread the combined tissue dilator–airway catheter over the guidewire and advance it into the skin incision. Following the curve of the dilator, advance the

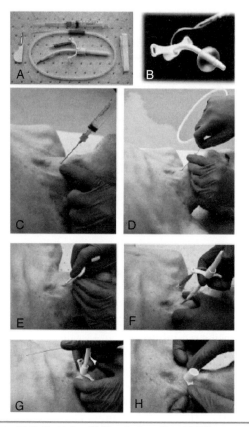

Figure 27.5 Key steps for the percutaneous/ Seldinger technique. Reproduced with permission from: *Manual of Emergency Airway Management*, 4th edition, editors Walls, R. M. and Murphy, M. F., *Lippincott Williams Wilkins*, 2012.

A) Kit contents. B) Cuffed tube. C) Needle insertion. D) Wire placement through needle. E) Small incision. F) Airway with dilator inserted with wire guidance. G) Airway inserted to the hub using a gentle twisting motion. H) Wire and dilator removed as one.

dilator–catheter unit through the subcutaneous soft tissue and into the trachea until the cuff of the catheter is flush against the skin of the neck. A slight twisting motion may be needed.

Step 6: Remove the tissue dilator and guidewire as a unit, leaving the airway catheter in the trachea.

Step 7: Secure the airway catheter to the neck with the "trach tape" provided in the kit or other appropriate means.

Issues for consideration

In a number of authoritative texts, the authors imply that finding the appropriate landmarks relevant to cricothyrotomy (i.e. thyroid cartilage, cricoid cartilage, cricothyroid membrane) is relatively straightforward. This may be true. However, in an emergency situation, possibly confounded by obesity or trauma, landmarks can be misidentified. Often the hyoid bone is confused as the thyroid cartilage, resulting in an initial incision that is too high. Several studies have highlighted this issue.[11–13] Particular care should be taken to recognize this pitfall. Bedside ultrasound has been proposed as an accurate adjunct for identifying the cricothyroid membrane.[14,15] While ultrasound may have a role in *planning* for an anticipated difficult airway, its role in the failed airway is unclear. Given the time required for setup, it may only steal away precious seconds in the setting of a failed airway. Correct anatomical identification is fundamental to the procedure and is of key importance for both initial skill acquisition and ongoing skill maintenance.

Seconds count

There are few occasions in clinical medicine when time is of such an essence – when seconds make a difference between life and death. In the case described at the beginning of this discussion, had the procedure taken much longer, the patient likely would have died or been left with severe anoxic injury. Therefore, the frantic search for equipment or a struggle to remember key functional steps in the procedure must be avoided. While numerous complications from cricothyrotomy are well recognized (i.e. hemorrhage, laryngeal injury, false passage, etc.), probably the most life-threatening consequences are attributable to the duration of hypoxia.

In this chapter, three approaches to surgical airway access have been described: RFST, the standard technique, and a Seldinger-based technique. No one method has been proven conclusively to be superior. Given the infrequency of this procedure, a trial with sufficient power to determine superiority is unlikely to ever be completed. Consequently, clinicians should choose a method and practice to maintain proficiency so that in a time of need it can be performed quickly and effectively.

References

1. Walls, R., The emergency airway algorithms. In R. Walls, Murphy MF, editor, *Manual of Emergency Airway Management*, 2012, Lippincott Williams & Wilkins: Philadelphia, PN, p. 22.

2. Bair, A.E., *et al.*, The failed intubation attempt in the emergency department: analysis of prevalence, rescue techniques, and personnel. *J Emerg Med*, 2002. **23**(2):131–40.

3. McGill, J., *et al.*, Cricothyrotomy in the emergency department. *Ann Emerg Med*, 1982. **11**(7):361–4.

4. Gillespie, M.B. and D.W. Eisele, Outcomes of emergency surgical airway procedures in a hospital-wide setting. *Laryngoscope*, 1999. **109**(11):1766–9.

5. Brofeldt, B.T., *et al.*, An easy cricothyrotomy approach: the rapid four-step technique. *Acad Emerg Med*, 1996. **3**(11):1060–3.

6. Holmes, J.F., Comparison of 2 cricothyrotomy techniques: standard method versus rapid 4-step technique. *Ann Emerg Med*, 1998. **32**(4):442–6.

7. Bair, A.E., *et al.*, Cricoid ring integrity: implications for cricothyrotomy. *Ann Emerg Med*, 2003. **41**(3):331–7.

8. Hill, C., *et al.*, Cricothyrotomy technique using gum elastic bougie is faster than standard technique: a study of emergency medicine residents and medical students in an animal lab. *Acad Emerg Med*, 2010. **17**(6):666–9.

9. Chan, T.C., *et al.*, Comparison of wire-guided cricothyrotomy versus standard surgical cricothyrotomy technique. *J Emerg Med*, 1999. **17**(6):957–62.

10. Cook, T.M., *et al*, Major complications of airway management in the UK: results of the Fourth National Audit Project of the Royal College of Anaesthetists and the Difficult Airway

Society. Part 1: anaesthesia. *Br J Anaesth*, 2011. **106**(5):617–31.

11. Aslani, A., *et al.*, Accuracy of identification of the cricothyroid membrane in female subjects using palpation: an observational study. *Anesth Analg*, 2012. **114**(5):987–92.

12. Elliott, D.S., *et al.*, Accuracy of surface landmark identification for cannula cricothyroidotomy. *Anaesthesia*, 2010. **65**(9):889–94.

13. Bair, A. E., *et al.*, The inaccuracy of using landmark techniques for cricothyroid

membrane identification: a comparison of three techniques. *Acad Emerg Med*, 2015. **22**(8):908–14.

14. Curtis, K., *et al.*, Ultrasound-guided, Bougie-assisted cricothyroidotomy: a description of a novel technique in cadaveric models. *Acad Emerg Med*, 2012. **19**(7):876–9.

15. Mallin, M., *et al.*, Accuracy of ultrasound-guided marking of the cricothyroid membrane before simulated failed intubation. *Am J Emerg Med*, 2014. **32**(1):61–3.

Communicating airway information: difficult airway letters and the MedicAlert National Difficult Airway/ Intubation Registry

Lorraine J. Foley, Vinciya Pandian, and Lynette Mark

Case presentation 1

A 71-year-old man with a history of thoracoabdominal aortic aneurysm is admitted to the hospital for aortic aneurysm repair and synthetic graft placement. His past medical history is significant for subtotal thyroidectomy 12 years earlier. He reports having dental trauma during the surgery but denies any specific knowledge of difficulty with intubation. Physical examination reveals full range of neck motion, surgical scar from thyroid surgery, good oral excursion, good mandibular profile, and good dentition. He is designated a Mallampati Class 2: faucial pillars and soft palate are seen, and the uvula is partially visualized. Prior anesthesia records from an outside hospital could not be obtained before the day of surgery. The anesthetic plan includes standard monitoring, an arterial catheter, and central venous access. The patient is induced with fentanyl and midazolam, and mask ventilation is easily established. Pancuronium is used for muscle relaxation. Several attempts with Macintosh and Miller blades fail to expose the glottic opening. Mask ventilation is successful after each attempt. Using a fiberoptic laryngoscope, the airway manager is able to visualize the complete glottic opening, tracheal rings, and carina, and the patient is intubated with a 7.0-mm endotracheal tube. Successful intubation is confirmed with continuous waveform capnography and bilateral breath sounds. Complications of the airway management include minimal soft-tissue damage in the oropharynx but no dental trauma. His aneurysm repair is uncomplicated, and he is extubated within 24 hours in the intensive care unit.

Issues with dissemination of difficult airway information

The case described above highlights the fact that comprehensive documentation in medical records is insufficient if the information is not easily accessible when it is needed. Dissemination of airway information is critical to preventing morbidity, mortality, and the potential liability exposure from failed airway management. Fewer than half of hospitals utilize electronic medical records (EMR); the rest still use handwritten records.[1] Despite the Affordable Care Act's increase in EMR implementation, older medical records are still stored on paper or as microfilm, sometimes off site. The challenge now is to integrate

Cases in Emergency Airway Management, ed. Lauren C. Berkow and John C. Sakles. Published by Cambridge University Press. © Cambridge University Press 2015.

multispecialty treatments and cross-reference critical information from numerous locations or sources to manage patients efficiently and safely.[1]

National guidelines and recommendations

To address concerns of patient safety and difficult airway management, the American Society of Anesthesiologists (ASA) organized a task force and published Practice Guidelines for Management of the Difficult Airway. These guidelines were initially released in 1993 and were last updated in 2013.[1] Specific recommendations for evaluation of the patient include examining previous anesthetic records, when available. Follow-up care includes documenting the presence and nature of the airway difficulty, informing the patient about the difficulty encountered, and following the patient for potential adverse events related to the airway difficulty. The Canadian Airway Focus Group also emphasizes the importance of clearly and accurately documenting every technique that failed and the technique that was successful to decrease the number of attempts during future intubations.[2] The Fourth National Audit Project[3] of the Royal College of Anesthetists and the Difficult Airway Society in the United Kingdom stresses the importance of not only assessing and documenting critical airway information but also seeking additional information from medical records, databases, patients, and their families before modifying the management plan to establish the airway successfully. Successful implementation of these recommendations requires a system by which critical difficult airway information can be documented consistently and made comprehensible and accessible to all healthcare providers despite geographical location and time of day.

National, international, and hospital-based airway registries

In response to the ongoing communication issues and the national guidelines and recommendations, in 1992, an anesthesia advisory council representing anesthesiologists, otolaryngologists, and risk managers joined with the nonprofit MedicAlert Foundation to establish the MedicAlert National Difficult Airway/Intubation Registry.[4] The MedicAlert Foundation had already been in existence since 1956 as a comprehensive medical identification service for over 6 million people worldwide and was endorsed by the ASA House of Delegates in 1979. The major objectives of the MedicAlert Anesthesia Advisory Council were (1) to develop mechanisms for uniform documentation and dissemination of critical information, (2) to establish a database to store and transmit patient information, especially airway-specific data, and (3) to determine through clinical practice if dissemination of clinical airway information could prevent future adverse outcomes and reduce healthcare costs. This national registry provides a mechanism whereby practitioners can record critical airway information uniformly and disseminate it easily while maintaining confidentiality according to the Health Insurance Portability and Accountability Act. It also provides a 24-hour emergency response service and a patient identification emblem/bracelet. When physicians need to obtain information, they can use the 24/7 live hotline through which the information will be relayed verbally or by fascimile. In 1994, we reported on our initial 111 patient enrollments into the registry and highlighted the benefits of enrollment: anticipation of a difficult airway resulted in fewer techniques attempted and a lower incidence of adverse outcomes. The Society for Airway Management (SAM) endorsed the MedicAlert National Airway/Intubation Registry in 1996.[5] Between 1992 and 2014, over 12,000 patients have been enrolled in this registry. There is a "Dear Patient" letter attached in approximately 12%

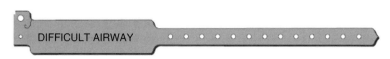

Figure 28.1 The Johns Hopkins difficult airway bracelet

of the registry from over 150 institutions that patients and healthcare members can access (see www.medicalert.org). Almost every American state is represented, with institutions comprising private, academic, and military practices.

With all hospitals requiring EMR, an in-house airway registry would be beneficial because all airway-related information would be easily accessible in one location. The Johns Hopkins Hospital multidisciplinary Difficult Airway Response Team (DART) program instituted a hospital-based airway registry that enables electronically communicated patient information to be accessed at any time.[6] The components of the registry include a visible blue "difficult airway" alert patient wrist band, an EMR "difficult airway" flag and note, and a web-based quality improvement database with immediate notification to DART oversight members (Figure 28.1). At discharge, the patient receives a difficult airway educational document. Additional patient follow-up includes a mailed "Dear Patient" difficult airway letter and recommendations for enrollment into the MedicAlert National Difficult Airway/Intubation Registry.[5] This process allows dissemination of airway information within the institution and provides the patient with specific airway-related medical information, should they choose to enroll in the MedicAlert National Airway/Intubation Registry.

Case presentation 2

A 48-year-old woman is brought to the emergency department by ambulance with signs and symptoms of asthma exacerbation. The patient reports that she does not have any significant past medical history except for asthma. She also reports having had a cholecystectomy 5 years earlier but cannot remember any anesthesia-related problems. Her husband recalls receiving a letter from her anesthesiologist about her airway but cannot remember the contents.

The patient appears anxious, restless, and dyspneic. Physical examination reveals a Mallampati Class 3, mouth opening 4 cm wide, and receding chin. She is using accessory muscles. Initially, her oxygen saturation is 92% while receiving 3 liters of oxygen via nasal cannula, but she becomes progressively hypoxic and delirious. She is induced with ketamine and is administered a neuromuscular relaxant in preparation for intubation. Direct laryngoscopy with a Macintosh blade reveals Cormack–Lehane grade 4. Direct laryngoscopy with a Miller blade reveals Cormack–Lehane grade 3. Mask ventilation becomes difficult. The practitioners place a supraglottic airway device but are unable to achieve ventilation and find themselves in a "cannot intubate, cannot oxygenate" situation. They perform an emergent cricothyroidotomy. The patient is stabilized and transferred to the intensive care unit (ICU).

After the patient arrives in the ICU, her prior medical records are obtained from storage. The anesthesia record for her cholecystectomy reveals that four attempts were made during intubation with both the Macintosh and Miller blades; all were unsuccessful. A video laryngoscopy was difficult but successful with only a partial view of her vocal cords. Mask ventilation was always successful between attempts at laryngoscopy. The anesthesiologist documented enlarged lingular tonsils and an unanticipated anterior larynx. Additionally, the anesthesiologist documented on the anesthesia record that the patient would be identified as a "difficult intubation" and receive a difficult airway management letter in follow-up care.

Issues with dissemination of difficult airway information

The case described above highlights a situation in which a previous anesthesiologist documented the difficult airway management and provided a plan for follow-up information to be mailed to the patient in a difficult airway letter. The fact that the patient's husband remembered the letter but not the contents suggests that he most likely did not appreciate the clinical implications of difficult airway management for future medical care plans. Therefore, it is important not only to send the letter but also to communicate the importance of alerting future providers of prior difficult airway management. Furthermore, if the hospital had had a hospital-based difficult airway registry, the emergency department providers could have accessed the patient's prior airway history, modified their airway management plan accordingly, and potentially avoided the need for the emergency surgical airway.

Difficult airway letters: to patients and to practitioners

Two main types of letters could be sent to disseminate information regarding difficult airways – "Dear Patient" and "Dear Practitioner."[4,7]

These letters should include the following information:

(1) Date and institution where the difficult airway was identified.
(2) Provider contact information.
(3) Patient characteristics on airway examination, body mass index, and other significant comorbidities.
(4) Type of difficulty encountered, such as mask ventilation, supraglottic devices, intubation, and extubation.
(5) Difficulties encountered with each unsuccessful technique and type of view seen.
(6) Successful technique with best laryngeal visualization.
(7) Implications for future care.
(8) Recommendations for registration with emergency notification service.

The two types of letters described above can further be classified into three categories: (1) Basic letter – difficult airway/intubation alert only, (2) letter with essential airway information, and (3) letter with essential airway information and attached medical record documents. Basic letters are generic and simply inform the patient or the practitioner that the patient has a difficult airway. Although this type of letter might be beneficial to the patient and non-anesthesia practitioners, anesthesia practitioners comment on the lack of any airway information and have even questioned their value. The letter with essential airway information discusses briefly why airway management was difficult and specifically comments on the ability to ventilate, what techniques failed, and what techniques were successful. The letter with essential airway information and attached medical documents may include scans of anesthesia records, surgical operative reports, and medical discharge summaries.

Difficult airway letter templates or guides are available on the websites of various national organizations, such as SAM, the Difficult Airway Society of the United Kingdom, the Danish Airway Society, and the Austrian Airway Society. In addition, the MedicAlert Foundation website has a specialty Difficult Airway/Intubation brochure and Difficult Airway/Intubation Registry database form, which was updated in 2014 by the SAM MedicAlert Task Force.

Summary

The consequences of difficult airway/intubation may include minor or major adverse events, hypoxic brain injury or death, risk of professional liability to the practitioner, and continued threat to patient safety if critical airway information is not effectively disseminated to the patient and future healthcare providers. The ASA Practice Guidelines for Management of the Difficult Airway recommends a written report or letter to the patient, communication with the patient's surgeon and medical colleagues, and considerations for a notification bracelet or equivalent identification device as components of comprehensive follow-up patient care. A difficult airway letter with recommendations for enrollment into the MedicAlert National Difficult Airway/Intubation Registry is an effective mechanism to communicate with patients and healthcare providers and promote patient safety.

References

1. J. L. Apfelbaum, C. A. Hagberg, R. A. Caplan, *et al*. Practice guidelines for management of the difficult airway: an updated report by the American Society of Anesthesiologists Task Force on Management of the Difficult Airway. *Anesthesiology* 2013; **18**(2):251–70.

2. J. A. Law, N. Broemling, R. M. Cooper, *et al*. The difficult airway with recommendations for management – part 1 – difficult tracheal intubation encountered in an unconscious/induced patient. *Can J Anaesth* 2013; **60**(11): 1089–118.

3. T. M. Cook, N. Woodall, J. Harper, *et al*. Major complications of airway management in the UK: results of the Fourth National Audit Project of the Royal College of Anaesthetists and the Difficult Airway Society. Part 2: intensive care and emergency departments. *Br J Anaesth* 2011; **106**(5):632–42.

4. L. J. Mark, L. A. Foley, J. D. Michelson. Effective dissemination of critical information: the MedicAlert National Difficult Airway/Intubation Registry. In C. A. Hagberg, editor, *Benumof and Hagberg's Airway Management*, 3rd edition. St. Louis, MI: Saunders, 2013, pp. 1094–105.

5. L. J. Mark, J. Schauble, G. Gibby, *et al*. The National Difficult Airway/Intubation Registry, MedicAlert Foundation. In J. N. Benumof, editor, *Airway Management: Principles and Practice*. St. Louis, MI: Mosby; 1996, pp. 931–43.

6. L. C. Berkow, R. S. Greenberg, K. H. Kan, *et al*. Need for emergency surgical airway reduced by a comprehensive difficult airway program. *Anesth Analg* 2009; **109**(6):1860–9.

7. T. L. Trentman, P. E. Frasco, L. N. Milde. Utility of letters sent to patients after difficult airway management. *J Clin Anesth* 2004; **16**(4):257–61.

Index